W9-BUE-028

Demanding Medical Excellence

Demanding Medical Excellence

DOCTORS AND ACCOUNTABILITY IN THE INFORMATION AGE

Michael L. Millenson

The University of Chicago Press
Chicago and London

Michael Millenson is senior analyst in the health and welfare consulting practice of William M. Mercer, Inc., a visiting scholar at Northwestern University, and an award-winning journalist.

The University of Chicago Press, Chicago 60637
The University of Chicago Press, Ltd., London
 Published 1997
Printed in the United States of America

06 05 04 03 02 01 00 99 98 97   1 2 3 4 5

ISBN: 0-226-52587-2 (cloth)

Library of Congress Cataloging-in-Publication Data

Millenson, Michael L.
Demanding medical excellence : doctors and accountability in the information age / Michael L. Millenson.
p. cm.
Includes bibliographical references and index.
ISBN 0-226-52587-2
1. Medical care—United States. I. Title.
RA395.A3M476 1997 97-16677
CIP

♾ The paper used in this publication meets the minimum requirements of the American National Standard for Information Sciences—Permanence of Paper for Printed Library Materials, ANSI Z39.48-1984.

Men began to hear with surprise, not unmingled with some vague hope of ultimate benefit, that . . . the comparative value of medical remedies and different modes of treatment of disease . . . might come to be surveyed with that lynx-eyed scrutiny of a dispassionate analysis, which if not at once leading to the discovery of positive truth, would at least secure the detection and proscription of many mischievous and besetting fallacies.
—Sir John Herschel, 1850

The quality of medical care is an index of a civilization.
—Ray Lyman Wilbur, M.D., chairman of the Committee on the Costs of Medical Care, 1933

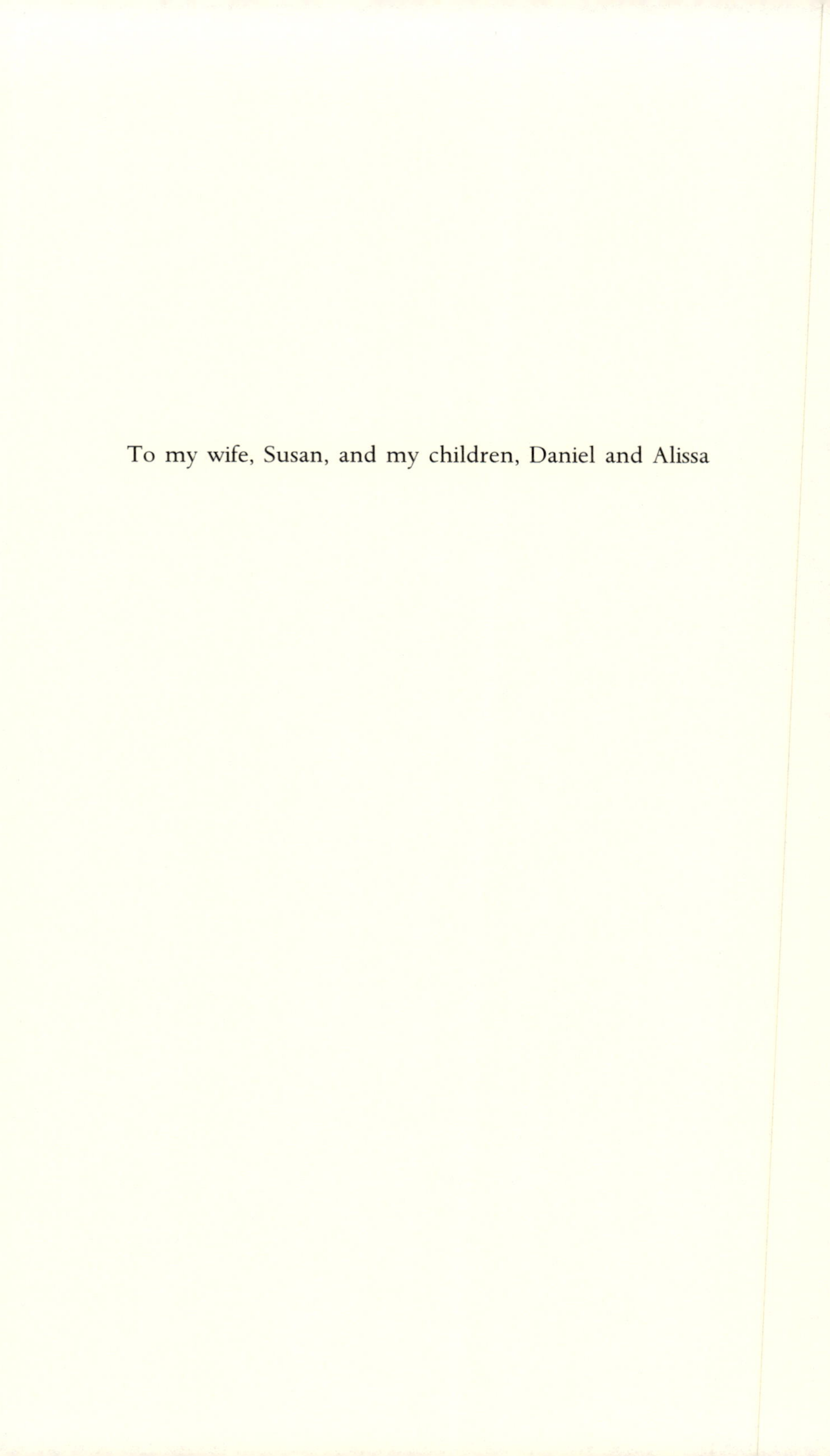

To my wife, Susan, and my children, Daniel and Alissa

CONTENTS

PREFACE

“God heals,” goes an old aphorism, “and the physician sends the bill.” Even in today’s world of miracle drugs and lifesaving surgery, the connection between the physician’s actions and the patient’s return to good health is often murky. The suggestion that one can quantify and compare clinical performance surprises many nonphysicians. It surprises a lot of doctors too.

I first delved into the quality measurement and management movement in 1986 as an Alicia Patterson Foundation Fellow on leave from my job as a reporter for the *Chicago Tribune.* The topic fascinated me. After all, affordability and access to care are important only if the care itself *helps.* I interviewed George Lundberg, editor of the *Journal of the American Medical Association,* who made an intriguing assertion: doctors should learn a lesson from industrial quality control. “The single most important thing that American medicine . . . should do is define quality indicators and follow them,” he said. I wrote up what I found, first for the Patterson Foundation and later for the *Tribune.*

I also became acutely aware that many physicians and hospital administrators disliked and distrusted quality measurement. The general public, however, barely knew it existed, which meant that those promoting the idea didn’t have much of a constituency. This book is an attempt to help redress that balance and bring the voice of the patient more fully into the debate over medical quality improvement.

In writing this book, I drew on nearly fifteen years’ experience observing the medical community at close range as a reporter for one of the nation’s largest newspapers. Just as important, however, were thousands of articles from the scientific literature, trade publications, and the general press, as well as an uncounted number of books. In addition, I interviewed many of the prominent experts in this field and spent time with many, many more physicians, nurses, patients, and others whose lives are bound up with the realities of everyday medicine.

Still, I am keenly aware that many of the assertions made here could be elaborated on and their pros and cons debated at great length. I am equally aware, however, that dwelling on the details of interest to clinicians and researchers is the best way to obscure the critical issues that are most important to patients. The largest barriers to systematically measuring and improving the quality of American medicine are not technical but cultural, as the pages that follow will make clear. To deliberately oversimplify for a moment, it is said that "where there's a will, there's a way." With quality measurement in medicine, it is the will that largely has been missing.

I am grateful to my many editors over the years at the *Tribune* for allowing me the freedom to go where my instincts and knowledge took me. In particular, Owen Youngman encouraged me to write a five-part series on medical quality issues in 1993 that the *Tribune* ran on page 1 and nominated for a Pulitzer Prize. My science writer colleagues Peter Gorner and Ron Kotulak provided me with a personal benchmark of proven excellence.

Stephen Crane, then with the Association for Health Services Research (AHSR), enabled me to turn a dream into a book by suggesting I apply for one of the Robert Wood Johnson Foundation's first Investigator Awards in Health Policy Research. This unusual award was designed to support research of broad public interest, not the mining of a narrow academic vein. Since the foundation does not grant money to individuals, only to nonprofit institutions on behalf of individuals, Edward F. X. Hughes, then director of Northwestern University's Center for Health Services and Policy Research, graciously granted me Visiting Scholar status at the Center. Teresa Waters, an economist who was the Center's associate director, was my invaluable guide through the thickets of academia during my two-year tenure there, while other Northwestern colleagues at the Center and the Kellogg School offered help and support in many ways. Jeff Erdman and Lisa Swirsky provided much-needed research assistance.

Robert Hughes, James Knickman, Robin Osborn, and the late Sol Levine—the individuals who came up with the idea of the Investigator Award and made it a working reality—inspired me to strive to combine intellectual rigor with the journalist's stock-in-trade of telling an interesting story. I am also grateful to my fellow Investigator Award recipients for thought-provoking criticism and comments.

I am deeply indebted to the individuals and organizations whose names you will read in this book for the gift of their time and to literally hundreds of others whom I interviewed too. I would like to single out for special thanks the people of the Intermountain Health Care System, particularly Brent James, and the Minneapolis–St. Paul medical and business community. Special thanks also go to some of the leaders of this field who gave particularly generously of their time: Donald Berwick, David Blumenthal, Robert Brook, Iain Chalmers, Mark Chassin, David Eddy, Paul Ellwood, Paul Sanazaro, Homer Warner, John Wennberg, and John Williamson. Thanks, too, to the Joint Commission on Accreditation of Healthcare Organizations for ongoing access to its excellent library resources and to *American Medical News* for access to its past issues. I appreciate those organizations that let me attend professional meetings without charge, particularly the Healthcare Forum and the Zitter Group.

Tom Moore, ace journalist turned health care author, was both a help and an inspiration. This book also builds on the writings of Richard Carter, Victor Fuchs, Uwe Reinhardt, Charles Rosenberg, Rosemary Stevens, and Paul Starr. I appreciate the sage words of advice on researching, writing, and revising this manuscript that came from from David Blumenthal, Diane Dubey, Judith Feinberg, Emily Friedman, Norbert Goldfield, Sheldon Greenfield, Kathryn Jandeska, David Kendall, David Lansky, Edward Lawlor, Susan Lieberman, George Lundberg, David Nash, Duncan Neuhauser, Alan Spiro, Scott Weingarten, and Sidney Wolfe. The flaws that nonetheless remain are of my own making.

During the time it took to write this book, I went from journalism to academia to the business world, joining the benefits consulting firm of William M. Mercer, Inc. This book owes its completion to the support of my Mercer colleague Arnie Milstein and, especially, to the consistent encouragement and support of Health and Welfare practice leader John Barton. My administrative assistant, Susan Hockman, has been an invaluable help.

It is important to note that none of my various employers was shown this book before it was accepted for publication, and none are responsible for its contents. The views expressed here are mine alone. I am indebted to my editors at the University of Chicago Press: John Tryneski, for patience, persistence, and assistance, and to Alice

Bennett, for yeoman's work in carefully editing a long manuscript in a short time.

This book began as an eighteen-month project and turned into a thirty-six-month marathon. It reached the finish line because of the support of friends and family, particularly my siblings; my father, who wielded a sharp copyediting pencil; and my wife, Susan, whose insights, assistance, and caring made all the difference in the world.

INTRODUCTION

A Different Kind of Revolution

With little fanfare, a gathering revolution is transforming the everyday practice of medicine. Owing more to laptops than lab coats, this is an information revolution, one that is beginning to yield answers to the most basic questions that haunt those who are sick: Who shall live and who shall die? Who will have pain and who will be free from pain? Who will become disabled and who will regain normal functioning?

The first fruits of this change can be seen at 7:00 A.M. on a gray November morning, when the cardiologists and cardiac surgeons of the Dartmouth-Hitchcock Medical Center converge on a conference room and shut the door. The heart specialists gather here at the same time every Friday to talk candidly about the treatment of patients at the Lebanon, New Hampshire, teaching hospital. This morning Douglas James, the veteran chairman of the cardiology department, has asked for time on the agenda to discuss a difficult decision. It involves a retired dairy farmer named Harold "Ray" Spackman.

Spackman was a native of New Jersey who moved to New England in the early 1950s to pursue his dream of farming. During most of his active years in agriculture, dairy farmers avidly consumed the same high-fat milk and cheese as their customers. Now the sixty-three-year-old was paying a price. He carried 279 pounds on a six-foot three-inch frame. His breathing was labored, and medical tests showed chronic lung disease, congestive heart failure, and coronary artery disease so severe that a heart attack loomed as an imminent danger. The most pressing question for Spackman's physicians was how to improve blood flow to his heart. One choice was angioplasty, in which a cardiologist clears the patient's arteries with a balloon-tipped catheter; the other choice was bypass surgery. In a twist on the typical hospital turf battles, cardiologist James advocated an immediate bypass, while William Nugent, the chief of cardiothoracic surgery, worried about operating on a patient with weakened lungs.

At many institutions, the debate over how best to treat Ray Spackman would have evolved into a clash of egos. The surgery and cardiology chiefs would have been pitted one against the other, each man's judgment implicitly on the line. But at Dartmouth-Hitchcock the discussion proceeded along a very different path, with profound implications for the way all medical decisions are made.

As part of his presentation, James took out a preprogrammed scientific calculator that is available to all the hospital's cardiac specialists. He entered Spackman's age, several aspects of his medical history, and some key measures of the heart's functioning. Then he pushed a button. The number that flashed on the screen showed the risk that Spackman might die during surgery or within thirty days afterward. The figure was not theoretical. It was based on the experience of Dartmouth-Hitchcock's heart surgeons, who regularly record the pre- and postsurgery condition of each bypass patient and enter it into a database. Moreover, the hospital carefully adjusts the mortality rate to account for how severely ill the patient is before treatment. For Spackman, the risk of death within thirty days of a bypass was 2.4 percent.

The next crucial piece of information comes from the patients themselves. Alone, with no nurse or doctor present who might influence the results, each heart patient answers a computerized questionnaire designed by Dartmouth-Hitchcock to elicit real feelings about the risks and the possible benefits of surgery. Spackman, a husband, father of five, and grandfather of eighteen, knew his situation was serious. In return for what surgery might accomplish for his life, he was willing to accept a 10 percent chance of death.

Although it was now clear that a bypass was low risk and Spackman was more than willing to take that risk, the most important question remained unanswered: whether surgery was the most effective and appropriate therapy. James felt it was; Nugent had his doubts. In seeking to resolve that critical issue, the heart specialists veered radically away from the "who can argue the most persuasively" model of medical decision making. Instead they turned their attention to a simple but highly dramatic chart. In graphic form it displayed the odds that Ray Spackman would still be alive five years after treatment.

The chart contained three separate curves. Each represented Spackman's probability of survival with a different therapy. All three curves started at 100 percent—the moment treatment began—then sloped downward as they progressed to the five-year mark. The calculations were based on the experience of North Carolina's Duke University Medical Center, which has tracked its patients' postsurgical lives for some two decades and validated its data against randomized clinical trials.

The striking differences in the three therapies could be seen with just a glance. When treated with heart medication alone, patients with symptoms similar to Spackman's had an average five-year survival rate of 9.4 percent—or less than one chance in ten. With angioplasty the rate jumped to 26.5 percent—about one chance in four. With bypass surgery, though, the average five-year survival rate increased to 46.2 percent—nearly even odds. Nugent looked at the information for a while, but there was not much to discuss. "OK," said the heart surgeon after a short time. "We'll do it."

Ray Spackman had nearly a 98 percent chance of surviving his bypass surgery, and he did. He also had an 80 percent chance of living for another year and a half, but he did not. The genial farmer died from congestive heart failure nearly eighteen months after his operation. Probabilities are not certainties. Nor does anyone expect a computer program to completely replace physician judgment, any more than computers in airplane cockpits have eliminated the need for skilled pilots. Nonetheless, the same laws of mathematics that give meaning to a baseball player's batting average or a sixteen-year-old boy's auto insurance premium are starting to dramatically improve medical decisions. At the same time, patients are gaining an unprecedented opportunity to evaluate those decisions by taking advantage of newly available, objective information about past medical performance.

Moreover, the stage is being set to explore questions that focus as much on maintaining good health or treating chronic illness as on curing acute disease. For example: Which hospital detects breast cancer at its earliest stages, and what type of treatments do its doctors employ most frequently? Which physician group provides the most reliable control of diabetes and its complications? Which health plan does the best job of helping asthmatics lead normal, productive lives?

The driving forces behind this transformation are social, economic, and technological, and they are closely linked to medicine's changing role in our society.

For centuries the physician's primary duty was to diagnose an illness and then track its natural course. Doctors did all they could to help the sick, but they did not have either the tools or the understanding of the body's workings they needed to consistently succeed. Although that situation began to improve in the mid-1800s, it was not until after World War II, just a little over fifty years ago, that biomedical research provided physicians with the weapons they needed to consistently win more of the battles against sickness and disease. Doctors were widely hailed as miracle workers, and "quality" care became synonymous with "more" care. More doctors. More nurses. More hospitals. More drugs. More diagnostic equipment. And of course ever more generous private health insurance and ever expanding Medicare and Medicaid benefits, so that more Americans could enjoy more access to more treatment.

For many years, a grateful public implicitly trusted that extra resources would automatically result in improved care. Gradually, however, cures once hailed as miraculous become mundane. Society stopped regarding all physicians with a tinge of awe and instead began to ask increasingly pointed questions about what we were buying for the more than $2 billion a day the nation spends on health care. Study after study has documented the routine use of unneeded and even dangerous treatments.[1] Harvard University researchers, for example, found that one-quarter of the heart bypasses, angioplasties, and catheterizations (measuring blood flow and blood pressure in the heart) performed on elderly heart attack victims are unnecessary. They could be eliminated with no effect on the patients' survival.[2]

As unsettling as the prevalence of measurably inappropriate care is the enormous amount of what can only be called ignorant care. A surprising 85 percent of everyday medical treatments have never been scientifically validated.[3] Although genetic engineering, organ transplants, and hormones that promise everlasting youth make front-page news, in an overwhelming number of cases the average doctor treating everyday ills simply does not know what works best.

Therapies that have not been scientifically tested can still be effective, but the gap between research and practice has real consequences. In the absence of reliable information, physicians' decisions fluctuate wildly. For instance, when family practitioners in Washington State were queried about treating a simple urinary tract infection in women, eighty-two physicians came up with an extraordinary 137 different strategies.[4] There are many, many similar examples.

"The perception we all want to have is that medicine is firmly based on reality, [that] our research enterprise systematically identifies important problems, and . . . [that] information is transmitted speedily to [doctors], who apply it unerringly," writes David Eddy, a physician and mathematician who has spent some two decades examining the scientific basis of physicians' decisions. "Unfortunately, the truth is that the practice of medicine is not based firmly on reality, . . . the transmission of research information into practice is precarious and the results are used selectively by practitioners."[5]

But if "more" isn't always better, then neither, automatically, is "less." There is increasing public concern that cost containment could be dangerous to health. At a time when "managed care" is becoming mainstream medicine, the "management" is still too often directed at cost alone. Some health plans have turned a blind eye to the hazards of pinching pennies, just as some fee for service doctors have long disregarded the harmful effects of unnecessary tests and surgeries.

Yet the spirited political debate over the financing of health care masks a more fundamental problem. The American population is aging, and the demand for new and more costly medical services is increasing. Whether we as a nation embrace fee for service or managed care, "medical savings accounts" or a completely government-financed health care system, the pressure to contain costs—in Medicare, in Medicaid, and in the insurance plans of employers—will not disappear. It will remain, and it will intensify. So too will the need for reliable information about the value of what we are buying.

If medical quality, like beauty, is in the eye of the beholder, then how can we judge between the doctor who advises bed rest for back pain and the one who recommends surgery? Between the hospital that provides therapy with a nurse who visits the patient's home and the one that insists patients remain hospitalized overnight? Between the health plan that discharges most new mothers within twenty-four hours and the one that waits two to three days? How, in other words, can we reliably distinguish between the rational use of limited resources and unethical rationing?

Back in 1840 the French physician Casimir Broussais wrote: "Is it possible that statistics should stop precisely on the threshold of medicine? That it be applicable to the duration of life, but not to the sick; that it serve to calculate the chances of life and death of the population in all social conditions, but be unable to calculate the chances of life and death of the populations of hospitals?" Nearly 160 years later, medicine is finally responding to that challenge. By adopting "the observation of clinical events under natural conditions,"[6] researchers are going beyond anecdote and, for the first time, reliably linking caregivers' actions with their effect on patients' health. In the process, they are opening the doors to the next medical revolution.

The goal of this new revolution is to systematically bring to everyday patient care the treatments that work best—not to replace the continuing revolution of biomedical discovery, but rather to complement it and make it whole. A health care delivery system characterized by idiosyncratic and often ill-informed judgments must be restructured according to evidence-based medical practice, regular assessment of the quality of care, and accountability. The alternative is a system that makes life and death treatment decisions based on conflicting anecdotes and calculated appeals to emotion.

Systematically measuring the outcome of patient care must inevitably lead to systematically improving it. Dartmouth-Hitchcock belongs to a consortium of five northern New England hospitals examining bypass surgery. In 1990 and 1991, after an intensive study of the link between processes of care and results, the hospitals undertook a series of seemingly small changes. The patient's breathing tube was removed more quickly. The size of sutures was reduced. The patient's heart was flushed with blood at a key point in the surgery. Although these types of technical refinements would never rate a mention on the evening news, their calculated purpose was to spread the "best practices" at each institution to all the others. The results were extraordinary. The death rate of bypass patients dropped by one-quarter. During a two-year study period in which rates were tracked for a scholarly article, the hospitals estimated they saved an additional seventy-four patients' lives.[7]

In the crowded offices of the Dartmouth-Hitchcock cardiothoracic surgery department, thirty-six separate charts are pinned up on a fabric-covered wall. The bar graphs and pie charts track everything from the number of consecutive error-free cases without major complications to the mean number of minutes bypass patients remain on a heart pump during surgery. The staff has nicknamed the display "the Wailing Wall." Each surgeon also receives a single page that sums up a long list of measures in an easy-to-read "instrument panel."

The analogy to aviation is deliberate. Like pilots monitoring their instruments, the Dartmouth-Hitchcock doctors, nurses, and support staff use their instrument panel to differentiate between normal ups and downs and unexpected events that signal real trouble. For example, the staff quickly homes in on a small upsurge in infections that might otherwise be dismissed as random bad luck. Instead, the change in the rate of infections documented on one of the instrument panel charts is traced to moving a protective curtain from one side of the operating table to the other. Nugent, the cardiothoracic surgery chief, says the instrument panel gives him a secure feeling of being in control. It is a change "from being reactive to being proactive, and from not knowing to beginning to know."[8]

This tracking of patient care borrows unabashedly from "continuous quality improvement" (CQI) techniques commonly used in monitoring industrial processes. Dartmouth-Hitchcock is a leader in adopting this approach, but it is far from alone in doing so. Even the Mayo Clinic, perhaps the most respected physician group in the world, has begun redesigning its patient care processes with the help of CQI. One group of Mayo clinicians, after working with the techniques, wrote glowingly: "[CQI] is an exciting development . . . [that] can genuinely enhance the art and science of medicine."[9]

In order to understand how medicine will be practiced in the future, this book digs into some little-known parts of medicine's past, examines some of the most promising developments of the present, and then looks ahead. This exploration is divided into four parts.

DOING THE RIGHT THING AND DOING THE RIGHT THING RIGHT

In the midst of an influenza epidemic in Victorian England, a London newspaper sent a reporter posing as a patient to the city's top medical specialists. Although the symptoms the "patient" described remained the same at every stop, the doctors' advice varied, as did the drugs they prescribed.[10] In the century since then, not a lot has changed. Researchers who evaluated Medicare data on the treatment of patients across the United States uncovered differences as distinctive as any from Queen Victoria's time.

"In health care markets, geography is destiny," concluded a 1996 report from Dartmouth Medical School's Center for the Evaluative Clinic Sciences. For example, 1.4 percent of elderly women in Rapid City, South Dakota, received breast-conserving surgery for breast cancer. In Elyria, Ohio, 48 percent did. An elderly patient with back pain in Fort Myers, Florida, was four times as likely to undergo surgery as a man or woman living in Manhattan. And a man with an enlarged prostate in Newark, New Jersey, was twice as likely to get a part of his gland surgically removed as if he lived in New Haven,

Connecticut.[11] The first section of this book examines how doctors make treatment decisions. It looks at both the choice of the most appropriate treatment ("doing the right thing") and the way that treatment is provided ("doing the right thing right").

The common public image of the doctor as scientist oversimplifies the relation between patient-care physician and researcher. In some cases, community doctors immediately apply new discoveries. At other times research results are not specific enough to be put to use in patient care. And at still other times, community practitioners continue to go their own way no matter what the research says, as chapters 1 and 2 illustrate.

Whatever treatment decision is made, errors in providing treatment have grown into a deadly serious problem. Many people believe they will be protected if their physician is "conscientious, hard-working [and] trustworthy," as a popular Sunday newspaper supplement put it;[12] the truth is more complex. As chapter 3 illustrates, treatment-related deaths and injuries are caused by a complex set of factors. Because the victims die one at a time, the public remains largely unaware that there are a chilling 180,000 treatment-related deaths in hospitals every year.

Chapter 4 goes inside one hospital to show that these medical mistakes are neither random, rare, nor inevitable. Patient by patient, problem by problem—drug reactions, hospital-caused infections, inappropriate blood transfusions—Salt Lake City's LDS Hospital has attacked treatment-caused injuries and deaths. One of the secrets of LDS's success is a custom-built clinical computer system that may serve as a national model for how to save patient lives.

Although consistency and carefulness in treatment are important, they must rest on a solid base of scientific knowledge. Chapter 5 tells the story of Gypsy Heuston, an Idaho high-school student who fell victim to a puzzling and often fatal disease known as ARDS. As a result of her illness, she was enrolled in a randomized clinical trial designed to test an experimental therapy. This chapter examines how researchers go about gathering scientific evidence on what works best and then put it into practice—and how in many instances practice precedes evidence.

As medical innovations proliferate, it becomes a greater challenge to keep up with the best possible practice. At Los Angeles' Cedars-Sinai Medical Center, the neighborhood hospital for glitzy Beverly Hills, Dr. Scott Weingarten has emerged as one of the nation's most astute developers of practice "guidelines" that point physicians in the same direction as the best medical evidence. It is hard, not very glamorous work. As chapter 6 shows, however, well-conceived guidelines can reduce unnecessary care, cut medical costs, and with a nearly complete lack of drama, save lives.

If objective measurement of medical treatment has been slow to take hold, it is in no small part because most physicians have fiercely resisted it, even when the efforts have been led by other physicians. The next section of the book shows the effect of that resistance on patient care.

THE TARNISHED HISTORY OF MEDICINE'S GOLDEN AGE

In 1965 the steadily rising death toll from auto accidents prompted Congress to hold its first hearings on automotive safety. Ford Motor Company chairman Henry Ford II was indignant. "We've always built safe cars," he declared. Congress passed landmark safety legislation anyway, and the golden age of the American automobile, when cars were built any way the carmakers wanted to build them, was over.

The golden age of medicine also ended when the public began to question whether the health care "industry" had grown too big, dangerous, and costly to entrust its oversight solely to those who worked within it. In this section of the book, chapters 7 and 8 chronicle the first attempts to hold doctors and hospitals measurably accountable for their actions.

There was, for instance, Ernest Amory Codman, a prickly surgeon who practiced at Massachusetts General Hospital in the early twentieth century. Codman called on hospitals to track their surgical successes and failures and to make those results public as a way of motivating improvement. Codman's "End Result Idea," not surprisingly, was regarded by most of his peers as eccentric or worse.

Yet even as late as the 1950s, efforts by a few physicians to establish an objective "medical audit" of hospitals did not fare much better. The great majority of doctors were complacent. "The man who knows the riddle of . . . [the human body] is a god," confided one physician to another in a best-selling 1954 novel about the making of a doctor. "That's what we are—gods. And the thing that holds us together as a group is our realization of this. We know how the public feels about us."[13] Back in real life, even a national study implying that there were tens of thousands of "excess deaths" in United

States hospitals failed to provoke any immediate reaction from the "godly" profession.

With the advent of Medicare and Medicaid in the 1960s, however, the federal government began actively examining the details of medical practice. In the 1970s corporate America started to join in. Chrysler Corporation, threatened by bankruptcy, sent its health claims to a physician-run company for a computerized analysis and uncovered case after case of inappropriate and ineffective treatment of its workers. Chrysler's crackdown signaled a willingness by big companies to treat medical care like any other service whose quality and price could be managed. By the mid-1990s, the era of accountability had arrived with a vengeance.

HOLDING MEDICINE ACCOUNTABLE FOR RESULTS

"Dear Health Care Manager," began a 1995 subscription solicitation for a newsletter called *Accountability News.* "Your organization's future now hinges on how well you can *prove* you're delivering high-quality, cost-effective care. Employers have developed an insatiable appetite for cost and quality performance data. . . . [M]anagers must now incorporate quality-based accountability standards, performance measures and reporting systems into their decision making and strategic plans. Those who don't [adapt] will be swimming against a tide that may wash away much of their market share."[14]

Accountability is fast becoming the new reality of a once-insular profession. New York State's public release of surgeon- and hospital-specific death rates from bypass surgery has caused controversy and saved patients' lives, as chapter 9 relates. In chapter 10, the state of Pennsylvania and Hershey Foods Company illustrate the impact of a one-two punch of publicly available performance data and impressive purchasing power. In Minneapolis–St. Paul, meanwhile, an assertive group of employers banded together and drew up a meticulous list of contract specifications that those who provide medical care are required to meet. Chapter 11 explores how the slogan of a physician who went from county medical society president to corporate medical director—"Specify, but verify"—is forcing the profession to measure the quality of its care.

Chapter 12 takes readers inside the Mayo Clinic, exploring how one of the country's premier medical organizations is reacting to these new pressures on medical practice. Using the tools of continuous improvement, Mayo is struggling to practice what one of its leaders calls "textbook medicine"; that is, the best scientifically justified medicine all of the time.

Ironically, becoming "too efficient" can boomerang. Chapter 13 examines what happened to a four-man family practice in a small rural town when it tried to eliminate unnecessary care. Its fate raises the question whether the "marketplace" will reward high quality or whether cost is all that matters. That is the fundamental challenge facing American medicine as it moves swiftly in the direction of "managed care."

THE PROMISE AND PERILS OF MANAGED CARE

Not so many years ago, the managers of health maintenance organizations (HMOs) were regarded as wild-eyed socialists seeking to undermine fee for service medicine. Now, like aging sixties radicals who have traded in a peace sign for a profit-and-loss statement, HMO managers stand accused of acting like health care robber barons who skim off profits for themselves by scrimping on services for their members. Yet despite the heated rhetoric, some sixty million generally contented Americans were members of HMOs by the end of 1996. For better or worse, HMOs have become the tool that employers and (increasingly) Medicare and Medicaid have chosen for the nearly impossible task of attempting to ration care while keeping everyone happy. Chapter 14 probes the origins and present-day workings of what has come to be called "managed care."

Chapter 15 then previews the coming "era of the patient." Just as the Protestant Reformation and the printing press shattered the monopoly of the priests, and so changed forever the average person's relationship with God, so too is information about the outcome of care altering the relationship between patients and physicians. Increasingly they share responsibility for better health, particularly in the case of chronic disease; this sharing is being accelerated by the enormous amount of clinical information now available through the Internet. If information is power, then shared information inevitably leads to shared power. "The systemic barriers are lowering fast," says family physician Richard Rockefeller, president of the Maine-based Health Commons Institute. "At this point, information is running downhill like water, and we're removing all the dams."

THE CARE PATIENTS DESERVE

The idea that medical treatment can be measured and managed still makes many physicians and nonphysicians alike deeply uncomfortable. It calls into question many of our assumptions about the mixture of art and science that goes into medicine. It requires a rethinking of physician professionalism and of the responsibility of patients. And it challenges those who would hold doctors, hospitals, and health plans accountable for results to hold themselves accountable for using the power of information ethically. Like any revolution, this one raises questions that do not yet have answers even as it renders many of the old answers obsolete.

In an often-quoted aphorism, the eighteenth-century French philosopher Voltaire held that "doctors are men who prescribe medicine of which they know little to cure diseases of which they know less in human beings of which they know nothing." Yet Voltaire also understood what sets the practice of medicine apart from other work and doctors apart from other workers. Physicians, he wrote, are "men who are occupied in the restoration of health to other men, by the joint exertion of skill and humanity, [men] who are above all the great of the earth. They even partake of divinity, since to preserve and renew is almost as noble as to create."

This book presents a picture of medicine that encompasses both of those views. The stories that follow tell of negligence and nobility, of a failure to learn from science and a fierce determination to suffuse everyday care with the best that science can offer. There are actions taken out of narrow self-interest, but there are also many examples of selflessness and deep dedication to the mission of healing.

Robert Waller, president and chief executive officer of the Mayo Clinic's parent Mayo Foundation, has spent more than a quarter of a century as a practicing ophthalmologist and administrator. Although he is quiet and conservative, Waller's commitment to excellence and to accountability in everything the clinic does comes through loud and clear. In conversation, he succinctly articulates the ultimate promise of this blending of traditional medical practice and the information revolution. "The goal is the best care possible for every patient every day," says Waller. "Our patients deserve nothing less."[15]

PART 1

Doing the Right Thing and Doing the Right Thing Right

CHAPTER ONE

Some Do, Some Don't

> Science is the knowledge of consequences, and dependence of one fact upon another.
> —Thomas Hobbes, 1651

There is an unsettling, if little known, truth about the practice of medicine. Even the best-trained doctors go about their work with an astonishingly shallow base of knowledge concerning the link between what they do and how it affects a patient's health. Whether the setting is a small town, a suburb, or the heart of a big-city medical center, study after study shows that few physicians systematically apply to everyday treatment the scientific evidence about what works best.

Why don't patients typically get the best possible care? And how should the practice of medicine change so that they do? The problem begins with the fact that physicians generally know little about the practices of doctors outside their immediate professional circle. Busy with their own patients, they mostly assume that similarly trained colleagues provide the same kind of care and get the same results. Rapid changes in the technology and economics of medicine, however, have persuaded some doctors and hospitals to take a fresh look at rituals of care that are often taken for granted. In Maine, eight hospitals decided to come together and track their treatment of patients with pneumonia or heart attack, two very common conditions that are also life threatening. The hospitals would then compare notes on what they found. The results in this one small state showed just how deceptive the surface similarities of American medicine can be.

On a dark and drab evening in late fall, an internist from one of the hospitals drove about an hour down the Maine coast to an old inn where doctors and pharmacists from the other institutions were gathered. Richard Kahn had spent twenty-two years as a family doctor in the small town of Rockport, but he still stood out from the crowd. Kahn's bushy gray beard made him physically unmistakable, while his animated manner cut through ingrained local reticence.

Chatty rather than taciturn, opinionated rather than reserved, the fifty-four-year-old internist occasionally liked to create a small stir. When a patient exhibited a bit too much faith in his healing powers, Kahn might take out a nineteenth-century brass fleam that he carried in his pocket. He would unfold the knifelike object and flourish the razor-sharp thumbnails on each blade tip that were designed to slice open a vein so the physician could practice therapeutic bloodletting. "This was considered good medicine," the amateur medical historian would explain as the patient eyed the blades warily. Or Kahn might pass on a former professor's sardonic attitude about the latest pharmaceutical miracle: "Use a new drug when it comes out, before it develops side effects."

Kahn was a veteran of medical committees; he served on a national committee of internists interested in medical ethics. He quickly signed up to represent Rockport's ninety-five-bed Penobscot Bay Medical Center in the examination of pneumonia and heart attacks. The first study results were to be unveiled at this evening's meeting. Each institution was identified by a code number to encourage candor, but the open display of sensitive clinical information still seemed a bit like undressing in public.[1]

It didn't take long for the first provocative nugget of information to emerge. All eight of the hospitals treated pneumonia with a class of antibiotics known as cephalosporins, which are similar in structure to penicillin. But though the hospitals treated the same kind of patients, the strategies their staffs chose for using these powerful drugs seemed like a medical version of "Goldilocks and the Three Bears." Some liked expensive and sophisticated drugs; some liked inexpensive, less-sophisticated drugs; and some liked a strategy somewhere in between. Unfortunately for patients, it was unclear which therapy was "just right."

At one end of the spectrum, the doctors at Hospital 3 relied heavily on the massive firepower of sophisticated third-generation cephalosporins. These broad-spectrum antibiotics are the assault weapons of the drug world, destroying almost everything in their path. That's reassuring for doctors who want to prevent the escape of whatever bacteria caused the pneumonia. But bacteria that do survive broad-spectrum antibiotics tend to become "bulletproof"—resistant to almost any antibiotic therapy at all. To prevent resistant bacteria from spreading throughout the population, medical experts strongly counsel judicious use of the most sophisticated drugs.

Despite this advice, the medical staffs at the eight hospitals took very different approaches in prescribing antibiotics. A pneumonia patient entering Hospital 3 for treatment was about twelve times more likely to receive third-generation antibiotics than a patient at Hospital 5, who was the most likely to get a somewhat older second-generation antibiotic. A patient who entered Hospital 8 was the most likely to receive first-generation cephalosporins. Yet at Hospital 1, pneumonia patients received no first-generation cephalosporins at all! Researchers looked in vain for any consistent pattern.

The treatment of heart attacks raised even more troubling questions. In a typical attack, a clot in the coronary arteries blocks the flow of blood, and the heart muscle, starved of oxygen, immediately starts to die. If doctors can quickly inject a drug to break up the clot, the victim's chances of survival rise dramatically.[2] Similarly, if doctors administer a drug to thin the blood, the odds drop that another clot will form and threaten the heart.[3] For individual medical reasons, not every patient can be treated this way. Nonetheless, the eight hospitals' uneven performance left some physicians and pharmacists shifting uneasily in their seats as they watched the numbers projected on a screen.

At one of the hospitals where the doctors seemed determined to be aggressive, about two-thirds of heart attack victims under age seventy-five got thrombolytics (clot busters)—nearly twice the rate of thrombolytic use at the least aggressive hospital. At the most aggressive hospital, some 94 percent of all heart attack patients received an anticoagulant. At the least aggressive institution, only 59 percent got a blood thinner. Just as with pneumonia, the remaining hospitals showed no discernible pattern.

These hospitals that looked so much alike to patients and staff varied enormously in the treatment they provided. But why? And what was the effect on patients?

The variation could mean that the researchers conducting the study were mistaken and that the hospitals each treated very different kinds of patients. This didn't seem entirely plausible, however, when one hospital was administering clot busters to twice as many heart attack patients or giving sophisticated antibiotics twelve times as frequently.

The variation could reflect the mix of doctors at each institution. A specialist is more likely than a generalist to keep up with the latest research and use the newest drugs and equipment. Some hospitals could have been using cardiologists to treat heart attacks or pulmonologists for pneumonia while other hospitals relied on generalists.[4]

The flaw in that theory was that the hospitals didn't neatly divide into the high-use and low-use groups typical of the gap between specialists and other doctors.

The third possible explanation for the variations was the most unnerving. The differences could result from physicians' "practice styles" or "preferences," the polite terms the medical community uses to describe treatment that varies because doctors vary. This constitutes not so much an explanation as a tautology. The words "style" and "preferences" have an innocuous ring. In our consumerist society, it seems sometimes that the Declaration of Independence implicitly blessed each citizen's right to life, liberty, and the pursuit of styles and preferences. The consumer who prefers pasta over pizza, however, affects only her own life; the doctor who favors one antibiotic over another affects the lives of her patients.

In Maine, the small organization coordinating the variation study for the eight hospitals did not have either the time or the money to ask many questions about how treatment differences ultimately affected the health of the patients. The study's entire budget came to $30,000, or about the cost of one hospital's buying one basic ultrasound machine. Put another way, the money spent examining the treatment of nearly one thousand people who were hospitalized with pneumonia or a heart attack amounted to some $30 per patient.

As the discussion in the Maine inn neared its end that evening, Kahn raised his hand to make a final point. The information on variations in treatment should be presented to hospital leaders, he declared. And it should be given to the federally funded "peer review organization" that oversees the cost and quality of the medical treatment provided to Medicare patients. "If you're just doing this" (here Kahn turned and gestured to the group of about a dozen people), "you're not accomplishing anything. The whole idea is to change behavior and make medicine better."

The entire purpose of medical treatment, of course, is to make patients better. If some practices or preferences are more likely to lead to that result, then physicians and hospitals should be pushed to adopt them. If some styles of treatment are less successful, they should be abandoned.

Discovering "what works best" in medicine, however, is slow and difficult work. The answers are not intuitively obvious, and the search is not very glamorous. There are no teams of physicians working frenetically into the night, and there are no dramatic moments of discovery that would look good on a movie screen. The only exciting thing that happens is that some people get well faster and some people who would have died go home to their families alive.

CURING PNEUMONIA

In the middle of 1989, the medical director of Pittsburgh's Forbes Health System received disturbing news.[5] According to an internal report, an unexpectedly large number of Forbes patients were dying.

A hospital, like a bank, depends for its existence on public trust. It's nice if the bank is open for business during convenient hours and the tellers are friendly, but a bank's basic purpose is to ensure that depositors get their money back when they need it. Similarly, though hospitals may sponsor "wellness fairs," their fundamental mission is to heal the sick. Patients joke about bad hospital food; bad care isn't funny.

The community served by Forbes was unaware of any problem. The information came from a private data company, Medi-Qual, that held a contract to analyze the cost and quality of the system's care. The issue was not malpractice; the information Medi-Qual provided dealt with much more subtle medical behavior. By examining several clinical measures indicating how ill Forbes patients were when they entered the hospital, Medi-Qual calculated an expected patient death rate. It then compared the number of expected deaths with the number that actually occurred. In addition, Medi-Qual compiled a national registry of its customers that showed which hospitals did the best job of reducing the ratio of actual to expected deaths.

The formula Medi-Qual uses to determine the expected deaths is far from exact. Some experts believe it does a poor job of accounting for the complex effect that sickness has on a patient before treatment.[6] Other experts, though, believe the formula provides at least a roughly accurate confirmation that a hospital is doing well or, conversely, a warning that the quality of its care is lagging. Forbes's medical director, Richard McGarvey, was well aware of both viewpoints. McGarvey decided to investigate on his own whether the numbers on his desk were telling the truth. To do that, he went directly to the medical charts of some patients who had died and read the scrawled notes detailing the story of their treatment in the hospital. When he finished, he called together Forbes's key physicians. "Maybe we can explain to the news media and you folks that we don't buy this comparison, but when I look at these charts, we're not doing things quite the way I remember talking about doing them in medical school," McGarvey told the group. "Let's see if we can improve things."[7]

The flagship of the Forbes system is the 353-bed Forbes Regional Hospital. Situated in the rolling hills of Monroeville, a prosperous middle-class suburb fourteen miles east of Pittsburgh, Forbes Regional is a teaching hospital that prides itself on state of the art treatment. But according to the Medi-Qual data, the largest cluster of unexpected deaths occurred on the floors where it treated pneumonia patients.

No hospital likes finding problems with its care. The typical first reaction is outrage and denial. The second reaction is to form up a professional posse to hunt down and "hang" the doctors or nurses responsible for tarnishing the institution's honor. Unfortunately for that approach, the Forbes task force couldn't find any obvious villains. At first glance, pneumonia care seemed to meet all the hospital's standards. Puzzled, the group went back and reexamined the situation in a different light, this time dividing the pneumonia patients into "high-risk" and "lower-risk" groups. Looked at from this new angle, a grim pattern immediately emerged.

The high-risk group included many of the "old-old"; that is, patients over eighty. They typically contracted pneumonia in the hospital or at a nursing home. Frequently they had serious underlying diseases such as lung cancer or an infection of the bloodstream. These high-risk patients were dying about as frequently as expected.[8] The lower-risk patients, on the other hand, generally started out younger and healthier. They usually contracted pneumonia out in the community, then entered the hospital as their condition worsened. It was these lower-risk patients who were dying at nearly twice the expected rate. During one twelve-month period, for example, ten lower-risk pneumonia patients were expected to die. Instead, eighteen did.

An average of one "extra" death every two months could easily elude the notice of busy physicians and nurses caught up in the daily patient-by-patient struggle against disease. Even if it attracted their attention, they might understandably attribute it to an unlucky run of patients who failed to respond to therapy. The task force suppressed the urge to "explain the adverse outcomes on the basis of demographical, clinical and life-style differences," as McGarvey and assistant medical director John J. Harper put it.[9] Instead, they followed McGarvey's example and randomly selected a number of medical records of pneumonia patients who died and an identical number of records of pneumonia patients who survived. What the reviewers found was a vivid example of the link between mundane medical processes and patient survival.

In its most severe form, bacterial pneumonia is a frightening disease. Microbes invade the lung's microscopic air sacs, causing swelling and inflammation. Patients run a high fever, and they endure attacks of coughing while trying to clear their clogged lungs of a fiberlike fluid. Their breathing becomes shallow, rapid, and painful, and their pulse rate soars. As the body's ability to take in oxygen and rid itself of carbon dioxide slowly diminishes, the brain may die or the heart erupt in violent fibrillation and then stop.

Physicians try to prescribe the type of antibiotics most suited to kill whichever bacteria are causing the pneumonia infection. One way of identifying those bacteria is to analyze a sputum sample from deep within the patient's lungs. A blood culture is even better: in addition to confirming the sputum results, a blood sample shows whether the infection in the lungs is spreading dangerously throughout the entire body.

Although the staff at Forbes Regional knew all this, the hospital wasn't well organized to effectively fight the war on pneumonia. Busy nurses seeking a sputum sample left a cup by the bedside and asked patients to fill it "when they could." What often ended up in the cup was useless saliva. Meanwhile, a blood sample might not be collected until the patient had already been in the hospital for a full day. Though blood and sputum tests don't always provide reliable information on the source of infection, the Forbes staff was unnecessarily flying blind.[10] Worst of all, some patients were spending ten to fourteen hours in the hospital without receiving any antibiotic therapy at all.

In the part of the country where Forbes Regional was situated, two virulent strains of bacteria called *Mycoplasma* and *Legionella* had been identified as causing nearly one-fifth of the cases of serious bacterial pneumonia. Yet the Forbes Regional staff rarely ordered the type of antibiotics known to kill those bugs. The task force did not speculate on the reason, but it may have been ignorance. The hospital's infectious disease and pulmonary specialists were called in by generalist colleagues to examine only about one-third of pneumonia patients.[11]

In late 1989, the unhappy task force turned in a report whose key recommendation was simplicity itself: "Patients admitted with a diagnosis of pneumonia should have all essential diagnostic studies completed and therapy initiated promptly." To emphasize the point, the hospital presented doctors and nurses with a "clinical path" that explicitly spelled out the steps the staff needed to take to improve care.

Nurses stopped leaving plastic cups on patients' trays; instead, trained respiratory therapists were dispatched to the bedside to obtain a sputum sample. A time limit was set for initiating antibiotics: doctors and nurses were told to do it within four hours. The clinical path "strongly suggested" use of drugs effective against the *Mycoplasma* and *Legionella* bacteria. And it "encouraged" attending physicians to call in a specialist if the patient didn't improve within forty-eight hours.

Eighteen months later, Forbes Regional measured the effect of these changes. The death rate remained about the same for those patients with the highest risk of dying from pneumonia, but the seriously ill patients who did survive were regaining their health and leaving the hospital more quickly. In lower-risk pneumonia patients, however, the critical path had a dramatic impact. Their mortality rate plunged. Only about one-third of the patients who were expected to die according to the Medi-Qual measurement actually did. Given Forbes's mix of pneumonia patients, that meant saving one extra life each month; before the critical path was introduced, one "extra" patient died every two months. In other words, eighteen patients were saved by one hospital from one illness. Nationwide, bacterial pneumonia causes nearly one million admissions to hospitals each year and is the nation's sixth leading killer.[12]

Like a consistent baseball team, the Forbes Regional staff could see the payoff for its efforts in the "won" column—not in games, but in lives.

HOW TO SURVIVE A HEART ATTACK

In the kitchens of rural South Carolina, a breakfast of biscuits, sausage, fried fatback, and a can of cola raises no more eyebrows than do an oat bran muffin and a glass of skim milk in a coffee shop in downtown Los Angeles. At the 475-bed Anderson Area Medical Center, the hospital staff resignedly refers to its community as the buckle of the heart attack belt. Figures from the federal Centers for Disease Control and Prevention back them up.[13]

Anderson serves about 150,000 people in a semirural area that mixes farms, forests, and increasingly, factories attracted by low wages and stable small-town communities. The hospital enjoys a favorable "word of mouth" reputation, which is fortunate for residents, since the next nearest hospital is more than twenty miles away. In the late 1980s, however, Anderson's complacency was shaken by two studies that raised harsh questions about how it treated heart attacks.

Statisticians rely on the law of large numbers to determine the likelihood that an event happened by chance. If a hospital treats three heart attack patients and has a mortality rate of 33 percent—meaning that one patient died—that one death could as likely be caused by a circumstance beyond the hospital's control as by shortcomings in care. If a hospital treats three hundred or three thousand patients, the odds that a 33 percent mortality rate is due to chance alone are much lower. At Anderson, one study found that nearly 40 percent more heart attack patients died during a one-year period than would be expected to die, while another study also showed mediocre results. The evidence seemed to point to poor care as the culprit, but the number of patients involved fell just short of reaching the usual statistical standard for "proof."[14]

There was an additional difficulty, one that continually crops up when hospitals try to examine their clinical procedures. The study where the hospital's heart attack treatment looked the worst was based on information from payment claims forms Anderson sent to Medicare. The form is standardized, and it can be read by a computer. By comparison, clinical information taken from patients' charts must be painstakingly and expensively abstracted by hand. The convenience carries a price, however. Because Medicare payment is based on the patient's primary diagnosis, hospitals may not bother coding all the other coexisting problems of an elderly patient, even if those other problems were important in whether the patient lived or died.

The greatest risk in using claims forms for clinical purposes, though, revolves around an arcane practice called "upcoding." Although ethical doctors and hospitals avoid outright falsehoods in specifying a diagnosis, many hospitals guiltlessly use sophisticated computer programs that search for the most plausible and well-paid diagnosis that fits the patient's clinical signs. Upcoding has cast a pall of suspicion over claims-form information.[15] Despite these concerns, the leaders at Anderson, like those at Forbes Regional, decided that arguments about less than perfect information were beside the point. The disturbing implications of two separate studies demanded that the hospital conduct an honest internal appraisal.

Although the northwest corner of South Carolina is a conservative, even isolated, area, Anderson's top leaders were men with an unusually broad national perspective. D. Kirk Oglesby Jr., Anderson's chief executive officer, was finishing a term as chairman of the American Hospital Association. Frederic Jones, the executive vice president for medical affairs, came to the hospital after a twenty-year military career that included serving as chief of cardiology at a large U.S. Air Force teaching hospital. Both men were savvy about game playing with claims forms, but they also knew there are clear clinical tests to establish that a heart attack has occurred. It is a diagnosis not easily coded as something else. Moreover, if a patient's final status on discharge from the hospital was listed as "dead," then the patient very likely was exactly that. An expert outside consultant called in to examine the claims data and patient records confirmed the bad news. About one in five heart attack patients entering Anderson Area Medical Center was dying there. The problem was not the data, but the care.[16]

Every year about one American in two hundred suffers a heart attack, for an astonishing rate of one heart attack every twenty seconds.[17] It is the chief cause of death in the United States. The key to survival is quick treatment. The interval between the time a heart attack sufferer comes through the emergency room door and the injection of a thrombolytic, clot buster drug is called the "door-to-needle time." Someone treated within an hour of feeling chest pain is nearly 50 percent more likely to survive than someone treated after the "golden hour" has passed.[18] Procrastination can be a fatal error; patients who receive thrombolytics more than six hours after their first symptoms have no better chance of living than patients who get no thrombolytics at all.[19]

At Anderson, the average door-to-needle time stretched to a molasses-slow 162 minutes, or more than two and a half times the then-national standard of sixty minutes.[20]

Jones, a tall, courtly man then in his late fifties, carefully pondered what to do next. After leaving the military he had moved to Anderson, he explained in a broad southern accent, because he was "married to a South Carolina girl." After a decade as the hospital's top physician, he'd learned that it was pointless to issue military-style orders to "shape up" to the independent-minded medical staff. Instead, Jones decided to coat some tough actions with a thick layer of southern charm. We're not out to get you folks, he reassured the doctors. We're all in this together. What we've got here is a "systems" problem, not a problem with any individual physician.

Of course the system was composed of individual components. Heart attack patients who made it to Anderson's cardiac care unit (CCU) fared as well as similar patients in other hospitals. But a person who arrived at the emergency room with chest pain often waited there untreated until his family doctor could arrive from the office and issue treatment orders. As a result, heart attack victims were dying almost in sight of that CCU "promised land." The emergency room doctors and nurses were reluctant to take matters into their own hands and administer thrombolytic drugs whose actions they did not understand and whose possible side effects they feared. Some of the generalists were similarly untrained.

To demonstrate the impact of this practice "style" and "preference," Jones gave each staff physician a confidential copy of his personal "batting average" for heart attack patients. Drawing on a computerized clinical database, the numbers attempted to adjust the death rate to take into account how sick the patients were before treatment.

The hospital also calculated the "team" results of three types of doctors: general practitioners, internists, and physicians on the hospital's teaching service. Unlike individual results, "team standings" were shared with the entire staff. One finding stood out: the patients treated by general practitioners were significantly more likely to die. Faced with this uncomfortable fact, many GPs quietly dropped out of heart attack care. To encourage others to voluntarily bench themselves, Jones finally required them to consult with a specialist when they admitted a heart attack patient to the hospital.

The medical center set up a clinical pathway for heart attacks that was similar to what Forbes Regional used with pneumonia. Just as at Forbes, the effect of standardizing care was dramatic. Anderson's "door-to-needle time" plummeted to thirty-three minutes, or less than one-fifth the waiting time in 1987. And the hospital's death rate from heart attacks dropped by half, from nearly 20 percent to 10 percent. Although the national average mortality rate was about 8 percent, Anderson discovered that many patients in its area delayed seeking treatment. To address that problem, the hospital launched an outreach campaign.

Because of the hospital's changes in its medical care, two heart attack patients a month who likely would have died at Anderson were leaving the hospital alive. Just as with Forbes Regional, there was no secret formula to account for the turnaround. Some doctors who should not have been treating heart attacks stopped treating them. Other doctors and nurses learned to treat heart attacks more effectively. Most important of all, the entire staff became more consistent at doing all the little things that Added up to excellent care. Medical director Jones calls it "systems thinking." It amounts to saving lives based on a very simple principle. Said Jones, "People knew what they had to do."

A LESSON FOR PATIENTS

> He who saves one life . . . is as if he saved the entire world.
>
> —Talmud, Sanhedrin 37:A

The stories of Forbes Regional Hospital and Anderson Area Medical Center are not unique. Similar opportunities to save lives are discovered at every hospital in the country. The proof comes from the medical literature and from the kind of candid conversations physicians and hospital administrators engage in when they are among their peers. To cite one well-known study, RAND Corporation researchers Robert W. Dubois and Robert H. Brook closely examined 182 deaths that occurred at twelve hospitals. About one in seven deaths from stroke, pneumonia, and heart attack were unanimously judged as preventable by a panel of three doctors independently reviewing charts. If the standard had been two of the three doctors agreeing, then nearly one in four deaths would have been ruled preventable.[21]

That conclusion seems well within the realm of possibility. In a study of relatively small Tennessee hospitals, for instance, Medicare patients with pneumonia waited an average of twelve hours before receiving any antibiotic therapy. Many of these vulnerable older patients never even had a blood culture performed.[22] Meanwhile, EHS Health Care, a large Chicago-area system, recounted at a medical conference a litany of difficulties with its pneumonia therapy that mirrored Forbes's experience. Seventy percent of pneumonia patients admitted from nursing homes were getting no antibiotics in the emergency room. The antibiotic prescriptions of those who did receive drugs were changed 80 percent of the time on the regular hospital floor, showing a high degree of uncertainty about treatment. And some of the hospital staff (to the surprise of the researchers) had no idea that the sputum sample was important.[23]

Persistent problems in treating heart attacks are documented even more clearly. In late 1993 the federal Medicare program analyzed the treatment of ten thousand elderly heart attack patients in four states to see whether physicians complied with the voluntary guidelines issued by groups like the American College of Cardiology and the American Heart Association. The results can best be described as dis-heartening.[24]

Fully one-fifth of heart attack patients who needed thrombolytic clot busters never received them. More than one-third of those who should have been instructed to take one aspirin daily to prevent further blood clots left the hospital without getting that potentially lifesaving advice. Patients whose medical records indicated they were not candidates for these therapies were excluded from the analysis.

The average door-to-needle time for administering thrombolytics in the four states was one hour. At the time the study was released in early 1994, the voluntary national standard was between thirty and sixty minutes. When the study was conducted, fewer than one in seven hospitals administered clot busters within a half hour after the patient came through the door.[25] In late 1996, the American College of Cardiology and the American Heart Association issued new guidelines saying that prompt medical treatment was so important that anyone suffering from a heart attack should be evaluated and referred to a specific pathway of care within ten minutes of arriving at the emergency room.

Researchers at the Mayo Clinic, world renowned for its treatment of difficult medical problems, told the 1995 meeting of the American College of Cardiology just how simple it would be to meet that half-hour heart attack treatment goal. First, the Mayo trauma unit prepared a "tackle box" for its emergency room, containing the equipment and drugs that doctors and nurses needed to begin heart attack treatment immediately. Then the clinic gave members of its trauma unit staff two pocket-sized cards to carry. The cards remind them when drugs should be given to heart attack victims, what kind of drugs different patients need, and what doses to administer. This approach worked not only at Mayo's sophisticated hospitals in Rochester, Minnesota, but also at community hospitals in small Minnesota towns like Lake City, Wabasha, and Austin.[26]

Meanwhile, although administering beta-blocker drugs to heart attack victims is one of the most scientifically substantiated of preventive medical services, just one in five eligible patients received the therapy when they went to the hospital, according to an analysis of four years of Medicare data for New Jersey. The consequences were grim: when other factors were controlled for, concluded Harvard's Stephen Soumerai and his colleagues in an 8 January 1997 *JAMA* article, those who did not get the beta blockers had a 43 percent greater chance of dying and a 20 percent greater risk of being rehospitalized for cardiovascular disease.[27]

SAVING LIVES FOR PENNIES A DAY

Here's how easy it would be to save literally thousands of lives. About 500,000 Americans die each year from heart attacks.[28] Use of the "tackle box" and pocket cards could save 2,500 to 5,000 of those people, the Mayo Clinic's Stephen Kopecky calculated. That estimate seems conservative.

One-quarter of patients hospitalized with a heart attack do not receive livesaving thrombolytics.[29] Sometimes there is an explanation. Doctors may think some patients are too old to benefit from the $6,000 a dose therapy because early clinical trials of the drugs raised doubts about the response of the oldest patients. But in a more recent trial, a man treated with a clot buster at age 110 was reportedly still going strong three years later. At other times, such as with the eight Maine hospitals, the reasons for failing to administer clot busters are not at all clear. According to a 1994 study, if hospitals and physicians simply followed professional society guidelines on thrombolytic drugs, some 12,000 lives a year would be saved.[30] And though the authors of the *JAMA* study on the poor use of beta blockers did not estimate how many lives would be saved by increasing the survival chances of four-fifths of elderly heart attack victims (not to mention the effect on younger patients), that number would surely be quite substantial.

As for pneumonia, it kills some 175,000 Americans annually. It is one of the most common reasons for hospitalization among the elderly, and it is the nation's leading cause of death from infectious disease. The death rate for just lower-risk patients who require hospitalization is about 5 percent;[31] other studies have also found a wide variation in how well hospitals perform in treatment of pneumonia.[32] If all hospitals treated it as consistently as Forbes Regional, a fair estimate is that the overall death rate from pneumonia would fall by one percentage point. That means 1,750 lives would be saved each year.

It is easy to view this type of calculation as depending on ideal conditions unobtainable in the real world, like those studies that say we would all live 3.7 years longer if we never ate another french fry. A laudable goal, perhaps, but not very practical. The changes discussed here are different. They are not theoretical; hospitals have already made them and shown they can be effective in saving lives. The changes are not complicated. All that is required to reap their benefits is an investment of time and money; for instance, choosing to invest $30,000 to study the quality of care instead of using the $30,000 to buy a revenue-producing ultrasound machine. Put another way, the only barrier preventing hospitals from saving tens of thousands of extra lives each year is the willingness of doctors and hospital administrators to change.

CHAPTER TWO

What Doctors Don't Know

One of the problems of the future is to educate the public itself to appreciate that very seldom, under existing conditions, does a patient receive the best aid which it is possible to give him in the present state of medicine.
—The Flexner Report, 1910

Consider for a moment a cautionary tale about American medicine: As part of a large study, researchers from the American Child Health Association picked a sample of one thousand eleven-year-olds from the New York City public schools. After finding that 61 percent of the children had already had their tonsils removed, the researchers sent the remaining children to a group of school doctors. The physicians duly reported that 45 percent of those students needed a tonsillectomy.

The other students, who had been told their tonsils did not need to be removed, were sent for a second opinion to different school doctors. These doctors examined them and concluded that 46 percent of the group needed a tonsillectomy. One more time, the remaining children who had been told their tonsils were all right—in fact, had now been told by two groups of doctors that their tonsils were fine—were sent to more doctors for another opinion. The new physicians concluded that 44 percent of the group needed a tonsillectomy.

By now, only sixty-five of the original one thousand children had not either had their tonsils removed or been told they needed to be removed. These grizzled veterans of the tongue depressor circuit were mercifully spared any further medical attention. The researchers decided that it was not the symptoms of the individual children that explained the diagnosis. "Variation is not so much due to the differences in the conditions of the children as it is to differences in the viewpoint and standards of the [medical] examiners," the researchers wrote.[1] Their study was published in 1934.

Skip ahead twenty years to the height of the Baby Boom. In the mid-1950s, children of insured workers had about a fifty-fifty chance of having their tonsils removed.[2] Yet an exhaustive review of the medical literature up to that time found no evidence that a tonsillectomy accomplished its purposes. "The continuance of the practice of indiscriminate T[onsillectomies] and A[denoidectomies] is indeed an enigma," the March 1958 issue of the prestigious *Journal of Pediatrics* noted plaintively.[3] Elsewhere a researcher who pointed out the absence of objective evidence justifying the procedure termed the tonsillectomy "an elaborate, institutionalized, cryptic ritual."[4]

Fast forward nearly twenty years once again, to the mid-1970s. Physicians now conceded openly that 50 to 80 percent of tonsillectomies were probably unnecessary.[5] This time, for a variety of reasons, the publicity finally began to have a significant impact, and the frequency of tonsillectomies began to decline.

Finally, however, skip ahead about two more decades, to the grandchildren and great-grandchildren of those New York City schoolchildren from the early years of the century. A 1991 study provided good news and bad news. The bad news was that a tonsillectomy was still the surgical procedure most likely to be performed inappropriately. The good news was that the situation had improved markedly in sixty years. Now only about one tonsillectomy in four was unneeded.[6]

The tale of the tonsillectomies contains a sad postscript. During the Baby Boom years of 1950 through 1955, some two hundred to three hundred children under age fifteen died annually from anesthesia, postoperative hemorrhaging, and other effects of tonsillectomies.[7] The surgery itself was probably unnecessary; these children's deaths were a tragic waste. This count of victims does not even include the children injured either physically (aspiration pneumonia) or psychologically. Because of the overnight hospital stay away from parents, some of the very youngest children (tonsillectomies were even performed on infants) suffered from night terrors, fears, and dependency for months or years afterward.[8] More broadly a part of the body that plays a role in protecting against infection and disease was needlessly removed for decades after medical researchers suspected or knew the tonsils' real function.[9]

One of the promised benefits of a tonsillectomy was preventing frequent ear infections, a condition known as otitis media. Ironically, a present-day treatment for that same problem may be used just as inappropriately. At present almost 700,000 children have tympanostomy tubes inserted into their ears each year as a treatment for otitis media. But more than a quarter of the time (27 percent) that treatment is inappropriate, according to a 1994 study in the *Journal of the American Medical Association.* Another 41 percent of the time the clinical indications are "equivocal."[10]

That means several hundred thousand children each year are having ear tubes implanted that offer no clear medical benefit, even though inserting the tubes places the children "at increased risk for undesirable outcomes" that can include permanent damage to the eardrum from repeated reinsertion of tubes.[11]

What happened with the tonsillectomy and the tympanostomy procedure that followed it was not an aberration. The same pattern of widespread use of unnecessary or ineffective surgeries has been repeated with hysterectomies, open-heart surgery, and treatment for ulcers, among many other conditions.[12] Even today women frequently undergo electronic fetal monitoring during labor even though there is no agreed-on evidence that it accomplishes anything other than increasing the chances that the baby will be delivered by the riskier methods of a cesarean section or forceps.[13]

"Much, if not most, of contemporary medical practice still lacks scientific foundation," wrote a commentator in 1993. "Some 'new' technologies have clearly harmed people. . . . Responsibility for this medical malfeasance lies primarily with physicians, although consumers have often demanded unproven technologies."[14]

For patients, the question is why physicians act this way. Do doctors decide on treatments based on their personal experience, or do they rely on studies in the medical literature? What role is played by the demands of patients and the seductive call of the latest technology? To what extent are physicians affected by where they trained and the specialty they chose? And increasingly important in this time of medical cost containment, Is physicians' judgment subconsciously swayed by the way they are paid? In other words, How does your doctor decide "what works best"? A review of the tangled roots of scientific medicine, and another look at the history of the common tonsillectomy, suggests some answers.

THE HEALER BECOMES A SCIENTIST

The ideal of physician as scientist long predates modern times. The Hippocratic oath hints at the physician's unique responsibilities as much by what it omits as by what it says. Although the fifth century B.C. oath contains a pledge of loyalty to "Apollo, the physician, and Aesculapius, Hygeia, and Panacea and all the gods and goddesses," these ancient Greek deities are presented neither as causing sickness nor as curing it.[15] Instead of appealing to the heavens for healing, Hippocrates looked for objective evidence about how each patient's illness might best be treated. " 'I believe that attention should be paid to all the details of the science [of healing],' wrote Hippocrates in a series of essays and aphorisms that led later generations to hail him as the Father of Medicine." Medicine was a science, because sciences dealt in facts, and there was factual evidence that a physician's ministrations could lead to "the complete removal of the distress of the sick."[16]

Physicians still turned for guidance to the writings of Hippocrates and his followers centuries after their deaths. The rational approach to disease prevention and treatment the Hippocratics so eloquently advocated, however, proved less durable than their founder's reputation. The medical rationalists' influence gradually declined as they were succeeded by priests, magicians, mediums, apothecaries, barbers, and other self-anointed healers. "The accurate descriptions of the Hippocratics," wrote one historian, "gave way to surmise, guesswork and unsupported inference."[17]

Since God's healing power was clearly proclaimed in both the Old and New Testaments, it could be dangerous to argue for a more earthbound model of disease and cure. Rationalism risked being mistaken for heresy.[18] In one example of the bond between religion and healing, the archbishop of Canterbury was legally able to award medical degrees in England as late as 1840.[19] (Bishops had an even more direct connection to medical therapy according to one folk belief, which held that whooping cough could be cured by drinking water from the skull of a bishop. Perhaps the desire to avoid such active participation in the healing process inspired the archbishop to start issuing medical degrees.)[20]

The respectful title "doctor," from the Latin word for "teacher," began to be applied to all sorts of healers in the fourteenth century, about the time Chaucer was writing his bawdy *Canterbury Tales.* If doctors of the time were truly teachers, the lesson plan remained highly idiosyncratic. Every physician seemed to propound a different theory about the cause and cure of disease. Although this began to change with the Enlightenment, even the most respected doctors of that time were not immune to fantastic theorizing.

For example, Benjamin Rush, a Quaker physician and signer of the Declaration of Independence, asserted that "Americans are tougher than Europeans [and] American diseases are, correspondingly, tougher than mild European diseases." An advocate of copious bloodletting as a standard therapeutic approach, Rush advised American doctors and their patients to approach treatment in a way that was "heroic, bold, courageous, manly and patriotic."[21]

In December 1799 George Washington, the father of American nationhood, got a chance to put Rush's theories to the test. Washington had gone for a horseback ride in the snow around his Mount Vernon estate. Though still vigorous in retirement, the sixty-seven-year-old former president and Continental Army commander developed a persistent fever and a severe sore throat. Doctors summoned to Mount Vernon wrapped the throat in poultices and gave him warm vinegar and molasses to gargle. To break the fever, the doctors decided on what Benjamin Rush might have called a "bold and patriotic" course of therapeutic bleeding.

> In a common technique of the time, the doctor sat next to the patient and placed a moderately tight ligature around the arm or leg above the area to be lanced. Once the veins were properly swollen and visible, the surgeon employed a lancet or small knife to make an incision. . . . Plunging the spear-pointed knife into a vein through an oblique incision created an orifice of about an eighth of an inch, generally sufficient to allow the flow of blood to gush out.[22]

Washington's physicians repeatedly drained his blood, but the patient failed to respond. Weakened and in great pain, Washington began to slip into unconsciousness. "I thank you for your attention" were his last words to those crowding around his bedside. "You had better not take any more trouble about me, but let me go off quietly. I cannot last long."[23]

Hippocrates had admonished doctors to "help or at least to do no harm." During the long dark ages of medicine, physicians seemed unable to comprehend that their well-intentioned attempts at curing the sick might be having the opposite effect. While British physician and essayist William Tully called the lancet "a weapon which annually slays more than the sword," advocates invoked the authority of medical tradition. Bleeding "has had the endorsement of each age and generation [of physicians]," argued one mid-nineteenth-century defender.[24] Pseudoscience validated a menu of similar grisly treatments.

"Paper after learned paper recounts the benefits of bleeding, cupping, violent purging, the raising of blisters by vesicant ointments [and] the immersion of the body in either ice water or intolerably hot water," a twentieth-century analyst commented. "All these things were drilled into the heads of medical students."[25]

By the middle of the nineteenth century, the physical sciences were making sweeping progress. Steam engines powered threshing machines, looms, power tools, railroads, and even a bus or two. A Western Union telegraph line connected New York and San Francisco, helping to put the money-losing Pony Express out of business forever.[26] But medicine remained oddly frozen in time.

A series of extraordinary breakthroughs finally burst the dam of stagnant medical tradition. In 1819 the Frenchman René Laënnec invented the stethoscope. The instrument provided important new clues in diagnosing disease by allowing doctors to hear previously unintelligible sounds emanating from the internal organs. In 1846, in the first public demonstration of surgery under anesthesia, a patient at Massachusetts General Hospital had a tumor removed from his neck after dentist William T. G. Morton anesthetized the man with ethyl ether. (About forty years later a young M.D. working in the Austrian province of Bosnia and Herzegovina reported that cocaine could be used as a local anesthetic. However, surgeon Sigmund Freud eventually decided his true medical talents lay elsewhere.)[27] In 1865 the English surgeon Joseph Lister demonstrated that washing the hands in a sterile solution, phenol, prevented the transmission of infection and disease during surgery. Lister's advocacy of what came to be called antiseptic surgery grew out of Louis Pasteur's theory that bacteria caused infection.[28]

Medical education too was evolving. "Therapeutic nihilists" championed the novel notion that it was better for a physician to do nothing for a patient than to provide a treatment that could be harmful. William Osler, a legendary medical teacher and humanist of the period, urged students at Baltimore's new Johns Hopkins University School of Medicine, "Weigh evidence and [do] not go beyond it."[29] By 1912 enough physicians were following that advice that "a random patient with a random disease, consulting a doctor chosen at random, had, for the first time in the history of mankind, a better than fifty-fifty chance of profiting from the encounter," in the frequently quoted phrase of Harvard biochemist Lawrence J. Henderson.[30]

To be sure, skeptics detected a difference between Osler's lofty vision and the reality of the local doctor's office. As playwright George Bernard Shaw put it in his 1913 introduction to *The Doctor's Dilemma:*

> I presume nobody will question the existence of a widely spread popular delusion that every doctor is a man of science. . . . To a sufficiently ignorant man, every captain of a trading schooner is a Galileo, every organ-grinder a Beethoven. . . . As a matter of fact, the rank and file of doctors are no more scientific than their tailors; or, if you prefer to put it the reverse way, their tailors are no less scientific than they.

Osler aside, medical schools of the era endorsed competing ideological agendas ranging from botany to homeopathy. The newly minted physician sometimes lacked even a high-school diploma. When doctors had little to offer patients other than a sympathetic ear, educational credentials were not critical, but the advance of scientific research made new demands on would-be physicians. The helter-skelter nature of medical education increasingly seemed like a painful anachronism. With the backing of the fledgling Carnegie Foundation, educator Abraham Flexner drew up a blueprint for wholesale change. Flexner visited 147 medical schools in the United States and 7 in Canada. He methodically scrutinized their curriculum and their facilities, discovering, for example, that one school hid empty laboratories behind locked doors with signs saying "Anatomy" and "Physiology." Flexner's final report minced no words. Chicago, with 15 medical schools, was called "the plague spot of the country." The medical department at the University of Buffalo was dismissed as "a fiction."[31] Other schools were "disgraceful" and "shameful."

Flexner's revelations sparked outrage among the public and the profession. His recommendations to upgrade and "standardize" medical education won the moral backing of the American Medical Association and the financial backing of the Carnegie and Rockefeller Foundations. The eventual effect on medical education was so powerful that the Flexner Report has been called the most important document in the history of American medicine.[32] The Flexner Report appeared in 1910. By 1930, only 76 of the 131 independent medical schools operating in 1910 remained.[33] Most of the survivors had forged an affiliation with a university, and all had pledged to follow a rigorously scientific curriculum.

Rabbinic legend credits the Abraham of the Old Testament with destroying the idols his father worshiped and becoming the first to embrace the worship of the one true God.[34] The Abraham of the Flexner Report triggered an analogous epic cultural shift in medicine, and his deeds gradually assumed a similar mythic cast. Flexner and his supporters permanently separated medicine from the most dubious practices of its professional forefathers. Flexnerians "insisted on the fundamentally scientific nature of medicine, on the pursuit of excellence and on the inadmissibility of ignorance, sham and fraudulent claims," wrote Jeremiah Barondess, president of the New York Academy of Medicine. Science and clinical practice became tightly bound together. "In a crucial conceptualization, [the Flexner Report] linked the good of the profession to the welfare of its patients."[35]

The timing of the Flexner Report was also fortuitous. By the beginning of the twentieth century, biomedical research began yielding the kind of tangible benefits that the physical sciences had begun to contribute years before. In the 1920s came the discovery of insulin as a treatment for diabetes mellitus and the use of liver as a cure for anemia, which until that time was fatal. By the mid-1930s, physicians could prescribe a few tablets of the new sulfanilamide drugs to vanquish infectious diseases that used to devastate entire communities.[36] The death rates for tuberculosis, typhoid fever, meningitis, measles, dysentery, and whooping cough plunged between 1900 and 1935 owing to a combination of better medical care and long overdue improvements in public health and sanitation.[37]

Lewis Thomas worked as an intern in Boston in the early 1930s. (Thomas would later become a respected medical researcher and historian.) In *The Youngest Science,* he provided an eyewitness account of the impact of these first "wonder drugs": "The phenomenon was almost beyond belief. Here were moribund patients, who would surely have died without treatment, improving in their appearance within a matter of hours of being given the medicine and feeling entirely well within the next day or so."[38]

Between 1936 and 1945, the death rate from pneumonia dropped by 40 percent. Then came penicillin, which was more effective than the sulfanilamides and posed less risk of toxic side effects. The first article describing penicillin's powers was published 18 August 1940 in the British journal the *Lancet,* but there was not much of an initial supply available to meet the immediate demand. The entire world inventory of penicillin in 1942 was barely adequate to cure one serious case of meningitis, and the drug was carefully hoarded for military use until the end of World War II. Yet by 1950, after just five years of commercial availability, penicillin was being prescribed by doctors for 60 percent of their patients.[39] By then "virtually everyone had heard of miracle drugs, and many people knew they owed their lives to them."[40]

As medical capabilities grew by leaps and bounds, the pseudoscientist lampooned by George Bernard Shaw faded from the public imagination and was replaced by a white-coated wonder-worker. Popular films like *Men in White* and *The White Parade* dramatized doctors.[41] A made-for-television movie commissioned by the American Medical Association, *A Life to Save,* was broadcast on an impressive 157 stations nationwide.[42] If real-life doctors sometimes failed to meet public expectations, in part it was because expectations were so high. Physicians, wrote one journalist in 1954, were supposed to be "on the one hand, a group of dedicated and white-coated scientists, bending over test tubes and producing marvelous cures for various ailments, and, on the other, equally dedicated practitioners of medicine and surgery, devoting themselves to easing pain and prolonging human life, without thought of personal gain and at considerable self-sacrifice."[43]

Reflecting this public faith in medical science, federal funding for biomedical research exploded twenty-five-fold in a decade, jumping from less than $3 million in 1941 to an astonishing $75 million.[44] Until the 1980s, the growth remained exponential.[45] Few questioned the worth of this enormous investment as breakthrough followed breakthrough. In 1953 James D. Watson and Francis H. Crick defined the structure of DNA, the molecular building blocks of life. In 1955 Jonas Salk announced that his vaccine against poliomyelitis had been proved safe and effective after a mass test on 1.8 million schoolchildren. Only three years before that momentous proclamation, a polio epidemic had struck more than 50,000 Americans, leaving 3,300 dead and thousands more crippled. Word of a safe and effective protection against this dread scourge was received by the public, remembered one newspaper editor, "like the news of a major military victory."[46]

The first cardiac pacemaker was implanted in 1959. In 1967 South African surgeon Christiaan Neethling Barnard removed the heart of a twenty-five-year-old woman killed in a traffic accident and transplanted it into a fifty-five-year-old man whose severe heart problems threatened his life. In 1969 British physicians helped produce a "test-tube baby" with in vitro fertilization.[47]

The pace of medical progress in these years was vividly illustrated by a comparison of the 1975 edition of *Cecil's Textbook of Medicine* with its first edition, from 1927. Editor Paul Beeson rated 60 percent of the remedies contained in that first edition as harmful, dubious, or merely treating symptoms. Only 3 percent provided fully effective treatment. In the intervening years, effective regiments had increased sevenfold, while the dubious therapies shrank by two-thirds.[48]

The sweeping changes in medical science were soon accompanied by equally important shifts in medicine's role in society. Before World War II, the limited effectiveness of the physician's armamentarium was matched by the limited ability of most patients to pay for treatment. In 1940, only about twelve million Americans, or less than 10 percent of the population, had some form of health insurance. Then, during the war, labor unions got around a government-ordered freeze on wages by bargaining for increased benefits such as health insurance. After the war, there was a benefits boom. By 1950 an astonishing seventy-seven million Americans suddenly had health benefits as employers continued to respond to a combination of union demands and favorable federal tax treatment.[49]

Improvements in the effectiveness of medical treatment meant that more sick people sought a doctor's care. The advent of widespread health insurance meant that more of those seeking care could pay for it. On 1 July 1966, much of the nonworking population was given the right to the same basic health benefits most workers enjoyed. That was the date that federally sponsored Medicare coverage for the elderly and the joint federal and state Medicaid program for the poor went into effect. (The legislation had been passed the year before.)[50]

Meanwhile, the government and private industry also opened their coffers to support training of new doctors and nurses and the construction or renovation of thousands of hospitals. By the late 1960s the biggest barrier to good care for most middle-class Americans was a doctor shortage. Quipped one magazine: "Time is the greatest healer. Considering how long it takes to get a doctor, this may be the best arrangement."[51]

Questions about the clinical quality of the care delivered by this mushrooming medical infrastructure were largely left for doctors to answer to their own satisfaction. The original Medicare legislation, for example, merely called on hospitals to guard against inappropriate care by setting up internal committees to review the work of their peers. That kind of hands-off approach by outsiders was one of the reasons that later generations of physicians would call this the golden age of medicine.

On closer inspection, though, this golden age was flecked with dross. There was a stark gap between medical image and medical reality, though it remained largely hidden. The idea that reform of medical education had transformed everyday medical practice into a standardized science was a myth. The belief that all physicians incorporated the latest scientific findings into their practice was untrue. And faith in physicians' policing themselves was grossly misplaced, as the futility of the repeated professional warnings against unnecessary tonsillectomies would demonstrate.

BEING POPULAR IS BETTER THAN BEING GOOD

The tonsils are a pair of oval masses at the back of the throat; the adenoids lie at the base of the tongue. Both are part of the body's immune system, helping to protect against upper respiratory tract infections. In children the tonsils often become inflamed, although the problem usually vanishes by age fourteen or fifteen. The tonsils are so accessible that even the ancient Greeks performed tonsillectomies, although they were cautious about reaching for the knife. They operated only when a severe infection and abscess on the tonsils led to pain, fever, and difficulty in swallowing.[52] Perhaps that is why the Romans appropriately described someone with an illness as a "patient," a word whose Latin root means "to suffer."

This professional consensus about the need for tonsils surgery persisted for some two thousand years. An 1885 handbook for British physicians advised, "It is comparatively seldom that an operation [to remove inflamed tonsils] is necessary. Children grow out of it."[53]

The operation to remove inflamed adenoids, meanwhile, did not come into regular use until the end of the nineteenth century. Some patients may have hesitated at the doctor's door when they found out what was involved. As late as 1892, a highly respected United States medical text recommended that physicians scrape out the adenoids with their fingernails.[54] But by the beginning of the twentieth century, the practice of surgery underwent a metamorphosis. With the introduction of anesthesia and aseptic surgery, the twin burdens of pain and a high risk of death were lifted from the surgery patient. As a consequence, the professional consensus about when it was advisable to operate changed just as radically.

In the years after World War I, tonsillectomies began to grow in popularity, helped by a new medical rationale for the procedure. A medical theory called "focal infection" suggested that bacteria spread from a focal point in the tonsils to the teeth and then throughout the entire body.[55] According to this hypothesis, inflamed tonsils were responsible for diseases ranging from rheumatism to pneumonia.[56] Newly trained otolaryngologists (ear, nose, and throat specialists) emphasized surgery to such a degree that a caustic observer characterized them as "carpenters in oto-laryngology."[57]

Whether medical specialists generally promote unneeded treatment or whether the increased number of procedures they perform reflects pent-up patient demand is still the subject of lively debate. Tonsillectomies clearly owed something to both. Specialists wrote articles praising the surgery as the latest medical treatment, and worried parents responded to those promotional pieces by pressuring their family physicians to keep up with the times.[58] The boom was on.

In the late 1920s tonsillectomies and adenoidectomies reached a level of popularity comparable to a dance craze. Tonsillectomies accounted for more than one-fourth of all United States hospital admissions. Children, particularly children of the growing urban middle class, were admitted to the hospital in droves.[59] By the mid-1930s, when the Flexnerians were ready to declare victory in standardizing the medical school curriculum, fully one-third of all operations performed under anesthesia in the United States were tonsillectomies![60] Even young doctors in training could see that something wasn't right. John Romano, an intern in Milwaukee during that period, later recalled: "There are ridiculous fads that go on in medicine. . . . [The interns] used to take out tonsils and adenoids. The group of us used to do fifty every Monday, imagine! You go in and scoop out the tonsils of these kids. I used to think, 'What the hell are we doing?' "[61]

J. Alison Glover, a British physician, attempted to answer that question by carefully analyzing tonsillectomies performed in England and Wales. His 1938 work supported the key role played by doctors' preferences and laid the basis for more far-reaching studies performed decades later. Glover reported

> striking contrasts [in the surgery rate] in areas apparently somewhat similarly circumstanced. . . . A child living in Rutlandshire or the Soke [District] of Petersborough is nineteen times more likely to un-

> dergo tonsillectomy than one living in Cambridgeshire. An Enfield child is twenty times more likely to have the operation than one in Hornsey. A child living in Bexhill would seem to enjoy climatic and cultural advantages at least equal to those of a Birkenhead child, yet he is twenty-seven times more likely to be submitted to operation. . . . In each of these categories, there are extreme variations in the operation rate, the extremes often being in adjacent areas.[62]

The tonsillectomy was touted as an effective method of reducing the chance of ear infections. So Glover examined children's medical records in a school district where a school medical officer had reduced the annual number of tonsillectomies from 186 to 8. The rate of otitis media (ear infections) actually went down. A larger region of the country reported the same kind of experience.[63] Although these studies lacked the careful controls that would have allowed Glover to claim "proof" of a cause and effect relationship, they raised troubling questions. At least eighty-five children under age fifteen were dying from tonsillectomies each year in England and Wales.

When one reads the proceedings of the 1938 Royal College of Surgeons meeting where Glover presented his results, it is obvious that many of his contemporaries shared his doubts. Scientifically controlled studies of the tonsillectomy's effectiveness were twenty years overdue, opined one surgeon.[64] Yet the first such studies did not appear until the early 1960s.[65] Even then, flaws in study design rendered the results inconclusive.[66]

It took until the 1970s for new research to confirm what had been widely suspected for decades: most tonsillectomies were unneeded. The appearance of good studies, though, was only one reason the tonsils boom finally fizzled out. Although science was important, it was not what ultimately changed doctors' behavior. After all, the science had been known for years. More important were unprecedented hearings held in Congress on the human and financial cost of unnecessary surgery. Tonsillectomies were one of the worst abuses.[67]

The legislators who dared to ask tough questions of the "men in white" turned for support to a new breed of researchers who were aggressively examining the scientific basis of medical care. These researchers, using tools unavailable to Glover and his predecessors, were shedding a disquieting new light on how doctors behaved in the everyday practice of medicine.

THE EMPEROR HAS NO CLOTHES

The year was 1969, and John E. Wennberg was eager to improve care for residents of rural Vermont. To do that, the thirty-three-year-old director of the state's new regional medical program embarked on a bold course. At a time when the average American's closest encounter with a computer was HAL in *2001, a Space Odyssey,* Wennberg decided to use the University of Vermont's sofa-sized mainframe to track the care of the entire state's 444,000 people.

As a college undergraduate, Wennberg had dabbled in philosophy, German, religion, and anthropology. Later he trained as both a physician and a public health epidemiologist. None of this provided any information whatever about dealing with computers. In his new job, Wennberg wanted to know how people's care was affected by where they lived within the state and by where physicians practiced. He wanted to know the influence of the patient's age, sex, and income level on treatment. And he wanted to know how well Vermont's hospitals were serving the community. Needing an expert to turn these detailed data wishes into computer commands, Wennberg turned to Alan Gittelsohn, his former professor of biostatistics at the Johns Hopkins School of Public Health.

Gittelsohn and Wennberg had been neighbors and friends in Baltimore. In their free time, they would spend many hours discussing ways to improve the delivery of medical care. The late 1960s were a time of national idealism. Given an opportunity to practice what he preached, Gittelsohn took a leave from Hopkins to join Wennberg in Vermont. He also recruited another former student, a restless math whiz in his early twenties named John Senning. Despite Senning's youth, his eclectic career résumé already included both computer work at an upstate New York hospital and punching cattle in southern Wyoming.[68] Thanks to the combined efforts of Wennberg, Gittelsohn, and Senning, Vermont medicine—and medical practice across the nation—would never be the same.

In those days before floppy disks and hard drives, working with computers carried a certain Wild West flavor. Gittelsohn and Senning wrote their instructions to the machine in a special programming language called FORTRAN. The process involved punching holes in cardboard cards to be read by the computer. Almost every day, the two men would bring their cards and heavy reels of computer tape to a large air-conditioned room beneath the kitchen of the university administration building. If it was late, the night-shift computer operator would roust his sleeping dog from under a big tape drive and boost one of the researchers' tapes into place. The tapes spun for hours as the computer analyzed information. The next morning the two men would return to carefully examine the results of the database management programs they had invented.[69]

The research team added information from U.S. Census Bureau surveys and insurance company claims forms to the tens of thousands of patient records from Vermont hospitals. Vermont, then as now, was the most rural state in the nation, its population largely scattered among several hundred small towns and villages. The researchers divided the state into thirteen hospital service areas. Fortunately for the comparisons they wanted to make, relatively few people moved into or out of the different areas or the state as a whole. Moreover, demographically residents of one area resembled residents elsewhere.

As the amount of information to be sorted grew more and more voluminous, the researchers invented data analysis techniques to examine the patterns of medical care. Finally, after months of stirring this massive data stew, the research team ordered the computer to spit out its conclusion. The men were stunned by what they found.

The biomedical research of the postwar years revolutionized what doctors could do to help patients, but the way doctors made decisions hadn't changed much since the times of Glover or the American Child Health Association. Physicians' preferences and practice styles still reigned supreme. Two out of every ten children growing up in one Vermont town had their tonsils removed by age twenty, for example, while in a nearby community the figure was seven out of ten. With the help of the computer, Wennberg could show that the problem was not limited to tonsils.[70]

Appendectomy rates varied threefold. So did the rates of prostate surgery. Hernia rates were about a third higher in the high-rate areas than in the low-rate ones. In town after town, there were large variations in the frequency of hysterectomies, mastectomies, the removal of hemorrhoids, and surgery for other common conditions.

The researchers turned to the medical literature in search of the "right" surgical rate for a particular disease or condition. They emerged empty-handed, unable to determine whether groups of patients who had fewer gallbladder or tonsils or hemorrhoid operations were healthier than those who had more surgery. But because surgery always carries a risk, the two men noted, the chances that too much medical care would hurt or kill a patient were "presumably as strong as the possibility [that] not enough" care would do the same thing.

Based on his training at Hopkins, Wennberg assumed that medical practice at the university hospital in Burlington would show a consistent pattern, while doctors in outlying areas might differ from this desirable norm. Instead, Wennberg discovered fluctuations everywhere. Glover's experience with tonsils in the England of the 1930s was being replicated in condition after condition in the American medicine of the late 1960s. There were no obvious clues to the "right" rate of surgery. To Wennberg, the extent of these variations represented a direct challenge to medicine's own sense of professionalism.

"What changed in my thinking was the concept that there was a center in medicine where there was a secure scientific basis," Wennberg said. "Everyone always knew there were outliers who were practicing erroneous medicine. What I began to see was that the problem was with the central tendency of [all physicians and hospitals]. *Everything* varied."[71]

Wennberg's insights did not interest the major peer-reviewed medical journals. Like Marley's ghost in Dickens's *A Christmas Carol,* the variations study crept in uninvited to rattle its chains and revive memories of the modern physician's prescientific predecessor, prescribing whatever therapy seemed like a good idea at the time.

At the University of Vermont School of Medicine, Wennberg's research on practice variations was received just as unhappily. Wennberg had been hired with the tacit expectation that he would link high-quality medical care for the region with more government funding for the medical center. Instead he implied that doctors and hospitals wasted the money they already received because of inexplicably high rates of hospitalization and surgery. Not long afterward, the medical school asked the federal government to audit Wennberg's program for possible violations of rules. When the auditors ended up praising the program instead of condemning it, strong hints were dropped by medical school higher-ups that Wennberg would still be wise to find another place to work. Thanks to a recommendation from one of the federal auditors, Wennberg ended up at Harvard. The job change turned out to be a stroke of good luck.

John Bunker was at Harvard on a sabbatical when Wennberg arrived. Bunker was a pioneer health-services researcher and a professor of anesthesiology at Stanford. He had seen the *Science* piece and discovered that it dovetailed with his own thinking. He promptly invited Wennberg to coauthor an editorial in the 6 December 1973 issue of the *New England Journal of Medicine.* An accompanying article in the journal documented different rates of surgery in Canada and Britain. The Bunker and Wennberg editorial addressed the broader issue of practice variation, but in a way that went well beyond the problem of financial waste. Here, in a prestigious clinical publication, the two doctors virtually accused fellow American physicians of killing patients with unnecessary procedures.

> There is evidence that rates for some . . . operations may exceed their therapeutic usefulness—that operations designed to decrease mortality may when performed in excess increase it. . . .
>
> [And] the evidence is strong that some operations are performed with a frequency in excess of documentable cost-benefit usefulness. How general is the phenomenon? Do more total operations lead to an increase in overall population mortality? There is some evidence to support this conjecture.[72]

Questions about the way doctors made decisions, once solely the province of a few mavericks, were starting to attract mainstream attention. Bunker asked Wennberg and Gittelsohn to contribute to an unusual book he was editing with Benjamin Barnes, another physician, and Frederick Mosteller, a statistician. The book explored an issue of increasing importance: How do we get the most from the resources devoted to medical care? The time-honored reply was to trust the professional judgment of each individual doctor. Bunker, Barnes, and Mosteller wanted to explore a different mental model.

The editors gathered men and women from a range of academic disciplines. They deliberately addressed the less heroic aspects of medical care, focusing on such issues as surgical fads, the quality of patients' lives after surgery, and the costs and benefits of specific surgical procedures. Sipping sherry or nursing a beer at the Harvard Faculty Club, the researchers would schmooze, break for dinner, and then continue their discussions during a formal presentation.

Like painters experimenting with different lighting and a fresh palette of colors, the Harvard group brought a new set of analytical tools to the study of what doctors do. Clinical expertise was combined with a dab of decision analysis, a splash of statistics, and a tinge of economic theory. The black-and-white image of "good doc–bad doc" was painted over with the variegated hues of professional uncertainty, cost trade-offs, and differing outcomes of care. The doctor-patient relationship was recast into a model that included the preferences of patients as well as physicians. The Harvard book, *Costs, Risks, and Benefits of Surgery,* appeared in 1977.

Wennberg's big break came a few years later, when his work attracted the attention of John Iglehart, a former reporter for the Associated Press and the *National Journal.* Iglehart had started a publication dealing entirely with the fast-growing field of health policy. He invited Wennberg to write the lead article for a theme issue of *Health Affairs* devoted to variations in medical practice.

The summer 1984 issue of *Health Affairs* debuted in July with a seminar for the news media and a visit to Capitol Hill to brief key congressmen and their staffs. Wennberg was also tapped as a speaker at a health policy forum for political insiders. "We didn't know medicine wasn't scientific until Wennberg made it come to life," recalled Judith Miller Jones, the forum organizer. "He made it real."[73]

Indeed he did. The prologue to Wennberg's article introduced him as someone who "has been driven by the notion that practice variations were important to identify and understand because they suggest a misuse of care." The article made it clear why Wennberg's views were so explosive: "Most people view the medical care they receive as a necessity provided by doctors who adhere to scientific norms based on previously tested and proven treatments. When the contents of the medical care 'black box' are examined more closely, however, the type of medical service provided is often found to be as strongly influenced by subjective factors related to the attitudes of individual physicians as by science."[74]

Wennberg went on to give everyday examples taken from his own work in Vermont, Maine, and Iowa. There was a 20 percent chance of a woman's undergoing a hysterectomy by age seventy in one market, a 70 percent chance elsewhere. There was a 15 percent chance of a man's undergoing a prostatectomy by age eighty-five in one town, a 60 percent chance in another. A child had an 8 percent chance of getting a tonsillectomy in one area and a 70 percent chance elsewhere. These were community data, not the work of one or two "bad" doctors. Congress, and the public, got the point.

A few months later, Wisconsin Democrat William Proxmire chaired a Senate hearing on variations in medical practice, with Wennberg as the lead witness. Citing the lack of research on medical outcomes as documented in *Health Affairs,* Proxmire declared: "We simply don't know if more is better. We do know, however, that more is terribly expensive and is pushing the nation's medical-care system toward a major crisis. . . . The question [is] . . . whether, in fact, we couldn't save immense amounts of federal money by investing a relatively small amount to standardize procedures and reduce unnecessary surgery."[75]

In 1984, 10 percent of the federal budget was going for health care, double the 1961 level. The Reagan administration had frozen Medicare reimbursement to doctors and hospitals, prompting widespread predictions that out-of-control costs foreshadowed the rationing of care as a way to save money. In this atmosphere, Wennberg's message to Congress held enormous popular appeal. In essence, he told the senators that there just might be such a thing as an economic "free lunch." As he put it in testimony to Proxmire's subcommittee on health appropriations:

> The extent of variation in reimbursements to hospitals under the Medicare program is such that if the low-cost patterns of care were the norm, we would not be faced with the pending bankruptcy of the Medicare Trust Fund, nor would we be now concerned with the specter that medical care must be rationed. For many medical or surgical conditions, the variations suggest opportunities to reduce expenditures under the Medicare and Medicaid programs without reducing the benefits of medical care.[76]

The revolution in thinking about medical practice had begun in the 1950s and 1960s, prompted by the work of men such as Johns Hopkins University epidemiologist Kerr White. (White is credited with popularizing the new term "health services research.") But it took Wennberg's research in the 1980s to bring this novel way of examining medical care to the attention of the general public. In the academic equivalent of a frog changing into a prince, Wennberg watched findings that had once seemed of interest only to the *Journal of the Maine Medical Association* turn up in popular publications as diverse as *Barron's, Cosmopolitan,* and *The New York Review of Books.*

"Wennberg . . . created the intellectual climate that allowed the rest to follow," said Duncan Neuhauser, another Harvard contributor to *Costs, Risks, and Benefits of Surgery.* "Before, [everyone thought] medicine was a science. There's one right answer, there shouldn't be any variation. What he was saying was, 'There is variation, it's big, and, by the way, there are cost implications to this.' "

Indeed, a 1980 article by Wennberg and his colleagues calculated that the United States would save $4.2 billion (in 1975 dollars) if the rate at which seven common surgical procedures were performed more closely resembled the low-usage parts of Maine and Vermont rather than the high-usage areas.[77]

A much-publicized analysis in the *New England Journal of Medicine* finally brought the relationship between frequent hospital use and quality of care right up to the door of the premier medical institutions in the country. In a 26 October 1989 article, Wennberg and colleagues compared the mortality rates of patients treated in Boston with those of patients treated in New Haven. Although Boston hospitals had far higher rates of admission and readmission after discharge, longer lengths of stay, and greater reimbursement, the death rates of the patients treated were nearly identical. What Wennberg did was adjust for whether the patients in New Haven, discharged earlier, were simply dying outside the hospital. "The lower rate of hospital use by Medicare enrollees in New Haven was not associated with a higher overall mortality rate," he concluded.[78]

Wennberg was not the only researcher in the early 1970s who was raising discomfiting questions about the scientific basis of medical practice. About a year after the first Wennberg and Gittelsohn article appeared, a young physician named David Eddy decided to illustrate the logical steps physicians took in managing patients with breast cancer. It was a hot topic. In the fall of 1974, the wives of both the president and vice president of the United States—First Lady Betty Ford and Second Lady "Happy" Rockefeller—were diagnosed with the disease.

Eddy's love of mathematics and logic had led him to Stanford University to work on a doctorate in engineering some years after he had already received his medical degree. But the logic he presumed lay behind medical treatment decisions was nowhere to be found. "My assumption was there was an orderly process, somewhat like a decision tree, where you weigh the pros and cons and choose the best [treatment] option," remembered Eddy. "That's how we buy a car or anything else."[79]

But as Eddy picked his way through hundreds of scholarly articles constituting a virtual forest of research, he could see no decision tree. Instead of careful studies demonstrating that a specific treatment produced a certain result, Eddy found only recommendations by experts. For stage 2 breast cancer, a physician should do this. For more advanced stage 3 cancer, the doctor should do that. Doctors were simply following rules of thumb garnered from other doctors,[80] with the original advice often based on flawed reasoning. Researchers' recommendations were frequently unsupported by data, resting instead on a foundation of questionable logic and even outright mathematical error.[81] "A close examination of the medical literature reveals a discouraging picture," Eddy wrote.[82]

Eddy's solid professional standing as a mathematician made his criticism of medical science difficult to dismiss. While still working on his doctorate, Eddy developed a mathematical theory on intermittent inspections that eventually won the highest award given in the field of applied mathematics. Within an extraordinary two years after receiving his doctorate, he was made a tenured professor at Stanford—the standard waiting period for mere mortals is a minimum of seven years. Still, Eddy's breast cancer commentary had little effect on patient care.

In a similar vein, in 1986 researcher John Williamson and his colleagues examined 2,696 citations in the medical literature related to the treatment of three important medical problems: bipolar disorder (the formal name for manic-depressive behavior); malignant melanoma, a form of cancer; and chronic rheumatic heart disease. Nearly two-thirds of the citations contained material that was irrelevant for use in clinical practice; 96 percent of the citations had information that the researchers considered not yet proved conclusively enough to be implemented.[83]

Other pathbreaking research exposed an embarrassing difference between how effective doctors thought their care was and how the patients felt about it. Robert Brook, at Johns Hopkins before joining the RAND Corporation, turned a critical eye on the care of three common conditions: urinary tract infections, high blood pressure (hypertension), and stomach ulcers. Medical specialists from Johns Hopkins Hospital and generalists from neighboring Baltimore City Hospitals reviewed the care of nearly three hundred patients who were treated for these conditions and then asked how effective they thought medical treatment had been in relieving discomfort and allowing patients to resume their normal activities.

The doctor's-eye view of medical care turned out to be filtered through a rose-colored lens. Physicians overwhelmingly believed their interventions were much more effective than they actually were. In eight out of the ten objective measurements, doctors estimated that patient health improved more than it really did. Moreover, the highly trained specialists' estimates of how patients responded to therapy were no more accurate than the estimates of the generalists.[84]

The insistent and sincere belief by physicians that what they do must be helping their patients could well be the best explanation for why doctors have shut their eyes for so long to treatment that does the opposite of what is intended. Instead of helping patients, it injures and kills them.

CHAPTER THREE

First, Do No Harm

> As to diseases, make a habit of two things—to help or at least to do no harm.
>
> —Hippocrates, *Epidemics*

On 23 March 1995, a page 1 article in the *Boston Globe* related the tragic tale of a young mother with breast cancer who was betrayed in her fight against the disease. The shocking nature of the story was magnified by the identities of those involved. The patient was a columnist for the *Globe* who wrote about health and medicine. And she was being treated at one of the nation's most respected cancer hospitals. Under a headline reading "Doctor's Orders Killed Cancer Patient," reporter Richard A. Knox wrote:

> When 39-year old Betsy A. Lehman died suddenly last Dec. 3 at Boston's Dana-Farber Cancer Institute, near the end of a grueling three-month treatment for breast cancer, it seemed a tragic reminder of the risks and limits of high-stakes cancer care.
>
> In fact, it was something very different. The death of Lehman, a *Boston Globe* health columnist, was due to a horrendous mistake; a massive overdose of a powerful anti-cancer drug that ravaged her heart, causing it to fail suddenly just as she was preparing to go home to her husband and two young daughters. The error was discovered only last month by Dana-Farber clerks [during a routine review of records], not [by] clinicians. . . .
>
> Dana-Farber officials still have no explanation for how such a thing could have happened, ascribing it merely to "human error."[1]

As if to underline the horror, an autopsy uncovered no visible signs of cancer. The previous weeks of painful treatment had succeeded, but the victory rang hollow. Another unidentified breast cancer patient who was given an overdose of the same drug as Lehman suffered irreversible heart damage.[2] "If this can happen at a place like Dana-Farber," one anguished medical expert asked, "what is happening in other places?"[3]

What indeed. Shortly before the disturbing facts behind Lehman's death emerged, a seeming epidemic of errors erupted among the nation's hospitals. In Grand Rapids, Michigan, a surgeon operating on a sixty-nine-year-old mastectomy patient removed the wrong breast. A New York woman died when a doctor mistook her dialysis catheter for a feeding tube and ordered food pumped into her abdomen. And in a series of incidents at Tampa's University Community Hospital, a fifty-one-year-old diabetic had the wrong foot amputated, a seventy-seven-year-old retired electrician died when a therapist mistakenly disconnected his ventilator, and a female patient got arthroscopic surgery on the wrong knee.[4]

Tragic though these individual episodes were, the more important issue was what they revealed about American medicine. Were they warnings of deep-rooted problems, or were they simply unrelated examples of inherent human imperfection? How common are deaths and injuries caused by medical treatment? And how preventable are they?

Much of the reaction to the spate of mistakes took a "no one's perfect" tone. A *Time* article, "The Disturbing Case of the Cure That Killed the Patient," called the frequency of medical errors "distressing," while reminding readers that "the opportunities for error have multiplied" because of the complexity of modern medicine.[5] The American Medical Association responded in a similar vein. "There are more than nine million physician/patient encounters every day in America," wrote AMA president Robert McAfee in a soothing letter to the editors of some two hundred newspapers. "An extraordinarily high percentage are positive. Some are miraculous. But isolated and sometimes egregious mistakes also occur."[6] Advice columnist Ann Landers printed a version of the same letter, signed by the AMA's chief staff member, surgeon James Todd, in a response to readers worried about their local hospital.[7]

Yet the central premise of the AMA leadership's argument was directly contradicted by the organization's flagship journal. An article titled "Error in Medicine" appeared in the 21 December 1994 *Journal of the American Medical Association* just a couple of months before the Lehman controversy broke out. The article specifically singled out professional complacency as a culprit in medical mistakes. "It is curious . . . that high error rates have not stimulated more concerns and efforts at error prevention," wrote Lucian Leape, a physician at the Harvard School of Public Health. *"Although error rates are substantial, serious injuries due to errors . . . are perceived as isolated and unusual events—'outliers'* " (emphasis added).[8]

An accompanying commentary in the same issue by David Blumenthal, also a Harvard researcher and clinician, was equally blunt. It declared: "Concerning medical error and its prevention, *the profession has, with rare exceptions, adopted an ostrichlike attitude. . . . Mistakes have been treated as uncommon and atypical,* requiring no remedy beyond the traditional. . . . [But a] large and growing collection of literature demonstrates that physicians' approaches to the management of medical error do not work well enough" (emphasis added).[9]

Although not mentioned in *JAMA*, an AMA scientific committee had issued a report specifically dealing with medication errors six months before. Based on a review of the medical literature, the report painted a picture far different from the reassuring portrait presented to the public by McAfee and Todd. The report concluded: "Medication errors expose patients to additional but preventable risks leading frequently to prolongation of hospital stay and, in some cases, contributing to morbidity [complications] and mortality. . . . *[They] are not rare events. . .* and they compromise the confidence of patients and the general public in the health care system. *Fortunately, most medication errors are preventable*" (emphasis added).[10] Like the *JAMA* articles, this report to the AMA's own Board of Trustees was never mentioned publicly by the AMA's senior officials.

Clearly, Betsy Lehman's death and the serious injury of the other breast cancer patient were preventable. Dana-Farber immediately took full responsibility for the mistake, even before a state investigation came to the same conclusion. The hospital's chief physician resigned as "a signal" of the institution's seriousness about change.[11]

If any good came of the Dana-Farber incidents, it was to highlight that the number one cause of medical mistakes is not incompetence but confusion. Although outright negligence and incompetence certainly exist, most treatment-related errors are caused by a poorly designed process of care that lacks safeguards to protect against anything less than human perfection. At Dana-Farber, for example, Betsy Lehman's physician mistakenly believed that the figure showing the total dose of the chemotherapy drug cisplatin over a four-day period was the amount of the drug to be given each day for four days. The resulting overdose led to Lehman's fatal heart damage.[12] The worst part of this mix-up is that it is not particularly unusual.

"The exact same thing that happened at Dana-Farber can [happen] and is happening at other hospitals around the country," said Michael Cohen, a founder of the Institute for Safe Medication Practices. "[Drug errors] happen every day, one or two times a day. Some of them may not be discovered, or some of them are discovered and not reported, but they're out there."[13] Indeed, a CBS News team from the show *48 Hours* reported seven cases where patients were accidentally given cisplatin instead of a less toxic chemotherapy drug, carboplatin.[14]

The frightening reality is that medical mistakes of all types are not unusual. Treatment-related injuries kill anywhere from two thousand to three thousand people every week, according to two major scientific studies—and that's just in the hospital. In a year, the medical casualty list includes more than three times as many Americans as were killed in the entire Vietnam War and more than four times as many as die annually in traffic accidents. It is the nation's leading cause of preventable fatalities. Apart from deaths, medical treatment will injure another 1.3 million people.[15]

That horrific toll may even be understated. Rather than relying on what physicians and nurses write down in the medical record—as most error studies have done—a 1997 study in the *Lancet* used trained observers to monitor care at an urban American teaching hospital. Based on what nurses and doctors discussed in clinical meetings, the observers tallied one serious adverse event—ranging from temporary physical disability to death—in about 18 percent of the patients. The more seriously ill the patient, the more likely that patient was to suffer some sort of treatment-caused harm.[16]

So why don't doctors and other caregivers pay more attention to errors? Before caregivers will act decisively, they—and the public—need to give up once and for all the comforting belief that the danger posed by treatment-caused errors either is unavoidable or hardly exists at all.

"THE PRICE WE PAY"

> I do not want two diseases, one Nature made and one Doctor made.
>
> —Napoleon Bonaparte

The year 1955 is indelibly imprinted in the annals of sports as the time the lowly Brooklyn Dodgers defeated the perennial champion New York Yankees to win the first-ever World Series for "Da Bums." In financial news, International Business Machines Corporation, a powerhouse in tabulating machines, shipped its first business computers to a few adventuresome customers. That same year, *JAMA* published a major article titled "Hazards of Modern Diagnosis and Therapy—the Price We Pay."[17] It encapsulated how doctors thought about treatment-caused injuries.

New York physician David Barr acknowledged from the start that "unfortunate sequelae and accidents attributable to sanctioned and well-intended diagnosis and therapy . . . could be regarded as one of the commonest conditions [in a hospital]." He implored colleagues to pay closer attention to the consequences of using the new drugs and techniques that flourished in the aftermath of the war. Common problems included "accidental drug intoxication" (which later would be called an adverse drug reaction), introduction of infection, and dangers from multiple procedures.

For all his concern, however, Barr could not see any solution to the problem aside from asking doctors to be more careful. In a defense of medicine that would be echoed time and again over the ensuing decades, Barr wrote: "These accidents, risks and dangers may be regarded as the price that we, as responsible physicians, must pay for the inestimable benefits of modern diagnosis and therapy. They are the hazards to which, with best intent and most correct practice, we must occasionally subject our patients.

Patients might be forgiven for thinking Barr a bit confused about who was doing the paying. Still, Barr's belief that patients were inadvertent victims of "the most correct practice" was typical. A prominent forensic medicine specialist complained in a 1954 issue of the *New England Journal of Medicine* that 50 to 80 percent of malpractice suits could be eliminated in physicians would only stop criticizing each other's *unavoidable* (emphasis added) errors.[18]

In 1956 the Yankees recaptured the baseball crown from the Dodgers in an exciting "subway series" rematch of the 1955 contest. IBM settled a contest of its own by promising the Justice Department it would sell computers outright to customers rather than using its market muscle to insist on lucrative leases. And in medical news, the *New England Journal of Medicine* followed *JAMA*'s lead in addressing the sensitive issue of "Diseases of Medical Progress." The list of various iatrogenic (treatment-caused) "diseases that would not have occurred if sound therapeutic procedure had not been employed" stretched on for pages.[19]

"Progress in every sphere of human endeavor creates new problems at each turn," concluded author Robert Moser, a major in the

U.S. Army Medical Corps. "At times, this may be discouraging, but it is never dull." Dull? Certainly not from the doctor's viewpoint.

However awkward Moser's conclusion sounds today, his and Barr's articles contained an important admission of responsibility. Since the 1910 Flexner Report on medical education, physicians steeped in the scientific method had seen themselves as protecting the public from the harm caused by quacks and impostors.[20] Barr, by referring to "correct practice," and Moser, by mentioning "sound therapeutic procedure," acknowledged that "scientific" physicians could harm patients too. It was left to Elihu M. Schimmel, an internist at the Yale University School of Medicine, to produce the first evidence showing just how many patients were being hurt.

Schimmel's examination of the medical service of Grace–New Haven Community Hospital yielded startling results. During an eight-month period, medical treatment caused some sort of complication in one out of every five patients! Moreover, 16 of the 240 "episodes" proved fatal, wrote Schimmel in a 1964 article called "The Hazards of Hospitalization."[21]

Schimmel, too, linked the risks to the benefits, but he was obviously troubled by the high incidence of injuries. Though he did not formally attempt to determine which were preventable, his descriptions of specific incidents speak plainly about medical practice of the time. A fifty-year-old woman with cirrhosis died when air infiltrated the soft tissues of her chest after a diagnostic procedure lacerated her esophagus. A patient treated with the blood thinner heparin died from massive bleeding caused by a previously undiagnosed kidney tumor. And three patients died from overdoses of digitalis, a common cardiac medication.[22]

Schimmel's appeal for increased watchfulness during treatment was lost in the excitement of medicine's technological explosion, symbolized by the computed axial tomography scanner. The CAT scanner assembled thousands of X-ray images into one extraordinarily detailed picture of the body's interior, revolutionizing medical diagnosis. (The scanner also represented the first medical advance traceable to rock 'n' roll, since the British company that developed the device started life as the record label for the Beatles.)[23]

The love affair with technology during the 1960s and 1970s eventually exacted a price. A 1981 article in the *New England Journal of Medicine* updating Schimmel's work found that one patient in three on the medical service of a university hospital was harmed by treatment, an increase of more than 50 percent from Schimmel's time. (The "medical" service omits surgery and obstetrics cases, among others.) No one tried to quantify whether the benefits of medical treatment increased 50 percent during the same period.

There was some good news. Although more patients were being hurt, fatalities fell to two deaths out of each one hundred complications, as opposed to the seven out of one hundred that Schimmel had noted. Author Knight Steel and his colleagues strongly urged doctors to do a better job of monitoring "untoward events,"[24] but this latest warning had no more effect than had the unheard cautions of the previous quarter century.

Both Schimmel and Steel examined care at just one hospital. In the 1970s a few researchers began to cast a wider net, motivated not by guilt over patient deaths but by alarm over rising premiums for malpractice insurance.

A great deal had changed in medicine and in the nation. The country as a whole was far more prosperous. The Dodgers had moved from the tough streets of Brooklyn to the easy living of Los Angeles. IBM had all but abandoned its interest in tabulating machines and was pushing computers out the door with one hand and raking in cash with the other. Many doctors had barely earned a middle-class living in the 1950s. In the 1970s, physicians were starting to enjoy the fruits of their labors.[25] Then, seemingly without warning, doctors' income and prestige were threatened by a malpractice "crisis." Premiums, particularly for high-risk specialties such as obstetrics, began to skyrocket. Experts argued whether the problem was poorer doctoring or better lawyering. With the backing of the California Medical Association and the California Hospital Association, a physician-attorney named Don Harper Mills launched the ambitious Medical Insurance Feasibility Study to try to find out the answer.

Mills undertook a research effort of unprecedented scope. He sampled 20,864 medical charts obtained from twenty-three state hospitals, all part of the search for "potentially compensable events"—a lawyerly term for treatment-caused injuries. Mills concluded that one patient in twenty was harmed by treatment. About four in a hundred of these "events" caused major, permanent disability, while almost ten in a hundred resulted in the patient's death. Although these percentages were small, they applied to nearly three million hospital admissions in California in 1974. That meant state hospital patients suffered 140,000 treatment-caused injuries, including 13,600 hospital-caused fatalities.[26]

To be sure, one-fourth of the deaths represented nothing more than a hastening of the inevitable. Mills cited a patient with terminal cancer who died prematurely from the effects of chemotherapy. Nonetheless, that still left 10,200 deaths that should not have happened.[27] If California's experience was typical, then hospital care caused about 121,000 premature deaths nationwide that year—or about 2,300 every single week.[28]

These were horrific numbers by any reckoning. Consider the protests over the Vietnam War that wracked the nation during this same period. In the nearly two decades that United States troops were involved there, about 58,000 Americans died, or fewer than half the number of deaths caused in just one year by medical treatment.[29] Deaths from traffic accidents, a national scandal, peaked at 54,589 in 1972.[30]

Mills reacted to this carnage by reaffirming his faith in physicians. He blamed the sharp jump in malpractice judgments on patients who naively thought that medical care was risk free. His themes were the familiar ones. "Society deserves the right to nourish great expectations from the advances in modern medicine, but *no one* [emphasis in original] should remain unaware that benefits and adverse risks [of modern medicine] are inseparable," wrote Mills in a 1978 article summarizing his findings.[31] "When *considering the circumstances* under which these risks [of treatment-caused injuries] arise, *their incidence rates are remarkably low*" (emphasis added).

In any event, Mills's professed interest was not in medical quality per se, but in *compensable* events.[32] From that viewpoint, Mills's study provided some good news: even when an "event" involved permanent disability or death for the patient, there was less than a fifty-fifty chance of "successful legal outcomes."[33] In other words, even "egregious" mistakes didn't necessarily result in large malpractice awards.

If the average patient had unrealistic expectations about the likely results of medical treatment, one reason may have been the doctors themselves. As will be discussed in chapter 15, it took years of lawsuits to force physicians to realistically describe the risks of treatment to patients in the first place. Moreover, there was an important cause of the malpractice "crisis" that could not be found by reviewing patients' charts. The social upheaval of the late 1960s and 1970s broke the medical code of silence that provided "maximum autonomy for the individual physician . . . and little criticism from peers."[34] One young physician actually burned his AMA membership card during the 1969 annual meeting of the group's House of Delegates. Physicians began testifying in courtrooms and before congressional committees about abuses. A new genre of kiss-and-tell books also contained scathing critiques.

In *Confessions of a Medical Heretic,* Robert Mendelsohn of the University of Illinois School of Medicine unabashedly advised readers of his favorites among the "dozens of anti-doctor books easily available."[35] Mendelsohn made his own contribution to the literature.

> Medical ethics are usually the opposite of traditional ethics. For instance, if you're in the operating room and somebody finds a sponge in the belly left from a previous operation, traditional ethics would make sure that somebody in the family found out about it. Medical ethics tells you to keep your mouth shut about it. The surgeon will say, "I don't want anybody to know about this," and if the nurse tells the family, she'll be out of a job.[36]

It is important to emphasize that it was public and congressional pressure that compelled organized medicine to address the issue of treatment-caused deaths and injuries. A two-year study by the American College of Surgeons and the American Surgical Association found that half of the nonfatal complications and a third of the patient deaths were preventable in the cases they examined—a disturbingly high figure.[37] As always, however, conducting studies and changing physicians' behavior remained two very different things.

SHINING A LIGHT INTO MEDICINE'S "SECRET CLOSET"

In 1971 there appeared on the scene a type of organization that was new to medicine. It was run by a doctor, but it was not tied in to the medical profession. It demanded government action, but it wasn't part of the government. The Public Citizen Health Research Group was set up by consumer crusader Ralph Nader, who had first gained fame by attacking the safety record of General Motors and the auto industry. Nader picked an aggressive thirty-two-year-old internist named Sidney Wolfe as HRG's first director. Since the organization had neither a big budget nor a large staff, Wolfe sought to magnify his impact through adroit use of the media—much as

Nader himself had done. The medical malpractice crisis was not caused by either lawyers or insurers, Wolfe asserted in testimony before a 1971 Nixon administration Commission on Medical Malpractice. "Something is wrong with the quality of health care in this country," he proclaimed.[38] Four years later, Wolfe told the AMA-sponsored newspaper *American Medical News,* "The health-care system is the leading cause of preventable deaths in this country."[39]

In the postwar years the news media's interest in matters medical was mostly confined to respectfully relating the latest clinical advances. But the social turmoil of the sixties and seventies changed journalism too. Estimates made in the mid-1970s that as many as 30,000 to 140,000 hospital patients suffered fatal drug reactions every year became big news.[40] Reporters who wanted to take a more critical approach to medicine could turn to Wolfe for help in finding the right scientific studies and then making them understandable to a lay audience. Medical writers began to imitate the aggressive tendencies of colleagues covering politics, the military, and even sports. "Thousands a Year Killed by Faulty Prescriptions," proclaimed a page 1 story in the *New York Times.*[41] Early in the *Times* story, a top AMA official admitted that the existence of a problem with medication errors could not be denied.[42]

The 1970s marked "the first time the public starts hearing the fact that medicine has a downside, not just an upside," recalled Wolfe, still feisty a quarter of a century later and still HRG's executive director.[43]

Not everyone was persuaded. Allegations linking medication misuse to thousands of patient deaths were "guesses" based on studies that were "incomplete, unrepresentative, uncontrolled and lacking in operational criteria," argued a critique in a 1975 issue of *JAMA.*[44]

Unfortunately, publicity in the popular press had no more effect on doctors' behavior than did publicity in the scientific literature. The evidence documenting frequent errors in hospitals continued to accumulate.

Researchers in California examined errors in prescriptions for small children who were very ill—by any definition, among the most vulnerable of patients. They discovered twenty-seven "potentially lethal" mistakes in a six-month period—"potential" because the methodology consisted of counting drug errors caught by pharmacists. The most likely error was an overdose to a child age two or under or to a child in the intensive care unit. "Only one death or serious injury to a child needs to be prevented to justify [better training of physicians]," the researchers pleaded in a 1987 article in *Pediatrics*.[45]

Similarly, pharmacist Timothy Lesar and his colleagues in Albany, New York, found "significant risk to patients from medication prescribing errors" when examining a large teaching hospital. There were roughly three errors in each one thousand medication orders, and more than half the mistakes could have harmed the patient if not caught, the researchers said.[46] The popular wisdom that errors are due to inexperience or a few "bad" doctors was contradicted by both the California and New York studies. Medical residents and more experienced attending physicians both made prescribing mistakes. "The risk for errors [is] widespread among prescribers and not the result of a small fraction of individual [physicians]," emphasized Lesar and colleagues in the 2 May 1990 issue of *JAMA*.

Seven years later, Lesar published a similar article. If anything, the situation had worsened. This time he and his colleagues found four errors per thousand medication orders, of which 70 percent could have harmed the patient if not caught (although in most cases the harm would not have been serious). Once more, the researchers emphasized the easy preventability of most of the mistakes.[47]

Over the years, doctors and nurses did at least begin speaking more openly about mistakes. "Medication errors are the skeleton in the closet of health care providers," lamented a 1988 article in the *Journal of Nursing Quality Assurance*. A 1989 headline in *Hospitals*, published by the American Hospital Association, read: "Drug Errors: Dangerous, Costly and Avoidable."

If anyone still believed that errors were "isolated," a painstaking study by Harvard Medical School researchers finally punctured that illusion. Like Mills's 1974 work, this effort too was undertaken because of concern over expensive malpractice judgments. The study's goal was to develop better estimates of the frequency of adverse events and negligence affecting hospitalized patients. In effect, the researchers were taking another cut at the question of bad doctoring versus better lawyering. Also like Mills, the Harvard researchers painstakingly reviewed a large sample of actual patient records, this time in New York State. Once again, what they discovered about patient care was deeply disturbing.

About one in twenty-five hospital admissions resulted in an injured patient, said Troyen Brennan and his colleagues in a 1991 article in the *New England Journal of Medicine.* (Like Mills, Brennan was an attorney and a physician.) Moreover, negligence was responsible for nearly one-third of the problems. About 3 percent of "adverse events" caused permanently disabling injuries, while nearly one in seven led to the patient's death. Medication errors were the most common cause of injury, accounting for 19 percent of all "adverse events," and two-thirds of the drug errors were judged preventable. Applying those percentages to current hospital admissions meant that roughly 23,000 patients died in American hospitals each year from injuries linked to medication use.[48]

The toll of patient deaths and injuries in New York documented by the Harvard researchers was depressingly similar to what Mills had found a full decade before in California. Extrapolated nationally, it translated to about 180,000 deaths and 1.3 million injuries each year owing to medical treatment.[49] "There is a substantial amount of injury to patients from medical management," the authors concluded in a triumph of academic understatement.[50]

Harvard Study coauthor Lucian Leape later became more blunt. He said: "Medical injury is . . . a hidden epidemic."[51]

The headlines given the Harvard study changed nothing at all. In a particularly pointed example, Leape participated in a study of drug errors at two of Harvard's own hospitals, Massachusetts General and Brigham and Women's. On 5 July 1995 another *JAMA* article from Harvard had this to say: "Adverse drug events [ADEs] were common and often preventable; serious ADEs were more likely to be preventable. Most resulted from errors [by physicians] at the ordering stage."[52] The researchers found 334 drug errors at the two hospitals in six months. "We use bar codes [to track] mayonnaise in the supermarket, but not for morphine in the hospital," Leape noted in frustration.[53]

Five months after the article appeared, a sixty-seven-year-old man in the Brigham and Women's intensive care unit died from a potassium overdose. A temporary agency nurse who lacked intensive care experience gave the man too much potassium in too short a time. The Joint Commission on Accreditation of Healthcare Organizations eventually lowered the hospital's accreditation status one notch, and hospital officials said they had reduced the use of temporary nurses and taken other steps to improve care.

There is no doubt that the overwhelming majority of doctors and hospitals abhor mistakes and try very hard to prevent them. In the light of that attitude, why do mistakes remain so prevalent? The answer requires looking at the practice of medicine from a different angle than usual.

MENTAL ERRORS

> Knowledge and error flow from the same mental sources; only success can tell the one from the other.
>
> —Ernst Mach, *Knowledge and Error,* about 1905

"Have you ever personally made an error that harmed a patient?" I asked a physician who writes eloquently about the need to improve the quality of medical care. The doctor hesitated. Promised anonymity, he recalled an episode of "mortification and shame" during his training.

> Yes, I did make such a mistake. I remember it vividly—every bit of it—and it later became the subject of an ego-bruising mortality and morbidity conference [where doctors at a hospital gather to discuss patient deaths and injuries]. It was a case where I made the wrong diagnosis on a very sick patient, began the wrong therapy, and the patient died. . . .
>
> If you have made a mistake, it's a bone-chilling experience, especially in a place that is intensely competitive and where you feel that your reputation is on the line every day anyway, as you do [working] in a highly pressured academic teaching hospital. There's this myth . . . that everybody else is perfect. I don't think we [interns and residents] thought once about getting sued. I think we thought everyone else would discover we were the frauds we thought ourselves to be.
>
> I felt awful about the error. It wasn't like I took off the wrong leg, but the fact was that it was within [my] power to make a decision, and a different decision might have prevented somebody's death.

"Have you ever personally made an error that harmed a patient?" I asked another physician who combines a community practice with research on health policy issues. He too hesitated, then spoke about a patient who died during his training period. The physician finished the story this way:

> I don't want my name attached to this. I'm not really sure why. It may be irrational, but it's [a] strong [feeling]. It wasn't that I was lazy. Laziness was the worst sin. One resident got called at 3:00 A.M. because

> a patient was having chest pain, a patient who "cried wolf" all the time. The resident didn't get out of bed to see the patient, and the patient had cardiac arrest fifteen minutes later and died. That's the kind of thing that's considered unforgivable. . . .
>
> I would be horrified to see my name in print with [my] mistake. You're just not supposed to make mistakes when you're a doc.

A young family physician named David Hilfiker received a great deal of publicity when he dared to write publicly about a mistake he committed while practicing in a rural Minnesota town. A pregnancy test that repeatedly came up negative turned out to be wrong. Hilfiker had not ordered a confirmatory ultrasound scan, in part because the patient would have had to drive many miles to the city. He ended up performing a D&C (dilation and curettage) that unwittingly turned into an abortion. Recalling the incident later, he wrote:

> Precisely because of its technological wonders and near-miraculous drugs, modern medicine has created for the physician an expectation of perfection. The technology seems so exact that error becomes almost unthinkable. We are not prepared for our mistakes, and we don't know how to cope with them when they occur.
>
> Doctors are not alone in harboring expectations of perfection. Patients, too, expect doctors to be perfect. Perhaps patients have to consider their doctors less prone to error than other people: how else can a sick or injured person, already afraid, come to trust the doctor?
>
> This perfection is a grand illusion, of course, a game of mirrors that everyone plays.[54]

The game begins early. Some technical and judgmental errors by interns or residents are expected, and they are corrected by the "attending" physicians who supervise trainees. The attendings follow a rule of thumb that medical sociologist Charles Bosk has called "forgive and remember." Even as certain mistakes are forgiven, the attendings remember them and closely observe the trainee to see whether similar errors recur. If the attendings "discern a pattern . . . and failures can no longer be considered random clinical events . . . [they] step up monitoring, become more dogmatic about the way they want work done and more critical."[55]

Certain mistakes are not easily forgivable, even once. They fall into the category of moral errors that cast doubt on the potential physician's trustworthiness, a characteristic much more important than technical skill. "Laziness"—putting some personal interest above the interest of the patient—is one example. Yet even "expected" errors carry an unmistakable stigma. They are rarely discussed with peers, particularly after a physician leaves training. There is an "absence of fallibility as a category in physicians' concepts of their profession."[56]

Unfortunately, the belief that "good" doctors don't make errors flies in the face of decades of research into why humans dealing with complex systems of any sort make mistakes. "Health-care delivery is usually *not* thought of as a system," writes Harold van Cott, a psychologist who worked with the National Academy of Sciences on human factors engineering. "Yet of all sociotechnical systems, it surely is the largest [and] most complex. . . . The good news is that 'many of the things that trigger or initiate human error can be changed.' "[57]

The field of human-error study got a series of spectacular assists during the 1970s and 1980s with the near-catastrophic accident at the Three Mile Island nuclear generating station; the explosion of a Union Carbide pesticide plant in Bhopal, India, which killed more than two thousand people; and the horrifying explosion of the space shuttle *Challenger* just seventy-three seconds after liftoff.

The rising death toll prompted researchers to systematically examine the thought processes that led to mistakes. The goal was both to prevent as many errors as possible and to keep the errors that did occur from causing harm. The factors that lead to human error are related to human thought processes, and they are as applicable in medicine as in industry.[58]

"All types of errors are rooted in the essential and adaptive properties of human cognition," writes James Reason, a behavioral psychologist at Britain's Manchester University. "The same adaptive mechanism that allows us to drive safely to work in a state of semi-wakefulness can come back to haunt us when the comfortable assumptions that let us operate on auto-pilot suddenly turn out not to be true any more."[59]

According to Reason, there are only two forms errors can take: skill-based slips and lapses, where an action does not go according to plan, and rule-based and knowledge-based mistakes, when the plan itself is inadequate to achieve its objective.[60] In health care, the different error types identified by Reason can be seen at work in that most common of miscues, the medication error.

Slips occur when the execution of a plan of action goes awry. For example, a slip of a doctor's pen turns "norflox," an abbreviation for the antibiotic norfloxacin, into "Norflex," the trade name for a muscle relaxant. At one hospital this error was discovered when a patient's spouse called the pharmacy to report that the patient was feeling weak and having hallucinations.[61]

A *lapse* is a mistake in the thought process, such as a brief bout of forgetfulness. For example, a doctor can write the correct drug name but the pharmacist can misinterpret it. As a result, the toxic cisplatin could be given in place of the requested carboplatin. A nurse might forget to check the drug dose she has received from the pharmacy against the correct dose on the order, or she might miscalculate the drug dose she is supposed to administer.

In a disturbing 1991 study, 110 nurses of varying experience levels took a written test of their ability to calculate medication doses. Eight out of ten made calculation mistakes at least 10 percent of the time, while four out of ten nurses made mistakes 30 percent of the time. Moreover, the error rate for dosages of drugs administered intravenously was "significantly higher" than for oral medications.[62] Similar studies of nurses and physicians in 1979 and 1983 found the same type of computation errors, even in a pediatric intensive care unit.[63]

I spoke to a Chicago woman who decided to become a nurse after her father was killed by an overdose of an experimental cancer drug. "If the nurses are friendly and smile and are neat, most people think it's good," she said grimly. "But everything could be clean as a whistle, and the nurses can't add."

In a *rules-based* mistake, the error appears not in the execution of the plan but in its very design. At Boston's Children's Hospital, a five-year-old boy suffering from seizures and other behavioral disorders was supposed to receive a behavioral drug with the brand name BuSpar. The pharmacist followed standard procedure and typed the first three letters of the prescription—*b-u-s*—into his computer. Because BuSpar was not in the hospital's formulary (an index of approved and commonly used drugs), the name of the antileukemia drug busulfan came up. No one had designed a rule to protect against this type of mistake. The hospital later said it believed the child would suffer no long-term effects, but other sources cautioned that busulfan could cause bone marrow failure or sterility.[64]

Finally, a *knowledge-based* mistake involves failure to acquire new knowledge in a novel situation that demands conscious analysis. In everyday life we all tend to practice "context-specific pattern recognition"; that is, we try to see if a new problem is similar to a problem we've resolved in the past so that we can apply a ready-made solution. The danger lies in the human tendency to avoid "cognitive strain," as Reason puts it. We can fail to recognize when the familiar response no longer works. Strong evidence is required to overcome a prior belief or theory.

So, for instance, the operators of the Chernobyl nuclear power plant in Ukraine continued with a planned reactor testing program even after gauges warned them the power was dangerously low. That deadly 1986 mistake sent clouds of radioactive fallout floating over much of Europe. Similarly, doctors and nurses who must regularly reassure frightened and sick patients can miss clear danger signals.

"The injuries inflicted by over-medication are to a great extent masked by disease," physician Oliver Wendell Holmes Sr. cautioned the Massachusetts Medical Society back in 1860. "How is a physician to distinguish the irritation produced by his blister from that caused by the inflammation it was meant to cure? How can he tell the exhaustion produced by his evacuants from the collapse belonging to the disease they were meant to remove?"[65]

Betsy Lehman was young, articulate, and far more knowledgeable about medical care than most people. Her husband, Robert Distel, was even a scientist employed by Dana-Farber. Despite all this, none of Lehman's caregivers took seriously the couple's protests that something was terribly wrong. Rather than stopping and analyzing Lehman's individual situation, the caregivers avoided "cognitive strain" and simply reassured the couple that chemotherapy is painful.[66]

Similarly, the mother of the five-year-old boy mistakenly given an antileukemia drug at Boston's Children's Hospital tried to tell nurses they were giving her son a different pill than he took at home. Despite the boy's vomiting and diarrhea, his mother's protests were ignored for five days until a nurse discovered the mistake on her own.[67]

The failure to perceive a new pattern was compounded in both cases by the psychology of "group think"; that is, when most members of a group are satisfied that all is well, other members tend to fall into line. At Dana-Farber, "the [medication] error . . . was a blunder compounded or overlooked by at least a dozen physicians, nurses and pharmacists, including some of the institute's senior staff," reported the *Globe*. "Along the way, they failed to respond to several warning signs, including Lehman's severe reaction to the medication, abnormal lab tests and electro-cardiograms indicating that her heart was in trouble."[68]

ERR AND ERR AGAIN

> The most fruitful lesson is the conquest of one's own error. Whoever refuses to admit error may be a great scholar, but he is not a great learner.
>
> —Johann Wolfgang von Goethe, *Maxims and Reflections*

On 26 May 1995 Vincent Gargano, a mail sorter from Chicago's northwest suburbs, began receiving chemotherapy for testicular cancer.[69] Encouraged by the knowledge that cancer of the testicles is curable in 80 to 95 percent of cases, Gargano sought treatment at the well-respected University of Chicago Hospitals. The forty-one-year old Gargano died in the hospital on 13 June. An attorney for the family charged in court papers that Gargano had been given four times the recommended dose of the drug cisplatin. The chemotherapy overdose destroyed his immune system and caused loss of hearing, severe kidney damage, and pneumonia that eventually led to his death. In response, the hospital suspended the physician responsible and issued a statement that said, in part, "We deeply regret this human error."

Gargano received the very same drug whose misuse had killed Betsy Lehman and triggered massive national publicity shortly before he began treatment. How could any physician or nurse, much less one at a major university hospital, not be aware of the potential harm from an overdose? How did the error still occur? That question leads to a broader one: why have forty years of scholarly studies and intermittent public scandals failed to make a significant impact?

One reason is that medical errors have remained largely invisible. An error committed in operating a nuclear power plant or commercial airliner is a great deal harder to hide. "The Federal Aviation Administration (FAA) works because when it fails it kills people a planeload at a time, and that's big news," noted Walter McClure, founder of the Minneapolis-based Center for Policy Studies. "Medical care kills people one at a time."[70]

The same month that Betsy Lehman died from a chemotherapy overdose, a commuter airline flight crashed in North Carolina. It was the second fatal commuter crash within a couple of months. Fearful travelers at one airport "refused to get on [commuter] planes," reported *USA Today*.[71] Yet while 1994 was the deadliest year for commercial aviation since 1988, three fatal commuter-plane crashes killed a statistically minute 25 passengers out of the 57.1 million who boarded a commuter flight that year.[72] Fatalities on commercial airlines claimed 239 lives, a tiny fraction of the more than 528 million passengers carried by commercial flights.[73] Measured by miles traveled, the safety of the commercial airline industry dipped from 99.9999 percent to 99.9961 percent.[74]

When a ValuJet Airlines flight plunged into the Florida Everglades in May 1996, the victim of exploding oxygen canisters that should never have been on board, the publicity led to a shake-up of the FAA. The National Transportation Safety Board had been pressing the FAA to tighten its standards on hazardous cargo for nearly a decade; the accident got the standards tightened.

"If you look at the aviation, space or nuclear-power industries, they're much more sophisticated in building systems that are error-proof, in their hardware and software, as well as their design of jobs and interactions," says Donald Berwick, president of the Institute for Healthcare Improvement, a nonprofit Boston group.[75]

The ValuJet crash killed 110 people. The annual death toll from the "hazards of modern diagnosis and therapy" remains more than a thousand times higher. Yet the Florida hospital that mistakenly amputated the wrong foot of one patient, did surgery on the wrong knee of another, and killed a third patient by removing his respirator was back in the news about a year and a half later after mistakenly giving a patient a drug to which he was allergic. The man had a heart attack and then lapsed into what was expected to be a permanent coma.

In medicine, mistakes are seldom discussed and lessons go unlearned. One respected observational study of drug errors by nurses concluded that nurses at a single hospital would make more than 51,000 errors in a year but report only 36 of them. "It is not easy to find the causes of errors," write George Di Domizio and Michael Cohen of the Institute for Safe Medication Practice, "and it is not professionally rewarding to build systems designed to reduce or eliminate errors."[76]

Some of the old self-protective instincts remain. In 1985 the *New England Journal of Medicine* estimated that 5 percent of the nation's doctors "ought not to be practicing medicine." That year, fewer than one half of one percent were disciplined. In 1995 fewer than 1 percent of doctors were disciplined, according to the National Practitioner Data Bank, and three-quarters of United States hospitals had not ever reported a physician disciplinary action since the data bank began.[77] Moreover, while consumers who are suspicious of their brokers can get their employment and disciplinary history from the National Association of Security Dealers, the medical societies have consistently fought against disclosing the names of physicians who have settled malpractice suits or been disciplined by a hospital.

Some doctor defensiveness is understandable. Although physicians consistently exaggerate the threat of malpractice litigation—few victims of mistakes ever file malpractice claims, and those who do typically receive modest monetary compensation—lawyers are quick to blur the distinction between malpractice and an avoidable error. Not all mistakes are automatically negligence, yet the two concepts are often used interchangeably. That could be seen during the controversy over Lehman's death, which came in the middle of an AMA campaign to persuade the most conservative Congress in a generation to place a federal cap on malpractice awards for pain and suffering. Trial lawyers and Consumers Union, the respected publisher of *Consumer Reports,* both seized on the Harvard medical practice study for their own purposes. They ignored both the distinction between negligence and preventable errors and the distinction between errors that occurred during the hospital stay and errors traceable specifically to a physician's action in the hospital. Instead of a reasoned discussion of medical mistakes, the public was treated to accusations that "negligent" doctors were killing 80,000 people a year.[78] Unfortunately, this kind of propaganda simply reinforces physicians' reluctance to address the error problem.

"Blaming the person does not necessarily solve the problem," argues human factors expert Marilyn Sue Bogner. "More likely, it merely changes the players in the error-conducive situation. "The error will occur again," added Bogner in the prescient introduction to her 1994 book *Human Error in Medicine,* "only to be associated with another provider."[79] In other words, effective change cannot come about because an individual doctor vows to do things differently. It is the system in which physicians, nurses and others work that needs to change.

There are signs that the medical profession may finally be close to acting on that insight. By 1996 federal tort reform was a dead issue as Republicans in Congress focused on the upcoming election.

In May 1996 the AMA announced a whole new approach toward medical mistakes. The group committed $200,000 to set up at National Patient Safety Foundation charged with funding research into error prevention and disseminating information on ways to prevent errors. That October, the AMA highlighted the foundation's planned activities at a national conference, cosponsored with other health care organizations, that was intended to dramatize the need for a systems-oriented error prevention approach. Among the invitees were many of the critics quoted in this chapter: Kenneth Barker and Michael Cohen on drug errors; Marilyn Sue Bogner and James Reason on system mistakes; and Lucian Leape to keep the spotlight brightly focused on the thousands of preventable deaths and injuries in hospitals.

The statements of AMA leaders about "isolated" mistakes were nowhere to be found. "Although experts agree that the error rate in medicine remains extremely low, now *even staunch tort-reform advocates say it's time to acknowledge that medical mistakes happen—are even common—* and to find answers rather than seek culprits," explained a page 1 story in *American Medical News* before the conference.[80] Nancy Dickey, chair of the AMA's board of trustees, explained the AMA's position: "We began to say, 'Isn't there something more we can be doing? We want to make sure we are doing everything we can to address issues of patient safety.' "

Martin Hatlie, a veteran AMA attorney, is the executive director of the new foundation. I asked him about the group's seeming 180-degree turn from "isolated mistakes" to acknowledging the existence of systemic errors. To his credit, Hatlie acknowledged that "people here were asking the same questions. Where is the consistency?" The approval of this new foundation by the AMA's board of trustees, said Hatlie, represented "an act of courage on the part of the AMA, that we're going to go forward and acknowledge as we haven't before that . . . a big number or a little number, errors are a problem. We are professionals. We have to do what's right. Physicians are accountable."[81]

Anyone who visits a doctor's office or is treated at a hospital can only hope that Hatlie is right. History suggests that continuing public pressure will be needed to make certain that the leadership of the AMA and its House of Delegates make good on their promises. Accountability must be to the public, not only to other professionals. In Connecticut, for instance, the state Office of Health Care Access published a consumer guide to hospitals that compared costs, mortality rates, and complication rates (including infections) in an understandable, color-coded chart. "Report cards" on managed care plans are starting to focus on error rates at hospitals as one important measure of quality.

Can the death toll from medical mistakes really be reduced? There's compelling evidence in the real world that a radical reduction awaits only the willpower to make it happen.

CHAPTER FOUR

Saving Lives, Bit by Byte

Every hospital should have a plaque in the physicians' and students' entrances: "There are some patients whom we cannot help; there are none whom we cannot harm."
—Arthur L. Bloomfield, M.D., about 1933

A patient trying to discover how well a hospital performs such basic functions as preventing medication errors and controlling infections is in much the same position as the patron of an expensive restaurant. Although the diners might thoroughly enjoy their meal, they remain ignorant of what goes on behind the closed kitchen door. The fish tasted good, but was it fresh? The vegetables looked attractive, but were the vitamins and minerals cooked out? The waiters hovered attentively, but did the cooks preparing the food remember to wash their hands? Similarly, the presence of distinguished physicians on the staff of a hospital does not necessarily prevent the medical equivalent of food poisoning—or worse.

Large numbers tend to turn a problem into an abstraction: "180,000 preventable deaths each year" out of "nine million physician/patient encounters every day." Although the problem of medical errors may be temporarily humanized—*this* man here who had the wrong foot amputated; *that* woman there who died of a drug overdose—the impression inevitably fades. There is no organized advocacy group to buy full-page ads with heartrending pictures of patient victims in the way that, say, groups combating drunk driving do. Yet patients' deaths and injuries do not happen nationally, they happen locally, one by one, and they can be effectively prevented that way. One of the best demonstrations of that truth is an initiative at Salt Lake City's LDS Hospital to prevent iatrogenic disease. Patient by patient, problem by problem—drug reactions, hospital-caused infections, inappropriate blood transfusions—LDS has shown that the risk-to-reward ratio of modern medicine can be changed if clinicians and administrators commit themselves to doing so.

LDS's program for monitoring adverse drug reactions is one of the nation's most highly regarded. When the initial results appeared in a 1991 issue of the *Journal of the American Medical Association,*[1] they were accompanied by an editorial from the Food and Drug Administration praising the initiative.[2] LDS officials privately believe their safeguards would have prevented the type of chemotherapy overdose that occurred at Dana-Farber. A separate LDS program halved the rate of infections suffered by patients undergoing surgery, another common hospital problem.[3] Meanwhile, if a patient's laboratory results indicate a pressing medical problem, the hospital's computer system automatically pages the nurse responsible for caring for that patient.

Of course none of this carefulness in caring guarantees that any individual patient will be cured. Even the most conscientious physicians providing the best treatment can be stymied by the limits of medical knowledge and the vagaries of human physiology. Yet LDS's accomplishment in shrinking the problem of treatment-related errors back to a human scale sends an important signal that should not be ignored. The theory of error prevention can be successfully put into practice. Mistakes that hurt or kill patients are neither random, rare, nor inevitable, and treating them as if they were is unacceptable. A program to reduce treatment-caused injuries and deaths can make a measurable difference in the lives of every person who enters a hospital trusting to return home safely again.

SAY NO TO DRUGS

> The complexity of modern medicine exceeds the inherent limitations of the unaided human mind.
>
> —David Eddy, M.D.

A little before eight in the morning, Stanley Pestotnik enters a locked basement office down the hall from the LDS Hospital loading dock and picks up a small stack of folded green-and-white computer paper. A clinical pharmacist who returned to school for a master's degree in computers and medical information, Pestotnik is passionate about policing drug use in the 520-bed hospital. In a few minutes, he'll start to walk his regular morning beat.

Every night the hospital computer scans the thousands of prescriptions ordered for or already being administered to LDS patients, then prints out an alert list of potential problems. And every weekday morning Pestotnik picks up the list and sets out to determine which alerts are the result of a computer programmed to be cautious and which pose a genuine threat to a patient's health.

From a clinical viewpoint, Pestotnik's mission is simple: to prevent patients from being harmed by their medications. In the health care world of the 1990s, however, that task is complicated by the harsh demands of economics. Even the most charitably motivated hospitals have always had to balance the conflicting demands of money and mission. Early nineteenth-century hospitals, for instance, professed to admit "only the morally worthy" and only those whose ills might reasonably be treated. Despite those high-minded declarations, "moral strictures could not well be applied to paying patients. . . . [T]he early hospitals were too hard-pressed for income. The Pennsylvania Hospital, for example, would admit incurable cases . . . and venereal, alcoholic and contagious cases as well if they could afford care."[4]

In time, health insurers took over the powerful role once reserved for wealthy individuals, with the federal Medicare program reigning supreme as the most influential health insurer of them all. When Medicare first started paying for seniors in 1966, it reimbursed hospitals in much the same way the Defense Department paid military contractors. Hospitals received a check based on their individual costs for each patient, plus an allowance for equipment and overhead. Not surprisingly, costs soared. The program's first two years cost twice as much as government actuaries had predicted, a pattern that only worsened. An alarmed congressional committee predicted in February 1970 that Medicare would cost taxpayers $16.3 billion in 1990. The actual figure turned out to be $109 billion.

It took nearly two decades for Medicare to throw out the old rules and deal hospitals a completely new hand. Starting 1 October 1983, the "cost-plus arrangement" was replaced with one that paid hospitals a fixed fee for each type of illness. The payment rate was based on the average time a patient needed to spend in the hospital for each condition. If a hospital's pneumonia patients, for example, generally went home within that time, the hospital made money. If they stayed longer, the hospital lost money. (There was some adjustment for truly catastrophic cases.)

This new system contained a glaring loophole. If a hospital deliberately admitted patients whose disease was mild, it could discharge them quickly and so guarantee itself a profit. To prevent that, the government began pushing for outpatient treatment, meaning no overnight hospital stay. Private health insurers, also bedeviled by soaring costs, followed the federal government's lead. Before 1983, the length of the average hospital stay had remained steady for seven years. Between 1983 and 1985 it slid 7 percent, even though only a third of hospitals fell under the new Medicare system in the first year of its phase-in.[5] Under pressure from insurers, hospitals also became choosier about whom they admitted. The rate at which Americans were hospitalized plunged by a third between 1983 and 1992—even without a return to reviewing potential patients' moral credentials.

Once a patient was admitted, moreover, there were sweeping changes in the pace of treatment. The average hospital patient was sicker, both because the less severely ill were treated as outpatients and because of demographic changes in the general population. Yet the hospital needed to discharge these older and sicker patients more quickly than ever. To escape from this squeeze, hospitals had no choice but to increase the intensity of therapy.[6]

By the end of the 1980s, the average hospital patient received fourteen medications, almost double the average when the decade began.[7] Severely ill patients frequently got more than thirty drugs. The medical chart of one such patient at LDS, for instance, listed antibiotics to combat an infection, gastrointestinal drugs to calm the stomach (at least in part because of side effects from the antibiotics), sleep-inducing drugs, and pain medications, among others.

Although additional medications can lead to faster cures, the trend concerns some prominent pharmacy researchers. "People are being treated extremely aggressively," cautioned Henri Manasse Jr., a veteran researcher into medication errors and the vice president for health sciences at the University of Iowa. "As the pressure to get people out of the hospital increases, you push the drugs a little harder . . . take it to the limit a little bit [in terms of dosage and frequency] to get faster results."[8] "There is heavy pressure to cure or improve the health of patients at the lowest cost," agreed William N. Kelly, chairman of Mercer University's Department of Pharmacy Practice. "Harming patients along the way sometimes seems secondary to these pressures."[9]

The explosive growth in the number and types of drugs the physician and pharmacist can choose from has only added to the risk. Physicians' prescribing errors have become an increasing source of risk to patients.[10] By the early 1990s, some nine thousand registered drug products were available in a dizzying array of dosage forms.[11]

When Stan Pestotnik arrived at LDS early one fall morning, the computer printout he picked up from the pharmacy office listed twenty-four potential adverse reactions to medications. That worked out to about six drug alerts for each one hundred patients occupying a bed the night before, a number that was close to the hospital's long-term average of five alerts per hundred patients.

In the early 1960s, at the peak of physicians' infatuation with the curative powers of the postwar "wonder drugs," medical leaders worried that doctors were not paying enough attention to potentially potent side effects. "Drugs can be standardized, but patients cannot," cautioned Hermann Blumgart, Harvard Medical School professor emeritus, in 1964. "The art of medicine demands adjusting the drug to the unique characteristics of the individual patient."[12]

At LDS, the computer system allows a physician to do just that. The hospital computer was first enlisted to improve drug prescribing in 1975, a year before two college dropouts in California set up shop in a garage and formed a company they called Apple Computer. The LDS system's capabilities have steadily expanded over the years. Each time a doctor enters a medication order into a terminal, the computer now examines scores of variables that would be next to impossible for any human to keep straight. For example, the system searches for interactions between the new medication and other drugs the patient is already taking; checks known allergies; examines laboratory results, such as the measure of kidney function, to see whether a drug was ordered in an appropriate dose; and even looks at the patient's diet. The computer also checks the prescribed dose against the generally recommended dose, looks at how frequently the drug is to be given, and makes certain the drug is appropriate for the disease.

Like physicians, the computer isn't perfect. For one thing, the program deliberately errs on the side of caution. A drug might trigger an alert when ordered even if it is never administered. Or a patient's complaint about a rash or stomach upset might wrongly be flagged as a drug reaction. Since no computer program can possibly anticipate all clinical situations, it is vital that LDS physicians be allowed to overrule the computer's recommendations. Indeed, what made the computer acceptable to the medical staff in the first place was an ironclad rule recognizing the superiority of the human mind in recognizing exceptions to the rules. All a doctor need do to override the computer is type an explanation into the terminal. The computer's task is detecting possible problems. Verifying those problems and trying to solve them still calls for the involvement of a trained human.

Pestotnik, alert list in hand, strides down the hallways and corridors of the hospital like a detective tracking down evidence of a crime. At one nursing station, he flips quickly through a patient's chart. At another, he stops doctors and nurses to ask a few quick questions about a patient's care. Sometimes Pestotnik even talks directly to patients—a rare event for hospital pharmacists, who are more accustomed to the supply lines than the front lines of patient care.

Those interviews follow a script carefully designed to determine whether an adverse reaction has genuinely occurred. "I don't want to put into your computer-stored medical record that you've had an ADE [adverse drug event] when you really didn't, because that could haunt you the rest of your life," Pestotnik explains. "They may withhold that therapy from you [in the future]."

At the first signs of real trouble, Pestotnik moves swiftly. One morning the alert list showed that a seventy-six-year-old woman had been receiving Narcan, a drug to reverse the effects of powerful narcotic painkillers. This was the second Narcan prescription in two days, which raised an immediate red flag. "This is one of our most sensitive indicators," Pestotnik says. "If Narcan is given, we determine why."

The medical chart told the story of a doctor struggling to walk a fine line between over- and undermedication. The elderly patient had suffered a stroke; she was originally given morphine to relieve her pain. When the morphine left her confused and lethargic, the doctor ordered Narcan as an antidote. But as so often happens with those who are sick and vulnerable, an effort to address one problem led to a different one. The woman began to show symptoms of an allergic reaction to Narcan, symptoms that were picked up by the LDS computer and passed on to the pharmacist as an alert. Pestotnik quickly checked the woman's condition, then telephoned her physician. In just a few minutes of private conversation, Pestotnik persuaded the doctor to cancel the Narcan ordered but not yet administered. The physician also agreed to replace morphine with acetaminophen, a painkiller more familiarly known by the brand name Tylenol.

No one can say for certain whether Pestotnik's intervention prevented the elderly stroke victim from becoming another casualty of the "diseases of modern medicine." The floor nurses or attending physicians might have acted similarly on their own initiative without the computerized alert. Still, Pestotnik noted: "If someone had continued to give [her] the drug and hadn't been aware of the adverse reaction, it might possibly have caused a respiratory arrest."

What is certain is that LDS consistently uncovers serious threats to patient health from medication use. More than nine out of ten of its alerts are judged clinically relevant and result in a change in therapy. About one in seven of the allergic reactions detected by the hospital is "severe,"[13] and researchers credit the system with occasionally preventing cases of actual malpractice.[14] Those results are precisely what one would expect from the research reported in medical journals for the past forty years.

"THIS IS THE PLACE"

It is partly serendipitous that this one hospital in a sparsely populated western state is a national leader in computer assisted patient care. No head of the medical staff or hospital administrator ever targeted that role. The credit largely belongs to an eclectic visionary named Homer Warner.

The phrase computer expert is often linked derisively to terms like geek, nerd, or wonk, as if to imply that the high priests of high technology must surely have achieved their position at the price of neglecting other aspects of their lives. Otherwise, why can't the rest of us figure out how to use our expensive microchipped machines? By any measure, Warner was cut from different cloth.[15]

Willard Richards, Warner's great-grandfather, trekked some fifteen hundred miles from Nebraska to Utah as part of the original group of Mormon settlers who fled westward to avoid religious persecution. Richards served as a close adviser to Brigham Young, the charismatic leader of that long migration and the man who molded the early Church of Jesus Christ of Latter-day Saints, as Mormons are formally known. When the group arrived at the edge of the Great Salt Lake in 1847, Young pronounced his people's exodus at an end with words that still resonate in the city he founded: "This is the place."

Homer Warner's father was a star receiver on the University of Utah football team. Homer also enrolled at Utah, in Salt Lake City, and eventually became the school's quarterback. After three years of studies, he applied to medical school and was rejected. He had been an indifferent student. Warner later acknowledged, "I liked football better than I did academics."

Rather than returning to his books, Warner volunteered for the wartime navy and trained as a carrier-based fighter pilot. Before he had a chance to see combat, however, World War II ended. Back in civilian life, Warner traded "top gun" for top grades and completed his undergraduate degree. This time he was accepted in an accelerated medical program at the University of Utah in 1946. He also began to study physiology, which deals with the physical and chemical processes of the body. He immersed himself in engineering and mathematics and eventually earned a doctorate in physiology at the University of Minnesota. Warner also trained in cardiology and internal medicine at Minnesota and at the Mayo Clinic. Recruited back to Utah, he established the state's first heart catheterization laboratory at the county hospital in mid-1953, a time when inserting a catheter into the heart was a bold new diagnostic technique.

After just a year, Warner switched to LDS, which was then called Latter-day Saints Hospital and was owned by the Mormon Church. He set up the state's second catheterization laboratory and began working with a group of hospital engineers on a project that would propel them into the national limelight. The group started assembling what they called a "circuit." Said Warner later, "When we built that first circuit, I didn't even know it was a computer."

His ignorance was understandable. In their modern form, computers were still new. The idea of using mathematical analysis to discern patterns of medical treatment was first proposed in seventeenth-century France by Blaise Pascal, who, when not discovering laws of physics or writing works of theology, helped invent modern probability theory. At age twenty-one, Pascal also invented the first simple digital calculator. It performed addition and subtraction with the help of dial wheels and a series of gears. But the construction of the first true commercial tabulating machine had to wait for the efforts of a diligent nineteenth-century American engineer named Herman Hollerith.

Hollerith was a man who disdained nonquantitative pursuits.[16] It is said that as a child he jumped from a second-story window to avoid a spelling lesson. After graduating from the Columbia University School of Mines in 1879 at age nineteen, Hollerith went to work for the Census Bureau. Here the development of the first true computer acquired its serendipitous medical connection. The bureau had recruited surgeon John Shaw Billings to help it prepare for its daunting decennial duty. Billings was already well known both as a gifted administrator and as the developer of *Index Medicus,* a monthly guide to current medical literature.[17] It was Billings who suggested to the young Hollerith that "there ought to be some mechanical way" of tabulating the millions of census questionnaires.

After months of working closely with Billings, by 1890 Hollerith was ready to enter into two contracts. The first was with the Census Bureau to use his Electric Tabulating System. The second, longer-term arrangement, was Hollerith's marriage to Billings's daughter. Thanks to Hollerith's machine, the 1890 census was completed in a third of the time of its predecessor, despite the addition of several questions. Hollerith, meanwhile, took advantage of his patents and a growing number of contracts to found the Tabulating Machine Company in 1896. After two name changes and a change in control, the company emerged in 1924 as IBM.

By the late 1930s and early 1940s, there were a series of breakthroughs. British mathematician Alan Turing helped design an electronic computer that was used to crack the codes used by Nazi Germany. The "Colossus" machine was the first to employ vacuum tubes as digital on/off switches in place of slower and noisier electromagnetic relays. The first all-purpose electronic digital computer, ENIAC (electronic numerical integrator and calculator) was completed at the University of Pennsylvania in 1946.

These early digital machines required large, heavily air-conditioned rooms in order to combat the heat given off by thousands of bulky vacuum tubes (ENIAC had 17,468 of them). By contrast, Warner's team of Utah engineers built a much smaller analog computer that fit into the constrained space of a hospital. Rather than translating information into the series of on/off pulses that form the backbone of data in the digital information age, analog computers represent information as electrical quantities. The relationships of those electrical quantities are then "computed" to calculate what the data mean.

One of the early computers built in Salt Lake City was inspired by the same mathematical principles that enable the tuner on a radio to amplify one channel while shutting out other frequencies. The research team used knobs, resistors, and circuits to assemble a device that "tuned in" to the electrical impulses involved in the beating of a patient's heart.[18] In an experiment, Warner put electrical transducers on the ends of catheters that he inserted into the patient's arteries. He used the impulses transmitted by the transducers to mathematically model the wave form made by the blood as the heart pushed it through the body and into the legs. That model, in turn, let him calculate the heart's pumping capacity and diagnose whether a patient had a problem that interfered with that capacity. Crude as these calculations were by today's standards, for its time Warner's work was extraordinary, groundbreaking research.

A young electrical engineer named Reed Gardner joined Warner's team in the late 1950s. Gardner, still at the hospital today, remembers a project in the early sixties in which he constructed computer monitors from the vacuum tubes of teletype machines. These custom-designed terminals eventually cost an extravagant $4,000 apiece, more than many of the new Fords Homer Warner's father sold at his downtown car dealership. But they were worth it. The computer provided critical, real-time readings of a heart-surgery patient's blood pressure, cardiac output, and heart rate that could not be matched in either speed or accuracy by nurses making the same measures manually. The innovation was immediately put to work with patients. "We didn't make any systematic studies about mortality," says Warner, "but we alerted people to situations [involving risk to patients] that they didn't recognize without [the computer]."

Elsewhere, other researchers pursued a similar agenda. A Palo Alto, California, anesthetist spoke of saving two people's lives during operations because of electronic monitoring. His experience was chronicled in a page 1 article in the 17 August 1959 *Wall Street Journal*. The story was headed, "Electronic Medicine: Scientists Press Work on Advanced Machines to Aid Medical Care. They See Automatic Nurses Watching Sick, Computers Helping Diagnose Illnesses."[19] One visionary from UCLA spoke of developing a master computer program "that anyone having access to a computer could use to analyze medical health data." If all went well, "each large population center in the U.S. might conceivably have one or more" medical computers.

Computers in medicine were not the only hot trend on page 1 of the *Journal* that day. There was a "wild proliferation" in America's large cities of "smarter look" coffeehouses serving espresso and cappuccino, an adjoining article informed readers. A Dallas coffee shop owner reported making back his investment in just two months.

Brigham Young, who as a Mormon abstained from any drink with caffeine, had chosen Utah as the site of his New Jerusalem in part because of its isolation from the outsiders who regarded the Mormon religion as apostasy. The state's vast unpopulated stretches made it a prime location for internment camps for Japanese prisoners of war during World War II and for top-secret military tests of nuclear weapons during the Cold War that followed. Homer Warner helped put Utah on the map in a different context. In the mid-1960s the

National Institutes of Health gave LDS a major grant that allowed the hospital to stop building its own analog computers and purchase a large digital machine. Other grants followed.

Warner "stayed awake nights trying to think of new ways to use the computer to solve significant problems," relates *Medicine in the Beehive State,* a history of Utah's medical community. (The state's nickname refers to the sober-minded industriousness of its first settlers.)[20] In the late 1960s, with the open-heart surgery procedure growing in popularity, Warner extended the computer's capabilities from the operating room to the patient's bedside.[21] Then a 1969 visit by Warner to an LDS intensive care unit changed everything. It provided the inspiration that would transform the LDS computer system into a powerful instrument for improving everyday care.

At the nursing station of LDS's cardiac intensive care unit, a monitor displayed a set of three lights—red, yellow, and green—for each recuperating heart surgery patient. When the green lit up, it meant the computer was taking readings. (At the time, monitoring was not continuous.) Red signaled an emergency, and yellow indicated a problem with one of the patient's clinical signs. As straightforward as that system seemed in theory, in practice it turned out to be dangerously ambiguous. Related *Medicine in the Beehive State:*

> [A] nurse [was] pumping up a blood-pressure cuff on the left arm of a patient who had a pressure-monitoring catheter in the right arm. A yellow light showed on the panel. The nurse was embarrassed when she saw [Warner] watching her and explained that she didn't know what to do next. They sat down at the computer terminal and looked at all the data in both the computer and the chart. They called the resident and jointly decided that the patient probably was having a cardiac tamponade [a blockage of the blood flow]. The surgeon on call promptly took the patient back to the operating room.[22]

Until he witnessed this close call, Warner had concentrated on expanding the computer's monitoring ability. Now he took the system in a very different direction. What was needed was not just a computer that provided more data, but one that could interpret the facts and turn them into immediately usable information. Although this insight was hardly new—science fiction writers had breezily taken such machines for granted for years—implementing it in real life posed significant technical challenges.

To begin with, researchers needed to put many more sources of clinical information into computer-readable form. Much like a human physician, the computer had to draw on a large amount of clinical knowledge if it was to correctly interpret the meaning of each patient's biological signs and symptoms. The LDS team, which was already expanding the computer database to include laboratory results and other measures, now broadened its effort.

A second barrier involved the state of the art of computer programming. In the late 1960s in Vermont, when John Wennberg and Alan Gittelsohn set out to analyze the variations in patterns of patient care, they were forced to invent ways of telling the computer what to do. The LDS team had to do the same thing. Warner, Gardner, and T. Allan Pryor, who had done programming for the early space program, developed a highly structured numerical coding scheme that put medical terminology into terms the computer could understand.[23]

Researchers confronted an even more difficult task after medical jargon was finally translated into computer code. Science fiction notwithstanding, computers don't think; they follow instructions. So the researchers had to compile a bits-and-bytes digest of a medical school education. This was the knowledge base that set forth the rules and relationships the computer would apply to all the pieces of patient information it received. Without a series of formal "if-then" rules—for example, if the heart beats so many times per minute, then the patient is experiencing fibrillation—the mass of stored data in the computer's brain was useless.

In Warner's view, physicians had three main tasks in taking care of patients: first, to gather and evaluate new information; second, to quickly access information already in the medical record; and most important, to evaluate all the information. Drawing on their knowledge of the medical literature and their experience in patient care, physicians needed to decide how to best manage patients' problems. The greatest unmet requirement for doctors was not more sophisticated diagnostic equipment, argued Warner, but better tools to help them interpret the information they already had.[24]

"The computer [is] a tool for facilitating and improving the physician's performance," he wrote. "Our challenge [as physicians] is to use this tool to the advantage of the patients we serve."[25]

To assemble a knowledge base that would allow the computer to understand clinical information, LDS researchers interviewed their medical staff on the "rules" they followed when treating patients with certain conditions. The researchers also painstakingly translated scientific articles into something a mainframe could get its circuits into. Jammed with notes from *JAMA* and nourished by the *New England Journal of Medicine,* the computer broke free of the limited role of simply informing the doctor that the patient had, say, a high level of blood gases. Instead, the computer could scan the medical literature in its memory and decide whether the likely cause of the high blood gases was metabolic acidosis—related to the digestive tract—or respiratory acidosis—related to difficulty in breathing. Both conditions can be life threatening, but they are treated very differently. By 1972 the LDS computer could interpret blood gas results and electrocardiograms. Meanwhile, in an experimental program at the University of Alabama Medical Center in Birmingham, a computer system began to administer blood if a patient's blood pressure fell below a certain level.

As computer capabilities improved, physicians' attitudes did not always keep pace. It was one thing for a doctor to tell the computer what to do; it was another for the computer to advise the doctor. In a 9 July 1973 *Wall Street Journal* article, "Doctors' Helpers: Computers Play an Increasing Role in Diagnosing and Recommending Treatment of Medical Problems," the former chairman of an AMA committee on computers noted enthusiastically that computerized medicine was spreading at "an unprecedented rate." But the article ended by acknowledging that "many physicians are openly hostile to the whole concept of computer medicine, fearing that the machine may one day usurp their duties."[26]

Eugene Stead, a physician-researcher at Duke University, conducted an informal experiment. A number of primary care physicians were asked to examine a computer generated medical history and a handwritten one generated by a human and pick which was better. The human history won overwhelmingly. The researchers then took the information from the handwritten history, reworked it slightly, and printed it out so it looked as if it came from the computer. Next the original computer generated history was rewritten by hand. When doctors were shown the new choices, they again picked the handwritten history by an overwhelming margin.[27] At LDS, the research group decided to give their computer system the friendly moniker HELP, emphasizing its role as a physician's assistant.

Gradually, HELP did help (and the system's name was turned into an acronym for Health Evaluation through Logical Processing).[28] When automated entry of prescription orders into a computer terminal began in 1975, about a quarter of all prescriptions at LDS stayed on paper. But by 1988, with a new generation of doctors and a new era of cost containment pressures, 99 percent of all LDS prescriptions were entered into a computer terminal.

LDS hospital researchers carefully identified thirty-five possible causes of an adverse drug reaction. Then they launched a campaign using the computer system to minimize or eliminate each one.[29] For example, antibiotics that were supposed to be gradually infused over the course of an hour were sometimes administered by harried nurses in fifteen minutes. A change in the computer's program to monitor intravenous drug infusions reduced the number of infusion-related reactions to zero.[30]

In 1990 LDS patients suffered just forty-one severe reactions to medications. Given the high rate of medication-caused injuries reported in the medical literature, LDS might have rested on its laurels, secure that the unfortunate incidents that did occur were "isolated." Instead the hospital chose to pursue continued systematic improvement of its care processes. By 1994 only nine LDS patients experienced adverse drug reactions. In other words, seven out of ten reactions were eliminated.[31] The Harvard research team examining adverse medical events had concluded that four out of ten errors in administering a drug could be prevented.[32] LDS's record thus surpassed their supposed ideal. When a drug reaction did occur, it was almost always of a type that could not have been anticipated.

LDS also targeted infections of surgical wounds. When a patient is being prepared for surgery, antibiotics are most effective if given no later than two hours before the procedure begins. Busy surgeons, though, can forget to order the drugs in time. With a computerized reminder system, the percentage of patients receiving their first antibiotic dose on time jumped from 40 percent in 1985 to 99.1 percent in 1994.[33] Meanwhile, LDS reduced its overall rate of wound infections by half, from nearly 2 percent to less than 1 percent.[34] Once again that accomplishment can be compared with that of the "ideal" low-error hospital. The Harvard researchers estimated that 70 percent of all wound infections could be prevented.[35] (LDS says its rate was lower than average to begin with.)

Everywhere researchers looked, they saw opportunities. In the mid-1980s the HELP system was expanded to automatically alert caregivers to potentially life-threatening lab results. In one group of patients the number of hours spent in a life-threatening condition dropped by a third. In another group, with a different and equally severe condition, it dropped by half.

"Before the HELP system was implemented, it might have taken weeks to discover errors in treatment," one LDS physician candidly reported. In one instance an elderly woman with a hip fracture received inappropriately prescribed oxygen therapy for two months. (Her low oxygen levels were due to anemia.)[36]

Once more, it is important to emphasize that these problems were not unique to LDS. According to the Harvard study, 40 percent of the injuries caused by inadequate monitoring can be prevented. In a few places, though, LDS seemed to be having extra trouble. A 1986 review by outside accreditors, for example, found that only one-fourth of the blood transfusions being ordered were clinically appropriate. The hospital responded by entering the proper clinical indications for a transfusion into the HELP system. The physician could always override the computer's warning that a transfusion was inappropriate. Overrides, though, were regularly reviewed by the hospital's quality assurance department, which could go the computer and call up data showing the patient's clinical signs at the time of the transfusion. Soon, 99 percent of blood transfusion orders met the hospital's strict new criteria.[37]

Reed Gardner, now LDS's director of medical informatics, compares the effect computerized monitoring has on doctors to the effect on drivers of knowing a police officer is using a radar gun. The radar gun "encourages" motorists to obey the speed limit, says Gardner dryly.

Meanwhile, a decision-support program put on the computer in 1986 took on the complex problem of delivering precisely the antibiotic most likely to be effective against a patient's infection. The bacteria in infections are highly specific. The prevalence of one strain or another varies from city to city, hospital to hospital, and even from one floor of a hospital to another. By tracking the prevalence of bacteria at LDS and recording which antibiotics proved effective against them, the hospital reduced the death rate of patients who needed antibiotics by more than one-fourth (from 3.65 percent to 2.65 percent). And at a time when rampant antibiotic overuse is giving rise to frightening problems with resistant strains of bacteria, as related in chapter 1, LDS cut its antibiotic usage to two-thirds of the national average.[38]

If reducing patient injuries and deaths does not provide the same prestige as isolating a new strand of DNA or developing a new surgical technique, few at LDS seem to care. Nor are they bothered that most patients haven't a clue about the efforts of their unseen protectors. "It's nice when patients tell me they feel better," comments

John P. Burke, a veteran Public Health Service epidemiologist and the hospital's chief of infectious disease, "but my real satisfaction comes from seeing when the numbers get better, from seeing lives saved on paper."[39]

THE SIN OF COMPLACENCY

> I know the past, and thence I will essay to glean a warning for the future, so that man may profit by his errors and derive experience from his folly.
>
> —Percy Bysshe Shelley

In 1967 a New Mexico radiologist named Marcus J. Smith published an unusual medical confessional. *Error and Variation in Diagnostic Radiology* neatly laid out for Smith's colleagues the types of interpretation errors to which radiologists commonly fell prey. What made this book different was that the author had carefully tracked his own cases and regularly referred to his personal mistakes as prime examples of what *not* to do.[40]

There was, for instance, the sin of complacency, which included "hobby-riding"; that is, focusing on a condition or organ in which the doctor has a particular interest and ignoring signs of other problems. There was the sin of "recency": the last patient I saw had pneumonia, so this patient's signs probably indicate pneumonia too. And there was the seductive spell of the "mythical malady," which caused a doctor to diagnose the faddish disease of the day instead of the patient's true ailment.

Smith recognized, years ahead of his time, that simply telling doctors to "try harder" to avoid make mistakes accomplished little. "An attempt has been made to avoid the quicksand of hackneyed advice such as 'keep your eyes open,' 'obtain consultations' or 'keep up with the literature,' " he wrote. Instead of indulging in clichés, Smith carefully divided radiology errors into six major categories and made systematic "recommendations for improvement and corrective action."[41]

The impact of this noble effort was nil. "Everything Dr. Smith said in 1967 applies equally well today," sighed Spencer Borden IV, a pediatric radiologist and consultant, as he showed Smith's work to a polite group of colleagues. "We in health care do not do a good job of looking at our mistakes."[42]

The word error is derived from the Latin *errare,* "to go astray," implying that the way to prevent errors is to stay on the right path.

But in the absence of a compass or road map, people may not even know they are lost. Or they may just not want to admit it. Like step one in the twelve-step recovery program pioneered by Alcoholics Anonymous, correcting many problems begins with admitting that they exist and that something can be done about them.

The failure to look unblinkingly at errors is not limited to medication mistakes. In August 1975 the federal Centers for Disease Control launched a formal Study on the Efficacy of Nosocomial Infection Control (SENIC) to address hospital-caused infections. The problem was big news after former President Richard Nixon nearly died from nosocomial pneumonia following vascular surgery at a California hospital in early 1974. About 15,000 people did die that year from all types of nosocomial infections, the CDC estimated then. (A nosocomial infection is one that originates in a hospital; presumably the mistake that nearly killed Nixon was one of those "compensable events" in researcher Don Harper Mills's database.)

Twenty years later the death toll from nosocomial infections has risen by nearly a third, to some 19,000 deaths, plus 58,000 complications. Yet the CDC has never even standardized the definition of a nosocomial infection or verified that different hospitals report information in a comparable manner. In other words, in nearly two decades the agency has never really tried to systematically understand the causes of nosocomial infections and then act to prevent them. Of course no newspaper columnist (or former president) has been killed by a nosocomial infection lately.

Nosocomial infections are "an ignored problem," charges Richard Wenzel, author of an authoritative textbook on infection control.[43] Adds Wenzel, a physician at the University of Iowa Hospitals, "It's easy to show we're over 50,000 deaths directly due to bloodstream infections in the United States, [even when] adjusted for the underlying disease."[44]

You don't need a computer to reduce treatment-caused deaths and injuries; you only need to carefully examine how you practice. In 1897 the Austrian physician Ignaz Semmelweis realized that new mothers attended by midwives had a much lower rate of infection than those treated by medical students. He discovered that medical students were going straight from the pathology laboratory to delivering babies without washing their hands. Semmelweis's observation was derided by colleagues, and he ended up in an insane asylum ten years later and died there. Nearly one hundred years later, doctors wash their hands only 14 to 59 percent of the time before seeing patients, said Duncan Clark, an emeritus professor of preventive medicine in New York City.[45]

When it comes to preventing mistakes, however, most hospitals don't even know how they are doing. Twenty hospitals were randomly sampled by two nursing researchers in a 1995 study to gauge the availability of data on errors in administering medications, patient falls, the occurrence of new decubitus ulcers (bedsores), nosocomial infections, and unplanned readmissions to the hospital (a common indication that something went wrong with the patient's care). Only two indicators—medication errors and patient falls—were collected consistently, noted the 1995 paper.[46]

To be sure, using a computer inarguably opens up untapped possibilities. In the late 1960s the National Institutes of Health sponsored a dial-in program in which physicians could ask a computer questions about drug therapy by using a touch-tone phone as a data entry device.[47] More localized computer monitoring "has been feasible and affordable for 12 years," fumes Auburn University's Kenneth Barker, a veteran medication-error researcher.[48] In 1985, a cardiologist at a Veterans Administration hospital in south Florida told the American Heart Association about preventing drug reactions with a program he wrote for the inexpensive microcomputer on his desk.[49]

Most industries have allocated 10 percent of their capital budgets for information systems; health care providers have spent just 2 percent.[50] Still, the use of clinical information systems is finally increasing. In 1991 about 3 percent of hospitals with more than one hundred beds had bedside computer terminals; in 1994 nearly 10 percent did. The annual growth in spending for all sorts of hospital information systems was projected to hit $8 billion in 1997, nearly double the 1991 level.[51] Boston's Dana-Farber joined the move to computerized drug ordering just a little too late. Its system was set to become operational a few months after Betsy Lehman died. Similarly, the Kaiser Permanente health plan in Denver installed an automated review of mammogram readings only after one of its radiologists was found to have missed the need for a follow-up physical exam in 259 breast X rays over an eighteen-month period. The offending radiologist was fired.[52]

The most sophisticated computer system will not lead to better care, however, unless caregivers are willing to act on the information they receive.

At Boston's Brigham and Women's Hospital one evening, Evan Rosen received a couple of unusual messages on his pager. On two separate occasions a computer in the sprawling medical center's laboratory dialed his beeper directly to warn him that the serum potassium level of one of his patients had fallen dangerously low. Serum potassium is a measure of a patient's kidney function. By chance, the alerts occurred on Rosen's first night of "call" duty as a resident. Fresh out of the University of Michigan Medical School, the thirty-year-old had already earned a Ph.D. at Michigan in molecular endocrinology before coming to the Brigham for further clinical training. As he walked around the hospital's busy coronary care unit, Rosen was grateful for the computerized reminder. "I found it to be very, very helpful," he said. "There are a lot of things going on at once, some of them more important than others. It's easy to get distracted."[53]

Some of Rosen's more senior colleagues have proved equally distractible, but not equally grateful for reminders. At Beth Israel Hospital, like Brigham and Women's a Harvard-affiliated center, researchers tested a computerized alert system that monitored elevated creatinine levels. Creatinine, like serum potassium, is a measure of kidney damage. When the alert system was turned off, patients who were receiving potentially toxic medications had a 45 percent greater risk of suffering serious kidney damage. "Computer-based alerts . . . prevent serious renal impairment [and] preserve renal function," researchers concluded.[54] Yet fewer than half (44 percent) of the Beth Israel doctors responding to a questionnaire issued by the research team said the alerts were helpful in care of their patients. In fact, a little more than a quarter of the doctors (28 percent) found the alerts "annoying."[55] Without the alert system, it took an extra *twenty-two hours* for doctors to adjust or discontinue toxic medications. One wonders whether the patients involved would characterize their suffering as "annoying."

In a medical culture that insists on the unattainable ideal of physician perfection, it is difficult for a doctor to stand up and demand that money be spent on preventing medical mistakes. Hospital administrators, too, share that reluctance to stare honestly at the flaws in the mirror. Moreover, although no hospital wishes harm to its patients, the cultural predisposition to view mistakes as inevitable and unpreventable meshes with an economic incentive that has traditionally pushed in the same direction. The patient who remains hospitalized an extra couple of days because of a treatment-caused injury does not receive free care as a way of making amends. The meter keeps on ticking.

In a 22–29 January 1997 article in *JAMA,* LDS researchers put dollar figures on the money involved in the average adverse drug reaction. At LDS, it increased a patient's hospitalization by almost two full days and increased the cost of the stay by nearly $2,300. There was also a significantly increased risk of patient death.[56] In that same issue of *JAMA,* David Bates of Brigham and Women's Hospital and his colleagues looked at two Harvard hospitals and concluded that preventable drug reactions led to extra patient care costs of $2.8 million in just one year at a large sophisticated teaching hospital.[57] But *whose* costs? Here Bates exhibited the same high-minded obliviousness as the physician-researcher in the 1950s who referred to treatment-caused injuries as the price "we [doctors] must pay" for medical progress.

"The substantial costs of ADEs (adverse drug events) to hospitals justify investment in efforts to prevent these events," wrote Bates in a formulation that was repeated in news stories about the study. In fact, the financial cost of drug reactions is overwhelmingly borne by health insurers and self-insured employers (absent provable malpractice), just as the physical price for mistakes is paid—as always—by the patient. Only as a growing number of hospital beds are filled with fixed-payment patients, whether from Medicare or from "managed care" plans, does the calculus change.

If that reasoning seems somewhat cold, it is a fair reflection of how investment priorities have been set by hospitals in the real world. Even at LDS, where millions of dollars and thousands of hours of staff time have been invested in reducing mistakes, several researchers confided to me that their work was not always greeted with unbridled enthusiasm by those responsible for the hospital's bottom line. Indeed, although media reports commonly referred to drug-error prevention efforts at Intermountain Health Care, as of the start of 1993 the extraordinary HELP computer system had been installed at only one other Intermountain hospital other than flagship LDS. But at that time, as health reform loomed and the number of fixed-payment patients at Intermountain grew sharply, the board approved $40 million to install HELP at all its hospitals.[58]

Certainly no one familiar with the technology of drug-error prevention believes that technological barriers have been the issue. "How long, Oh Lord, must this continue?" read a note posted by a University of Michigan biomedical engineer to an Internet news group shortly after Betsy Lehman's death became public. "In 1974 we had an on-line patient-record system that flagged unusual lab results or unusual . . . prescriptions, and that was at a vet[erans] hospital. That's 21 years ago. . . . Isn't it time that basic computerization be part of the expected, and required, care at medical facilities?" The note continued: "That humans make 0.1 percent errors on prescriptions may be forgivable; that hospitals don't take obvious actions to protect themselves and patients, well within state-of-the-art, is not."[59]

CHAPTER FIVE

State of the Art

Medicine aims to cure that which is perceived, treatment being based on judgment rather than on ill-considered opinion.
—Hippocrates

For most of human history, both the sick who sought healing and the caregivers who tried mightily to provide it knew that success was elusive. "One cannot really have confidence in doctors and yet cannot do without them," sighed the eighteenth-century German poet and playwright Johann Wolfgang von Goethe. Even well into this century, doctors prided themselves above all on their skill as diagnosticians. The doctor did not always possess the weapons to fight effectively against disease, but he could at least chart its natural history and let the patient know what to expect. The physician's role was "to cure sometimes, to help often, to comfort and console always."[1]

Medicine resisted the constraints of scientific theory. Most physicians remained securely convinced that what they saw with their own eyes in their daily work provided the most reliable evidence of whether a particular therapy worked. The English philosopher and essayist Francis Bacon criticized this "empiricism" as early as the seventeenth century, to no effect.[2] The trap of "spurious correlation," that is, a false assumption of a cause-and-effect link between two events, did not seem to have been well understood. Although the eighteenth century was Europe's Age of Reason, medicine held itself cautiously apart. "In medicine, all, or almost all, depends on . . . a happy instinct," said the French physician Pierre-Jean-Georges Cabanis in 1788. Quantitative reasoning was a distraction. "The certitude that is found [in medicine is] most often that of an artist," Cabanis declared.[3]

The advent of the randomized clinical trial (RCT) in the years immediately after World War II marked a great divide in medicine's evolution from art to science. Although the art remained—as it always would and should—for the first time the demands of objective evidence claimed an unchallenged place at the patient's bedside.

As beneficial as that was for society, rigorous scientific testing of new therapies carried a price. It was individual patients who volunteered to be assigned a therapy at random so that medicine could find out which treatment worked best.

A SUDDEN BRUSH WITH DEATH

The town of Rupert is a small farming community in the southern part of Idaho. It ranks as an urban center mostly by contrast to the expansive fields of sugar beets, potatoes, and grain that surround it. Restless teenagers looking for a little more excitement head south on Route 24 to Burley, home of potato-processing giant Ore-Ida. There, cars filled with teens go cruising on the main street of that marginally larger municipality.

One cool Friday evening in early spring, eighteen-year-old Gypsy Heuston finished closing out the cash register at the bowling alley in Rupert and hurried to meet a group of friends. Gypsy was athletic and outgoing; a member of her high school's bowling team, she also displayed the strong-willed temperament of a classic redhead. Sometimes the trait manifested itself as ambition: the Minidoca High School senior wanted to be the first in her family to go to a four-year college. At other times the willfulness came out as defiance. Gypsy enjoyed pushing her parents' 1:00 A.M. weekend curfew to the limit and maybe a bit beyond. It was a point of pride never to come home early.

This Friday night, though, Gypsy made a rare exception to her own rule. A little before 10:00 P.M. the teenager shocked her mother, Jeanette, by walking into the house and going straight to bed.

Despite that unusually early bedtime, Gypsy's parents had to shake her awake on Saturday morning. Even then the teenager lay half-dazed, wheezing and coughing, gasping to her mom that she couldn't breathe. Jeanette and Dennis Heuston immediately put their daughter in the car and sped to the emergency room of the small local hospital.[4] "It's pneumonia," said a general practitioner on call for emergency duty. He added that Gypsy's parents should bring the girl back for treatment of her lungs every four hours. Dennis Heuston immediately responded with an alternative treatment plan. "This is my daughter," he said vehemently. "You're going to admit her, or you're going to feel my boot where the sun don't shine." The doctor decided to accede to this second opinion.

In the hospital, antibiotics normally used to fight pneumonia produced no improvement in Gypsy's condition. Her breathing grew increasingly labored, while her parents grew more and more frantic. A worried nurse who was a family friend telephoned a lung specialist. He hurried to the hospital, examined Gypsy, and then turned solemnly to Dennis and Jeanette. Their daughter was suffering from a condition called ARDS. Her lungs were under sustained attack, and there was little the local hospital could do to stop it. If Gypsy wasn't transferred quickly to a more sophisticated facility, the specialist told the stunned parents, she could die.

On Monday morning a helicopter from LDS Hospital flew in from Salt Lake City to pick up Gypsy. While a portable breathing device forced air in and out of her lungs, the semiconscious teenager was lifted carefully onto a stretcher and placed in the copter's cabin. Jeanette, a security guard at Ore-Ida, sat protectively beside her daughter. Gypsy's sixteen-year-old brother and her father drove to Salt Lake City. Dennis Heuston, a thirty-nine-year-old former trucker with a history of two heart attacks and five back surgeries, flipped on the emergency flashers and raced through the normal three and a half hour trip in two hours flat.

As Gypsy was taken to the hospital's shock-trauma intensive care unit, Jeanette and Dennis Heuston tried to fight down their panic. They had only one question for the doctors and nurses: "Will you be able to save her?"

CAUSE AND EFFECT MEDICINE

The scientific method did not have an easy time putting down roots in everyday medical practice. For example, as recently as 1941, a young British medical student named Richard Gordon was astonished by the current therapy for pneumonia. When his class visited a hospital, Gordon found himself cast backward in time: "An immaculately blue-dressed, crisp-aproned, frilly-hatted ward sister demonstrated . . . 'dry cupping.' As elegantly as sewing samplers, she raised egg-sized mounds of patients' skin in wine-glasses vacuumised by heat, this being her favored treatment of lung congestion. . . . [O]ur current textbook still recommended the seventeenth century practice of bleeding and 'the application of six leeches over the liver.' "[5]

Of course, during this same period doctors in the United States were still prescribing arsenic and strychnine for anemia during pregnancy and for "low sex drive," and tablets made of dried hog kidneys were given to people thought to be "allergic" to cold or heat.[6]

Yet there were always some doctors capable of seeing beyond the conventional wisdom of their age. One of the most important in the establishment of scientific medicine was a member of the influential Paris School of Medicine, Pierre-Charles-Alexandre Louis. In the 1820s Louis applied what he called the "numerical method" to a careful study of typhoid fever. Louis was able to draw a connection between mortality and how long the person had lived in Paris. He also charted the victims' ages, concluding that "youth is a necessary condition for the development of the typhoid affection."[7] Louis's next step was even more daring. He directly challenged the usefulness of that most ancient of medical practices, bloodletting.

In Louis's world, bloodletting still occupied a place of honor. A British medical journal begun in 1828 chose the *Lancet* as its name to signal its scholarly intent. For those squeamish about submitting to the knife, there were always leeches. The gentle action of the blood-sucking worms made them particularly popular for treating women and children. During the French Revolution, leeches even acquired a political patina. Leeches and bloodletting were said to be in harmony with political liberalism, because they acted by "relieving the patient from oppression" as opposed to the mere treatment of symptoms.[8] France alone was importing more than forty-one million of these patriotic and medicinal slugs every year.[9] The word leech had at one time been a synonym for doctor, and not in an uncomplimentary sense. "To leech" meant "to cure."

Undeterred by either etymology or empiricism, Louis set up an experiment to test bloodletting's therapeutic powers. One group of patients with either pneumonia or inflamed tonsils was bled; the other group was not. Louis then evaluated whether bleeding made a measurable difference in the patients' eventual recovery. In Louis's view, "The edifice of medicine reposes entirely upon facts, and . . . truth cannot be elicited but from those [facts] which have been well and completely observed."[10]

Louis's conclusions constituted a sharp rebuke to expert medical opinion. In an 1835 book titled *Research on the Effects of Bloodletting*, he wrote that the patients who were bled not only remained sicker for longer, they had a higher death rate.

Not surprisingly, outraged leech users questioned Louis's methods. The Spanish-born, French-educated Benigno Juan Isidoro Risueño D'Amador, for example, warned that mathematical calculations threatened to substitute "a uniform, blind and mechanical routine for the action of the spirit and individual genius of the [physician] artist."

Nonetheless, Louis's work opened the way for an increasing number of scientific studies linking treatment with outcome.[11] Still, it was another full century before the first scientifically rigorous, randomized clinical trial of a medical therapy.

THE GOLD STANDARD

The design of the randomized clinical trial (RCT) had none of the drama of discovering a new drug or surgical technique. Yet in terms of its enduring impact on patient well-being, few events have been more important. Opinion and empiricism did not disappear, but proponents of a new therapy, no matter how distinguished they might be, now needed to produce factual evidence that it worked. Although various types of studies could be cited, the RCT became recognized as the gold standard of evidence.

For all the influence of the RCT, it was born as much of financial desperation as scientific curiosity.[12] The father of the randomized clinical trial was not a physician, but an economist. In 1946, when Britain was still devastated by the just-ended world war, streptomycin was being hailed by its United States developers as the first effective treatment for the often fatal scourge of tuberculosis. The British Royal Exchequer, however, had only enough money to buy a small quantity of this expensive new antibiotic. British medical experts worried that the evidence for the drug's effectiveness came from observing an uncontrolled series of patient cases and so might be flawed. Fearful that buying the drug might mean squandering precious financial resources but knowing that not buying it could cost lives, the British government turned to its Medical Research Council to investigate streptomycin's effectiveness. The council, for its part, looked to a forty-nine-year-old professor named Austin Bradford Hill to lead the Tuberculosis Trials Committee.[13]

Hill had himself contracted tuberculosis while stationed in the Middle East during World War I. During a long period of recuperation, he earned a degree in economics through correspondence courses. On its completion, Hill took a job with the Industrial Fatigue Research Board, a semi-independent body under the Medical Research Council. There he trained in epidemiology and became a protégé of a physician named Major Greenwood, who was an early leader in the use of biostatistics. Hill went on to become a professor at the University of London and director of the Research Council's Statistical Research Unit.

In designing medicine's first randomized clinical trial, Hill ventured far afield—or perhaps into the field. He was inspired by a book demonstrating how the laws of chance could be used to eliminate bias in agricultural experiments. By randomly planting different grains in different plots of land, wrote R. A. Fisher in *The Design of Experiments,* farmers could be certain that any resulting differences in yield reflected an "objective" and real difference in grain productivity.

Following this fertile furrow of logic, Hill set up a statistical series of random sampling numbers to determine which patients in the tuberculosis trials would receive which therapy. He concealed his exact methods even from the trial's clinical investigators. Hill also worked to reduce variation among the patients being tested. The British government had bought only enough streptomycin to give to exactly fifty people, while a control group would get a placebo. Hill chose his study participants carefully. All had to be suffering from acute progressive bilateral pulmonary tuberculosis, a type of TB for which the only known treatment was bed rest. Patients had to be from fifteen to thirty years old. Again, the intent was to eliminate extraneous factors that might influence the outcome.

The trial's results validated Hill's meticulous attention to detail. Streptomycin saved lives. After six months, fourteen of the fifty-two patients in the "control" group receiving only bed rest had died (27 percent). By comparison, just four out of fifty patients had died in the experimental group receiving both bed rest and streptomycin (7 percent). When the researchers examined the odds that this difference was simply a random event, no more indicative of the true state of affairs than a warm, sunshiny day piercing the gloom of a London winter, the probability was less than 1 percent.

The tuberculosis trial also demonstrated that miracles can still be accompanied by side effects. A significant number of patients became resistant to the antibiotic, allowing their disease to worsen; others suffered an adverse drug reaction. However, some differences that empirically might appear important proved not to be. For example, the average temperature of the streptomycin patients was lower than that of patients receiving just bed rest. A lone doctor observing that change in a single patient might have concluded that the drug was responsible, but an analysis showed the temperature difference was not statistically significant. There was no reason to treat patients differently because of it.

When the tuberculosis trial results appeared in a 1948 issue of the *British Medical Journal,* the randomized trial was almost immediately recognized as a breakthrough. Critics were not silenced, but the argument that a physician deserved the total freedom of an artist was irreparably weakened. Hill went on to conduct pioneering clinical trials that highlighted the dangers of tobacco. His work led to his being knighted by the queen and hailed by colleagues as the greatest medical statistician of the twentieth century, even though he held no degree in either medicine or statistics.

The randomized trial did not eliminate the need for expert clinical judgment, nor was it intended to. Instead, it placed clinical judgment within a new scientific framework. "Statistical methods may be no substitute for common sense," noted D. D. Reid, a former colleague of Hill's, "but they are often a powerful aid to it."[14]

A CALAMITOUS DISEASE

"Common sense" was clearly an inadequate basis for treating a medical problem as complicated as the one that had left Gypsy Heuston fighting for her life. "Common sense," after all, argued that Gypsy most likely had pneumonia—a misdiagnosis that could have killed her; she was fortunate to have been seen quickly by a specialist who recognized her disease. Still, her prognosis upon reaching LDS remained guarded. Doctors estimated her chances of recovering at just fifty-fifty.

Effective treatment for ARDS, even in the waning decade of the twentieth century, remains a very iffy proposition. It is just one of a long list of conditions on which medical researchers work unnoticed. No children walk in ARDS marathons and no entertainers wear ARDS ribbons. But by seeking treatment at LDS Hospital, Gypsy Heuston found herself drawn into the struggle against the disease.

The researchers who in 1967 first cataloged the set of symptoms that constitute ARDS called it adult respiratory distress syndrome. The bland "respiratory distress" hardly does justice to ARDS's calamitous impact. The tiny air spaces of the lungs fill with fluid, creating much the same effect as drenching a stack of sponges: when the water becomes heavy enough, the bottom sponges in the stack collapse. The collapse of the air spaces, or alveoli, diminishes the lungs' ability to transfer oxygen in and carbon dioxide out. If enough air sacs are destroyed, the body stops functioning and the patient dies.

One reason effective ARDS treatment remains problematic is that the physiological mechanisms of the disease remain a mystery. Physicians know how it is triggered, but not exactly how it works. Shocks to the body from other medical problems, such as pneumonia, trauma, or a severe postsurgical infection, frequently are the precipitators of ARDS, but in Gypsy's case there was no obvious cause. Moreover, ARDS patients are generally young—the average age is just thirty-three—and over the years they have gotten younger. This youth trend prompted a name change for ARDS to *acute* respiratory distress syndrome, but the new label didn't alter the discouragingly high mortality rate. At the beginning of the 1980s, the 10,000 to 15,000 people annually who contracted the disease had about a 60 percent or greater chance of dying.[15]

In the early 1980s, ARDS researchers in Milan, Italy, reported startling progress. The Milan team said they had boosted the survival rate of the very sickest of ARDS patients from the 9 percent reported by American researchers in the mid-1970s to a dazzling 77 percent. The technique they used was called "extracorporeal [outside the body] CO_2 removal." It addressed one of the key drawbacks of conventional ARDS therapy. ARDS patients who are kept breathing on mechanical ventilators are subjected to a high volume of oxygen (because the oxygen absorption of their lungs is inefficient) at a high pressure (because their lungs have trouble expanding). The ventilator therapy is not a cure; it is designed to buy time until patients' own lungs can fight their way back to health. But conventional ventilator therapy also carries risks. Although oxygen is vital to life, it is also a potent toxin. Too much can destroy the cells lining the lungs, mimicking the damage wreaked by ARDS itself.[16] Moreover, maintaining high pressure on the airways can lead to overexpansion and injure whatever healthy portion of a patient's lungs remains.

The Italian researchers tried to circumvent these hazards by placing next to the ARDS patient's bedside a machine that imitated the functions of the human lung. The patient's blood was removed and circulated through this artificial lung to infuse oxygen and remove carbon dioxide before being returned to the body. Although the artificial lung cannot be used continuously, even intermittent use allowed doctors to reduce the stress on patients' own lungs.

The report of success in Milan caused immediate excitement, but the results were based on observation of an uncontrolled series of patients. Before a therapy such as extracorporeal CO_2 removal ($ECCO_2R$) could be adopted for widespread use, it needed to be subjected to a randomized clinical trial.

In this instance there was a financial as well as scientific incentive for close scrutiny. $ECCO_2R$ therapy cost many thousands of dollars more than the traditional approach. At a time of increasing pressure to contain costs, pulmonologists needed to reassure hospital purchasing departments that $ECCO_2R$ represented a genuine advance.

The National Heart, Lung, and Blood Institute put up nearly $1 million to fund a clinical trial of $ECCO_2R$; LDS Hospital, recognized as a leading pulmonary research center, was chosen as the trial site. When the sickest ARDS patients entered LDS, they would be assigned randomly either to conventional ventilator treatment or to $ECCO_2R$. When enough patients had been treated, researchers would compare the groups to see whether the choice of therapy made any difference in outcome.

So it was that on 12 April 1991 a computer at LDS Hospital used a random-number program to pick the therapy for Gypsy Heuston. With the consent of her parents, the gravely sick teenager from Rupert became patient 29 in a scientific exercise aimed at determining what ARDS treatment worked best.

FACING FACTS VERSUS "BURNING WITCHES"

Alan Morris, director of the pulmonary research unit at LDS Hospital, never met either Gypsy or her parents. Like LDS epidemiologist John Burke, who confessed that his real satisfaction came from "seeing lives saved on paper," Morris was first and foremost a researcher.

A New York City native, Morris entered Yale Medical School in the early 1960s after studying chemistry at Princeton and biophysics at the University of Paris. The scientific method was his passion. Acting on hunches and getting emotionally involved only represented seductive invitations to commit the unforgivable sin of bias.

Temptation was ever present. Some physician would write to a medical journal asserting that his last twelve patients had responded to some new therapy, and there would be a rush to embrace it. Another doctor would pronounce the work "promising," and the rush would turn into a landslide. It happened. Morris, though, felt only scorn for those willing to be whipsawed by medical fashion.

Responsible clinicians understood that only a randomized clinical trial provided protection against the biases, beliefs, and blunders that constantly threatened objectivity.

A visitor asked Morris whether historical controls—comparing what happened to a present group of patients with the outcome for a similar group of patients treated in the past—might at least provide a strong hint about a treatment's ultimate worth. Morris quashed the suggestion, unhesitatingly ticking off factors that could contaminate the comparison. "The historical controls were with different ventilators, different antibiotics, different drugs for supporting heart pressure. . . . I can go on and on and on. . . . [Historical controls] are unreliable for comparison." What about the value of expert medical opinion? The question evoked a mixture of sarcasm and outrage. "Louis the Sixteenth received purgatives 1,100 times," Morris harrumphed. "The history of medicine is littered with therapies that were enthusiastically endorsed by the best practitioners of the day and then subsequently abandoned and demonstrated to be not only useless but sometimes harmful."

Then what about a comparison with "standard practice"? Responded Morris, "The argument that the practice patterns and the standard behavior of the day should be the arbiter of the correctness [of medical treatment] flies in the face of those who were appalled by the burning of the witches in Salem, Massachusetts." In case a visitor still did not quite get the point, Morris underlined it: "Clinical trials provide the best and most credible evidence likely . . . to lead to action, to change."

Morris's colorful characterization of medical miscalculation is substantially accurate. The postwar advent of the randomized clinical trial tempered, but by no means tamed, the impulse to provide treatments justified by little more than gut feeling and good intentions. The healing power of penicillin and other antibiotics contributed to a surge of medical optimism. To a doctor concerned more about an individual patient than some abstract scientific good, it might seem unethical to withhold a possibly beneficial therapy until the conclusion of a randomized trial. The British investigation of streptomycin took two years from study design to publication of results. That was lightning fast in scientific terms but meant a possibly deadly delay for an individual tuberculosis patient. Besides, the trial eventually confirmed that streptomycin worked. That the trial also produced important information about drug side effects and dosage levels could seem less important—not unlike the present-day argument about randomized drug trials for AIDS or cancer.

Postwar critics of the RCT attacked it for a smorgasbord of sins. It allegedly replaced humanistic and clinical values with mathematical formulas; degraded patients from human beings to "bricks in a column, dots in a field or tadpoles in a pool"; and led to the elimination of the doctor's responsibility to each individual patient.[17] Defenders responded that though the RCT was not the only way of advancing therapeutic knowledge, it was certainly a very important way. As for the ethics of using a "control" group, practicing physicians implicitly did the same thing already; the "controls" consisted of the doctor's impressions of what had happened to previous patients with the same disease. In that sense, all therapy is experimentation.

It took until the early 1960s for the RCT to win full acceptance. It is important to note that what ultimately carried the day was not an appeal to the intellect of doctors but an emotional public. It involved a West German sleeping pill called thalidomide.

Throughout United States history, tragedy and drug regulation have danced a tight minuet, with tragedy leading and regulation following close after. The original Pure Food and Drugs Act of 1906 was passed in response to problems with food safety that were dramatized for the public by the chief chemist of the U.S. Department of Agriculture, Harvey W. Wiley. In 1902 Wiley organized a group of volunteers called the "poison squad," who experimented on themselves by eating small amounts of suspect substances. The squad's efforts to embarrass Congress into action paid off when Upton Sinclair's muckraking novel *The Jungle,* a tale of the stomach-turning practices of the meatpacking industry, turned the issue of food safety into a national scandal a few years later.

Separately, a 1905 series of articles in the influential *Collier's Weekly* focused public attention on the uselessness—or worse—of drugs being peddled to a vulnerable public. Reporter Samuel Hopkins Adams revealed that formula sold as soothing for infants achieved its effect by using powerful opiates. And he reprinted burial notices of people who had testified to the healing powers of various potions, only to die from the disease they had supposedly cured.[18] Adams followed up the series with a similar exposé the next year.

The 1906 law that Congress passed in reaction to these abuses was primarily aimed at unsafe food, but it also required drug labels to be accurate. By 1930 the agency charged with enforcing the law, the

Agriculture Department's Bureau of Chemistry, had evolved into a separate Food and Drug Administration (FDA). Still, it took another thirty years for Congress to require that new drugs, like food, actually be safe. Once more, tragedy captured lawmakers' attention.

The advent of the sulfanilamides in the 1930s was the curtain raiser for later generations of wonder drugs. Although this class of drugs was first synthesized in 1908, their therapeutic value went unnoticed for years. When it was finally recognized, patent protection had expired. As related in chapter 2, the therapeutic properties of the sulfanilamides seemed like magic. In one dramatic public demonstration of their effectiveness, President Franklin Roosevelt's son was cured of a dangerous streptococcal infection with an experimental sulfa medication. Only twelve years before, the son of another president, Calvin Coolidge, had died as a result of "blood poisoning" brought on by a tennis blister.[19] Intense competition broke out among the big drug companies to see who could sell the most sulfanilamide pills. An editorial in the 2 October 1937 issue of the *Journal of the American Medical Association* warned enthusiastic physicians that there was a narrow line between a therapeutic dose of the new medication and a highly toxic one, but the clamor for the drug continued unabated.

A small pharmaceutical firm in Tennessee, the S. E. Massengill Company, decided to exploit a market niche bigger companies had neglected. It developed a version of the drug that could be taken in liquid form. Massengill's one-gallon bottles of Elixir Sulfanilamide contained 10 percent sulfanilamide, 15 percent water, small amounts of saccharin and coloring agents, and 72 percent diethylene glycol, a solvent and moisturizing agent. Before shipping this mixture to physicians, the drug company's laboratory carefully evaluated the appearance, flavor, and fragrance. But Massengill never bothered to test the drug's safety.

Physicians eagerly prescribed the pleasant-tasting, easy-to-swallow liquid for everything from sore throats to syphilis. During a four-week period in the fall of 1937, 353 patients, many of them living near Tulsa, Oklahoma, received Elixir Sulfanilamide. Within weeks almost a third of them were dead: 105 people died from diethylene glycol poisoning. As stunning as this mass poisoning was, even more deaths were avoided only because some patients stopped taking the medication their doctors had recommended after they were sickened by their first few teaspoonfuls.

In those days the FDA had no legal authority to seize the drug just because it was killing people. However, it happened that the label on the Massengill medicine bottles omitted the presence of the diethylene glycol. The FDA quickly jumped on this error as the legal basis for seizing 228 out of the total 240 gallons of elixir that had been produced. Had all that elixir been consumed, it is estimated that four thousand people would have died.[20]

Once more a highly visible tragedy prompted a congressional response. In December 1937 a physician member of the Senate proposed amendments to the federal Food, Drug, and Cosmetic Act that authorized comprehensive regulation of pharmaceuticals. By the summer of 1938, President Franklin D. Roosevelt was signing the bill into law. Now new drugs not only had to be labeled correctly, they also had to be demonstrably safe. Regulation of effectiveness—a requirement that the drug do what it was supposed to—had to wait another quarter of a century for yet another dance with death.

The sedative thalidomide was widely sold without prescription in Europe, South America, Australia, and Japan during the late 1950s. It did what it promised: it put people to sleep. But in 1961 scientists discovered to their horror that 7,000 to 11,000 women who took thalidomide while pregnant gave birth to children with shortened and malformed arms and legs or with no arms and legs at all.[21] Haunting pictures of the thalidomide babies appeared in magazines and newsreels and on the fledgling television news. In 1962, responding to public anger, Congress passed the Kefauver-Harris amendments to the Food, Drug, and Cosmetic Act, finally requiring drugmakers to prove that a medication was not only safe but effective. More directly relevant to thalidomide, drugs were also required to carry labels disclosing when they should not be used—for example, by pregnant women—and listing their potential side effects.

In submitting evidence to satisfy these rules, drugmakers were required by law to produce data collected from "adequate and well-controlled investigations, including clinical investigations." FDA guidelines emphasized that no drug would be approved unless it underwent a clinical trial whose protocol was approved by the FDA and whose results were reviewed by the agency and critiqued for accuracy and completeness. Objective evidence had dealt empiricism a resounding defeat.

The new law had limits. It did not apply to surgical procedures or to medical devices, for example. Devices were first regulated by the FDA in 1976, and surgical procedures remain largely unregulated still. With devices and, particularly, procedures, Congress and medical groups were reluctant to hamper a physician's freedom to innovate. Even the 1962 amendments permit an individual physician to prescribe any FDA-approved drug for any purpose, no matter what the official label says, an exemption used today for experimentation in treating fatal diseases. Professional ethics and a fear of malpractice litigation provide the only constraints.

In a health care system founded on a strong belief in individual rights, these seeming loopholes served as a legitimate safety valve. They enabled doctors to take whatever action they thought necessary to treat individual patients without having to wait for cumbersome government approval. The constant challenge to physicians,

however, was distinguishing between responsible innovation and recklessness.

Perhaps the most famous example of the risks of relying on each doctor's judgment involves the lobotomy. In 1936 Portuguese neurologist Egas Moniz and Swiss physiologist Walter Hess developed a method of severing the connection between the frontal lobes of the brain and its emotional centers. This simple procedure produced an extraordinary calming effect on patients who were psychotic or otherwise mentally disturbed. Moniz warned that the surgery should not be used except where other methods had failed, but enthusiastic practitioners embraced the frontal lobotomy anyway. The more adventuresome could even "cure" the mentally ill in their offices by inserting a thin blade into the skull through the bony case of the patient's eye and then rotating the blade until the proper area was severed.[22]

By the time Moniz and Hess shared the Nobel Prize for medicine in 1949, thousands of lobotomies were being performed every year. Yet by the end of the 1950s, careful studies revealed what had somehow escaped the notice of many practicing physicians for two decades: the procedure severely damaged the mental and emotional lives of the men and women who underwent it.[23] "Lobotomized" became a popular synonym for "zombie," and the number of lobotomies being performed dropped to near zero.

Just a few years after the lobotomy craze fizzled out, a burst of enthusiasm greeted another apparent miracle treatment, this time for ulcers. University of Minnesota researcher Owen Wangensteen reported in 1962 that "gastric freezing" relieved the symptoms of a patient suffering from stomach ulcers. For the first time physicians could eliminate stomach acid without surgical removal of the stomach, wrote Wangensteen and his colleagues in the *Journal of the American Medical Association.*[24]

The *JAMA* paper was carefully subtitled "A Preliminary Report of an Experimental and Clinical Study," but such caveats could not suppress the excitement over gastric freezing. In an era when "the man in the gray flannel suit" was likely to be holding a martini in one hand and reaching into his pocket for an antacid pill with the other (one-tenth of all Americans suffered from stomach ulcers), gastric freezing became an instant hit. The treatment was ballyhooed in the pages of *Time,* and a manufacturer of refrigeration equipment who had worked with Wangensteen rolled out the first gastric freezing device shortly afterward.

Unfortunately, the first physicians to adopt the technique were not always as careful about clinical indications as Wangensteen, nor were they as skilled. Reports began to surface of problems ranging from perforation of the patient's lower esophagus to an occasional death. Swenko Corporation of Minneapolis sold some 1,200 gastric freezers at $1,500 each in the first year, but demand rapidly dwindled as the reports of side effects multiplied. A careful randomized clinical trial of gastric freezing got under way in 1963. Six years later, when the procedure was already extinct, results of the gastric freezing trial were published in the peer-reviewed *New England Journal of Medicine.* The verdict was negative.[25]

In their excitement over the therapeutic explosion following World War II, too many physicians forgot that trying to help patients and actually helping them are not the same. The warnings of the late nineteenth-century "therapeutic nihilists" who preached that a physician should do nothing rather than embrace a treatment that could cause injury were disregarded as outmoded advice from a bygone era. Physicians, and their patients, had to relearn the painful difference between intuition and information.

Pediatrician William A. Silverman witnessed the near-miraculous effect of penicillin on sick newborns when it was a new drug and he was a new doctor. At a New York Academy of Sciences conference, "Doing More Good Than Harm," Silverman reflected: "The spectacular results of penicillin reinforced a 'magic-bullet-like mentality': there was preoccupation with a solitary target—the hoped-for benefit of treatment. The narrow view overlooked the ever-present risk of injury by 'friendly fire' in medical warfare: there are usually multiple, and, too often, harmful effects of treatment."

In one example, premature infants were placed in high-oxygen incubators for long periods to reduce the chance of brain damage. Only after that treatment became commonplace was it realized that too much oxygen can cause blindness. Other well-meaning interventions also exacted a heavy price. Concluded Silverman:

> One hapless scenario was re-enacted over and over: an exciting proposal, based on findings in pre-clinical studies; a leap to widespread clinical application; belated recognition of the possibility of disastrous complications; and evaluation by controlled clinical trial, if it took place at all, long after the unevaluated treatment was in general use.
>
> We can see now, in hindsight, that immature human patients have played a risk-taking role, not unlike the function assigned to canaries carried underground by coal miners. Repeated treatment disasters involving the highly vulnerable babies have given early warning to all of medicine: The practice of adopting treatments for widespread use before they are subjected to rigorous comparative trials is very dangerous!

SAVING THE LIFE OF A CHILD

At LDS Hospital, Alan Morris was acutely aware of the fiascoes of gastric freezing and lobotomy. More to the point, he knew from hard personal experience the gap that could separate a researcher's private hopes and the hard evidence of a clinical trial. Early in his career, Morris was a principal investigator in a multiple-hospital study of a different type of extracorporeal treatment for ARDS, one less elaborate than the new technology he was now testing. That study consumed several years, hundreds of hours of work, and hundreds of thousands of dollars of research funds, only to conclude that the experimental treatment was no more effective than the traditional one.

The whole purpose of a clinical trial is to determine cause and effect. Sometimes the relationship is as easy as watching an apple fall from a tree and then positing the law of gravity. Most cause and effect relationships are more subtle. Scientists are supposed to avoid jumping to conclusions, but modern researchers still fall prey to a variety of sins. On the one hand, some researchers exaggerate the effect of a new treatment by failing to control for which patients are allowed to enter the trial or why some patients drop out early.[26] On the other hand, they can underestimate the effect of an intervention on patients' health by including so few patients in a trial that it takes an enormous impact to produce a statistically significant conclusion.[27]

One unavoidable bias is the assumption that something is worth investigating in the first place. Some researchers, faced with ambiguous results, resort to the same statistical contortions practiced by politicians confronting an anemic public opinion poll. Politicians call it "spin." The academics wink knowingly at "data dredging"—searching for the numbers that look good. Morris would have nothing to do with any preconceived conclusion. With the attention to detail of an artist putting the finishing touches on a painting, he set out to design a clinical trial that would prove precisely duplicate what the Italians had done and beyond reasonable doubt either that $ECCO_2R$ worked better than conventional ventilator therapy or that it did not.

Testing a new procedure is more complicated than giving two groups of trial patients different pills. The $ECCO_2R$ procedure in particular was difficult and dangerous. Nurses had to insert thick catheters into veins in the patient's leg to channel the blood out to the artificial lung. Some patients required a tube into each lung. There was a constant threat that contamination would cause a new infection in patients who were already extremely sick, not to mention the chance of mechanical failure of the artificial lung. These risks were worth taking only because the possible benefit was so great.

To make sure its skills were up to par, the LDS team of doctors, nurses, and respiratory therapists carefully provided a total of 271 hours of high-tech pulmonary treatment to seven sheep.[28] Morris's plan for guiding patients through the "control" arm of the trial—the traditional ventilator treatment—presented a much greater challenge. Morris had already taken pains to duplicate the "experimental" procedures used by the Italians, but usually the "traditional therapy" arm of a trial allows individual doctors to treat patients however they normally would. Instead, Morris herded together the independent pulmonologists who practiced at the LDS shock-trauma unit and tried to get them all to agree to do things the same way.

Morris's reasoning went this way. When new drugs are tested, it is relatively easy to disguise who is receiving the experimental medication and who is getting a placebo. But when testing a large artificial lung, it was obvious which therapy was going to whom. The risk in this kind of "open" trial was that clinicians eager for a new therapy to succeed might inadvertently give the experimental patients extra attention that by itself could affect the outcome. To prevent that, LDS would write a protocol spelling out every detail of treatment. However, the logical Morris quickly discovered for himself the same problem that David Eddy had found when, as mentioned in chapter 2, he sought the decision tree governing how doctors treated breast cancer. A treatment regimen that appeared on the surface to be orderly and scientific quickly dissolved into a series of individual "rules of thumb" used by each physician.

To understand the problem, take just one instruction in the treatment protocol for ventilator therapy: "maximize PEEP" (the "positive end expiratory pressure" recorded when a person breathes out). That common instruction might seem clear enough, but it quickly becomes evident that "maximize" means different things to different people. Like instructions to "optimize the upbringing of your children or optimize the taste of the roast," noted Morris, "nobody's going to complain about them—they're conceptually quite compelling. But they're not executable."

The LDS staff had suddenly come face to face with the problem of physician practice variation. As individual doctors, they had broad discretion. Each could form a personal definition of what it meant to be "severely ill" or even what it meant to have true ARDS. In the absence of obvious malpractice or incompetence, no one would question their choices. But when the physicians tried to reach collegial agreement on which approach was best supported by the medical literature, discussion became dissension and peer review degenerated into peer rebuke.

"The meetings would go on a couple of hours once a week, at least," recalled one observer. "They couldn't find articles [to support their views]." "They said, 'You're wrong, you're wrong,' " remembered another person. "And they all came back the next week, and I think one of them brought an article, and it was sort of flaky. And they said, 'Gee, we really don't know [what works best], do we?' And then they went through this process of developing protocols." Or as a paper by the team later put it: "The major problem in creating the protocols was obtaining clinician agreement on protocol logic and their commitment to utilize it clinically."[29]

Step by step, the staff of the LDS shock-trauma unit forged a consensus on best medical practice. They agreed on how frequently patients needed to be monitored, on the settings of ventilators, and on the logic clinicians would employ in making decisions. Then, when the group thought its hardest work was over, the physicians discovered that their lofty conception of patient care omitted some crucial bedside details.

"They had never asked for nursing input," recalled Vicki Spuhler, head nurse of the shock-trauma unit "They tried to implement the protocol, and they couldn't even run it 40 percent of the time. The logistics of their decisions had never been discussed. . . . They didn't know what it meant to make . . . a change and then watch the patient's response, because the physicians don't do that, nurses do." Physiological theory didn't always work out in practice. So, for example, an instruction to remove a breathing tube when the blood gases reached a certain level meant that patients could be going through extubation when they should be sleeping. Let them get through the night, then extubate, the nurses argued. The doctors meekly gave in.

Eventually a chart running to more than forty pages and containing a total of 840 specific therapeutic recommendations was positioned by each patient's bedside. Doctors, nurses, respiratory therapists, and others all contributed. The group decided that the ideal of reaching the "right" therapeutic decision in each foreseeable instance was unattainable. There were too many things going on. Researchers counted 236 categories of clinical variables that might affect each patient.

As the protocol grew more complicated, the LDS research team programmed it into the HELP computer terminals by each bedside. There was, as usual, one basic rule. Consensus or no, any clinician was free to override the instructions at any time on behalf of any patient. Gradually, as real-life situations highlighted problems, the protocol evolved. Within four months, compliance rose from under 40 percent to more than 90 percent.[30] The LDS staff finally decided to reduce the PEEP oxygen pressure by a third in an attempt to limit damage to the lungs.

For Morris and the rest of the LDS staff, this experiment in standardization of care involved high stakes. They had spent thousands of hours developing the protocol. For Gypsy Heuston, the stakes were higher. By the luck of the draw, she was not chosen to receive the experimental $ECCO_2R$ therapy. Instead, Gypsy would be getting the traditional ventilator treatment, standardized by the new protocol. The stakes for Gypsy in this randomized clinical trial were her life.

Some patients enrolled in a clinical trial want desperately to receive the experimental treatment. If something is "new," they believe, it must also be "improved," whether it's a detergent or a medical treatment. Dennis Heuston says he and his wife didn't give the choice of therapy for Gypsy a second thought. "All we were caring was they could do something for her," he said.

Gypsy could not express an opinion. The teenager was last fully conscious when doctors in Idaho began placing a breathing tube down her throat. Then, once she arrived at LDS, doctors deliberately prevented her from waking up. In the sickest of ARDS patients, the amount of oxygen in the blood hovers at a level barely adequate to prevent permanent damage to internal organs. Should a patient flex a little finger or try to talk, the motion diverts oxygen to the muscles and threatens oxygen starvation elsewhere. As a result, the sickest ARDS patients are carefully placed into a near coma while (if all goes well) the remaining healthy cells in their lungs reproduce and the ability to breathe unassisted gradually returns. While this slow process works itself out, patients remain almost motionless, day in and day out, as nurses and doctors monitor their vital signs and tend the ventilator that keeps them alive.

By grim coincidence, James Pearl, Gypsy's pulmonologist, was also treating another Idaho teenager suffering from ARDS. Tami Robbins, who was flown to LDS Hospital about six weeks before Gypsy, was one of the youngest ARDS patients on record—only fourteen years old.[31] She was also one of the sickest ARDS patients then being treated by LDS. After Pearl gave Tami's family a candid assessment of their daughter's chances on her arrival at the hospital, they promptly nicknamed him "Dr. Death." Tami and Gypsy were similar in where they lived, their ages, and the physician treating them, but they were separated in one crucial way. Gypsy was getting the conventional therapy. Tami was chosen to receive the experimental $ECCO_2R$ treatment.

In the family waiting area at the hospital, Patty and Ken Robbins and Jeanette and Dennis Heuston sat and talked about Idaho, their kids, and this horrible disease. Was it a chemical spray in the bowling alley that had affected both girls? Something on the crops? No explanation seemed to fit. One topic the parents did not discuss, however, was which therapy for ARDS might work best.

The Heustons virtually lived at LDS Hospital, speaking regularly to their daughter as if she was awake, hoping that at some level she knew they were there and realized how much they cared. After six weeks, when the doctors became convinced that Gypsy was going to live, they let her wake up. Coming out of her coma, Gypsy struggled to remove the respirator. She tried to talk, but her throat, raw from the intubation, would not allow any words to come out. Scared and frustrated, Gypsy saw her father and grandfather standing anxiously at the end of her bed. "I remember everybody asking me, 'Gypsy, Gypsy,' getting me to turn my head so I knew where I was," she recalled.

"Asleep" though Gypsy had appeared to be, some of what was said to her during those long weeks had gotten through, transmuted into bizarre semiwaking dreams, a constant parade of nightmares. There was one exception, one remark that had made it through so clearly that Gypsy remembered it later. Someone (it had been her father) had called out to her, "Wake up, Gypsy, there's a good looking [male] nurse taking care of you."

Tami Robbins still remained in a medically induced coma. By coincidence, the two girls turned out to know each other. Though separated by four years in age and forty miles in distance, they had competed against each other on their high-school bowling teams. The staff brought Gypsy in a wheelchair to see Tami, but there was, not surprisingly, no response. Still, "Dr. Death" had turned into an optimist. Tami was going to make it, pulmonologist Pearl told the Robbinses.

Gypsy returned home in late April; Tami was discharged in early May. About that same time, LDS stopped enrolling new patients in the ECCO$_2$R trial. Forty ARDS patients had participated, and the original trial design had called for sixty. But an ethical problem prevented the hospital from implementing its original plan. The sticking point was not that the experimental ECCO$_2$R therapy was working so much better than the "control." Rather, it was the opposite. The older, less expensive, less painful, easier to implement ventilator treatment turned out to be saving many more lives than anyone had expected.

Historically, 9 percent of severely ill ARDS patients on ventilator therapy survived. In the LDS trial nearly 44 percent lived, or four times the historical experience. Just as surprising, about the same percentage of ECC0$_2$R patients survived, or half the survival rate reported in Milan. The trial result was highly significant from a statistical viewpoint; the odds that it had occurred by chance were only two in ten thousand.[32]

Not only did the ECCO$_2$R therapy fail to save any more patients' lives than the ventilator treatment, it kept patients in the hospital just as long. In fact, the average treatment cost for an extracorporeal therapy patient came to $97,000 (excluding the basic room charge), or $19,000 more than for a patient receiving mechanical ventilation. Given the 10,000 to 15,000 patients who contract ARDS annually, adopting the new therapy would add more than $200 million to the nation's medical bill without in any way improving the quality of patient care, LDS researchers calculated.[33]

Why, despite LDS's best efforts, had the hospital failed to duplicate the Italian results? One possibility was differences in the type of patients treated. More of the Italian patients contracted ARDS after suffering some traumatic injury, and those ARDS patients tended to have a higher survival rate than patients whose condition traced back to another cause. Aside from that theory, researchers could only speculate about unspecified "differences in our two clinical environments."[34]

The more compelling question was why the survival rate with mechanical ventilation had apparently quadrupled. Walking the floor of the shock-trauma unit, pulmonologist Pearl was inclined to credit the standardized protocol. Clinicians, he acknowledged, still have a tendency to work by gut feeling. They reason that " 'the last time I did this it worked, so I'll do it again.' But in fact that may not be the best thing for this patient." The protocol, representing a consensus of experts, persuaded Pearl and his colleagues to make fewer changes in the parameters of patient therapy.

"The protocol removes a lot of the subjectivity that can sort of interfere [with treatment]," agreed nursing supervisor Polly Spuhler. "You get emotionally involved with these folks . . . you immediately feel compelled to [change the therapy]. The computer has taught us to wait it out a little bit."

Marin Kollef, a nationally recognized ARDS expert at the Washington University School of Medicine, was more cautious. The ARDS mortality rate has been falling nationally, Kollef noted. And though studies with other diseases have shown that protocols can improve care, LDS could not demonstrate that its protocol was responsible for these ARDS results.[35]

LDS's Morris agreed. "There are no data yet describing the effect of computerized protocol control on patient outcomes," he said. Then why had the LDS staff continued to use the computerized protocols? "Because they make care easier, they coordinate care, and they set up a set of standard orders that operate twenty-four hours a day." And the effect on the lives of ARDS patients? "There's a good probability this approach will effect favorable changes in patient care," Morris grudgingly conceded. "What that probability is . . . we'll have to see."

As of early 1997, more than four years after the $ECCO_2R$ trial ended, the computerized ventilator protocols developed at LDS Hospital were undergoing a randomized clinical trial at ten hospitals around the country. Though the trial was not complete, LDS researchers said there was "virtually identical performance" in consistently implementing the protocols at places where the doctors had no input in designing them.[36]

The $ECCO_2R$ therapy is still used in Italy. Every so often, LDS gets calls from American hospitals eager to try it out in this country. Meanwhile, a breakthrough ARDS treatment remains elusive, although the mortality rate for ARDS patients who contract the disease in the aftermath of an infection has been gradually declining as present treatments are refined.[37]

Gypsy Heuston and Tami Robbins fought their way back from the brink of death with the help of skilled and caring nurses and doctors as well as high-tech equipment. But the battle took a toll. Tami, once active and athletic, developed asthma and heart problems. Her lungs retained only 40 percent of their former capacity, and her voice became hoarse and raspy. "She'll never be really healthy again," her mother, Patty, said sadly.

Gypsy, meanwhile, "was a totally different girl after all this happened," said her father, Dennis. "She had to learn to read and write and learn to walk again." She also seemed more uncertain intellectually. One thing that remained unchanged, though, was Gypsy's strong-willed temperament. Before her catastrophic encounter with ARDS, she had accumulated enough credits to graduate from high school. Although she left the hospital just a few weeks before her scheduled graduation ceremony, Gypsy was determined not to pick up her diploma in a wheelchair. Driving a hard pace in rehabilitation therapy, she was able to walk across the stage without even the help of crutches.

Shortly after graduation, Gypsy met a "cute guy" and got married that fall. A few years later they had a baby girl. In the hospital, doctors told Gypsy that her breathing was just fine.

A couple of years later, Gypsy was working as an assistant manager at a local gas station and convenience store, and she was taking a bookkeeping course by mail. She was grateful for the care she received at LDS and for her husband and her child, but she also knew that other doors that had once seemed open to her were now closed. "I probably would have gone to college, yeah," Gypsy said. "I wanted to go to medical school really bad." If ARDS hadn't intervened, "I probably would have."

CHAPTER SIX

State of the Science

> If the study of the history of medicine teaches us anything, it is that clinical judgment without the check of scientific controls is a highly fallible compass.
> —Arthur Shafer, M.D., about 1982

The high-rise towers of west Los Angeles' Cedars-Sinai Medical Center loom over a visitor, their soaring bulk a symbol of the prestige and prosperity of modern medicine. Cedars's origins were humble enough—a couple of modest buildings for influenza and tuberculosis patients in the early part of the century—but the hospital's founders had an eye for opportunity. As hospitals evolved into places where patients were healed as well as housed, Cedars grew into one of the largest medical centers in the western United States. The main hospital building and its adjoining twin towers contain more than twice the interior space of the United States Capitol.

Cedars is nationally recognized for its academic affiliation with the UCLA School of Medicine and for leading-edge biomedical research. Locally, the hospital is equally renowned for its attention to the lifestyles of the sick and famous. Buildings such as the Steven Spielberg Pediatric Research Center testify to close ties to the entertainment industry, many of whose most prominent members live just a short drive away in posh Beverly Hills. More broadly, the medical center prides itself on offering thoughtful amenities for a discriminating clientele. Every patient enjoys a private room, while mealtime brings "a wide selection of fine food," says a hospital brochure. More than eight thousand paintings, sculptures, and other art objects are distributed throughout the hospital, for "therapeutic purposes," under the watchful eye of a full-time art curator. And for those who demand extra special attention, luxury suites are available for $1,600 per day, a trifling $600 more than the average room price.

The gloss doesn't faze Scott Weingarten, director of the hospital's Center for Applied Health Services Research. Outgoing, with an easy and breezy manner, the thirty-something internist has put down small-town roots in this archetypal region of rootlessness. Weingarten was born at UCLA Medical Center, grew up in nearby west Los Angeles, and then attended the University of Southern California. He chose UCLA for medical school and stayed at Cedars for his internship, medical residency, and a fellowship. If karma counts, the tanned and energetic Weingarten is at one with his environment.

Weingarten's job, though, is no day at the beach. As head of "applied" research, he shoulders responsibility for a daunting task. He must regularly inform fellow physicians that the way they practice medicine seems to deviate from the scientific literature. Even in laid-back Los Angeles, that sort of implicit rebuke raises hackles—or worse. "Colleagues are not always glad to see me," Weingarten admits.[1]

Yet Weingarten has managed to thrive in this highly charged environment. Aware that high-powered specialists "do not want to hear from an internist telling them a better way to do neurosurgery," he checks his ego at the door. In appearances before colleagues, he purposefully plays the self-deprecating primary-care "doc." He is not the one asking them to change; the medical literature is making the demand. He is only an intermediary, gently prodding colleagues to follow a "clinical pathway"—essentially a series of guidelines for care—that takes their practice where the evidence ineluctably leads. "The advice needs to be good, [because] docs will challenge it," Weingarten says. "It all depends on the science."

In four and a half years, Cedars has produced thirty-five of these clinical pathways. More impressively, Weingarten and his coworkers have persuaded hundreds of notoriously independent physicians to meld their medical practices into at least a loose clinical harmony. As the pathways have slowly taken hold, care has become more consistent and more predictable; every patient covered by a clinical pathway is likely to receive a well thought out treatment plan. The cost of treating many conditions has dropped, sometimes significantly, but the quality of patient care has been maintained or even improved. Weingarten can make that assertion because he carefully measures his results. "My job is to improve the quality of care and the cost effectiveness of care in a demonstrable manner," Weingarten says, and he reels off a partial list of areas where the medical center has done precisely that: asthma, hip fractures, pneumonia, kidney transplants, pediatric heart defects.

A bare-bones summary of what Weingarten does sounds unexceptional: examine the medical literature; help doctors practice according to the best scientific evidence; and then analyze the effect of the changes on patients. Yet Weingarten and his colleagues have become minor celebrities within a segment of the medical community. Phone calls, letters, and speaking invitations flood in from around the country. A drug company distributed a videotaped interview with Weingarten to customers nationwide, and community hospitals in several states are testing whether a software version of the Cedars guidelines, marketed by a for-profit Cedars subsidiary, can work for them.

The accolades are well-deserved. It's one thing to rhetorically urge physicians to practice medicine according to the best scientific evidence or even to develop a guideline tied to a single randomized trial, as LDS Hospital did with ARDS. But to integrate evidence-based medicine into everyday practice, as Weingarten has done at Cedars, is an unusual accomplishment that serves as a model for the practice of medicine in the Information Age.

PUTTING SCIENCE INTO PRACTICE

Knowledge is not the same as action. No one can predict how, or even whether, medical evidence will change a particular doctor's decisions about patient treatment.

"The publication of discovered truths in medical journals, as well as their presentation in teaching and continuing-education programs, should educate physicians, change their beliefs and influence their behavior," concluded a commentator in the *New England Journal of Medicine*. "Unfortunately, competing forces—society's interests, patients' real or perceived demands, financial incentives, and fears of embarrassment or accusation of malpractice, to name just a few—also have a powerful influence on behavior. When these forces push in a consistent direction . . . new information may lead to rapid changes in behavior. When the forces are in conflict, however, new information is less likely to change behavior."[2]

This gap between the scientific evidence about what works best and the care patients receive calls into question the fundamental basis of the modern physician's authority. Your doctor may follow the results of one study, disregard the findings of a second, and be unaware of a third. The doctor in the office next door may have a totally different reaction. While the public worries that doctors' decisions may be influenced by financial incentives, ignorance and inertia are actually much more serious threats to patient health. Recent clinical advances in treating diabetes, asthma, congestive heart failure, and three other common conditions were not used by one-fifth to one-half of the physicians polled in one random survey. The doctors, whose ranks included primary care physicians and physician "opinion leaders," either did not know about the newer treatments or had not begun using them.[3]

The relationship between science and medical practice is complex. Science informs practice, but is just one influence on it. Many, perhaps most, patients believe otherwise, however. They think that "medical science, medical research and medical practice are identical, or worse, hierarchically arranged," writes medical sociologist Ann Lennarson Greer. In reality, "medical practice does operate under the umbrella of medical science, but medical practitioners do not take practice directives from medical researchers."[4]

Limited knowledge need not stand in the way of decisive action.[5] "Physicians flip-flop dramatically, and with unabashed confidence," observed Sherwin Nuland, a Yale School of Medicine professor and respected medical author, in the *New York Times*.[6]

Some caution is understandable. Scholarly articles are often written in arcane language that provides few clues about how to apply the results.[7] Important caveats may be discreetly omitted to spruce up an article for publication, or the results can be analyzed in a way that tilts them toward favorable findings.[8] There are also large "gray areas" of medical practice where studies provide little guidance. Meanwhile, the methodologically fastidious can even fret about the studies that were conducted but never written up because the results were negative. This is known as the "file drawer problem."[9] Finally, there is the ever-present worry that a treatment trumpeted in this month's issue of a journal will, like some once-fashionable diet craze, be discredited as a fraud a few issues later.

With all these worries, it's small wonder that the community physician busy with the pressing problems of patient care adopts a variety of coping mechanisms. When he feels insecure, he typically chooses among several options:

> One, he muddles through; two, he seeks a "sidewalk consultation" from a colleague; three, he seeks a formal consultation (frequently to document the fact that a consultation was secured for regulatory medical-legal reasons); or four, he consults the medical literature, mostly in the form of medical texts [textbooks] and ready references [i.e., reference books] . . . . Rarely, he goes to the current medical literature.[10]

Even when the evidence in the scientific literature is clearly written, unambiguous, well-publicized, and important, large numbers of doctors still do not respond. One of the clearest examples involves the treatment of heart attacks.

Few medical problems have as high a public profile as heart attacks. They strike the working class and executives, women as well as men. They are both deadly and common. During an eight-month period in 1988, reports of three important clinical trials on heart attack treatment appeared in prominent medical journals. The findings had life and death implications, and the intense media attention they received reflected this.

Two of the studies announced dramatic good news. According to one, the simple and inexpensive act of taking a small dose of aspirin every day could prevent an initial heart attack in many patients at high risk from this deadly disease. A second study, looking at the role of aspirin in treatment, concluded that regularly taking aspirin after a heart attack significantly increased the chances of survival. The third study sounded a warning. It cautioned heart attack victims taking a widely used class of drugs called calcium antagonists that this type of medication actually diminished their chances of survival.

Three years after these studies appeared, a separate group of researchers examined the medical records of some 2,200 patients to see how their physicians had responded. The long time span gave the cautious practitioner an opportunity to conclude that the heart attack trials represented a genuine clinical advance that applied to the kinds of patients community physicians treat. Sure enough, the professional and public attention made a measurable difference. More patients at high risk of a heart attack started taking aspirin. More patients who did suffer an attack got aspirin afterward. The use of calcium antagonists slid.[11]

Nonetheless, there remained a substantial number of physicians who either didn't hear the news, didn't believe it, or never got around to acting on it. More than a quarter of heart attack victims (28 percent) still were not being given easy to administer aspirin therapy. A third continued to receive calcium antagonists.[12] The researchers had no explanation for this lag.

In early 1997, years after these studies on aspirin's benefits first appeared, two advisory committees of the Food and Drug Administration recommended that aspirin makers be allowed to label their bottles with the information that aspirin could prevent a heart attack in some people. The agency was expected to consider granting similar permission for an advisory label that aspirin could also prevent a major stroke.[13]

Other medical breakthroughs have seeped even more slowly into everyday patient care. Take ulcer treatment. In the early 1980s, Australian gastroenterologist Barry Marshall began publishing a series of papers proffering a startling thesis. At a time when the medical community overwhelmingly believed that painful stomach ulcers were caused by stress, cigarette smoking, and similar environmental factors, Marshall attributed ulcers to an infection, a bacterium called *Helicobacter pylori*.

The prevailing medical wisdom held that no bacterium could survive for long in the acidic environment of the stomach, and at first Marshall's research group could not prove otherwise. It failed in repeated attempts to infect the stomachs of rats, mice, and pigs. Marshall, though, refused to give up. Joining the long tradition of physician self-experimentation, he drank down a pure culture containing one billion *H. pylori* organisms. Sure enough, he got sick. He then wrote an article reporting on his illness.[14]

A subsequent randomized trial demonstrated that a combination of antibiotics and bismuth (the active ingredient in Pepto-Bismol) could eradicate *H. pylori*. Since other drugs treated only ulcer symptoms, Marshall's ulcer clinic in Australia was mobbed by patients after news of the trial results appeared in 1988 in the widely read British journal the *Lancet*.[15] Yet in the United States, home of the "best medical care in the world," Marshall's research created barely a stir.[16]

Of course, Marshall's proposed cure for a chronic disease did not pass completely unnoticed. In 1991 American researchers reported similar results in the *Annals of Internal Medicine*.[17] Three years later experts convened by the National Institutes of Health endorsed antibacterial ulcer therapy as a standard treatment.[18] Marshall eventually moved to the United States, and in October 1995 he received the prestigious Albert Lasker Clinical Medical Research Award. It cited his "revolutionary research [that] dispelled the darkness surrounding a painful chronic disease."[19]

Seven years after Marshall's work first appeared, most United States gastroenterologists were finally testing ulcer patients for *H. pylori* before therapy. (What seem to be ulcer symptoms can be caused by other diseases, including stomach cancer.) There's a catch, though. Most ulcer patients are treated by their primary care physicians, not by specialists. Diagnosis of the *H. pylori* bacterium requires extra, often invasive, testing, and there is no consensus on the drug therapy that follows. Without a clear and easy therapy choice, many nonspecialists have simply avoided the problem. By one estimate, in early 1996 fewer than one in ten internists and family physicians in the United States treated ulcers with antibacterial therapy.[20] This despite the fact that the *Annals of Internal Medicine,* the publication of general internists, concluded back in 1991: "A strategy that includes eradication of *H. pylori* should be the first choice for the initial treatment of duodenal ulcer disease," since it is cost effective and also produces a lower recurrence rate.[21] The FDA's approval in 1996 of several simple drug treatments for ulcers may finally change common therapy.

Evidence about other treatments has also evaporated before it can reach patients. If a pregnant woman goes into labor prematurely, giving steroids increases the chances that the newborn's lungs will function properly. The evidence is clear; yet large numbers of obstetricians still do not do it.[22] Sometimes the evidence is there only if someone looks for it. As early as 1973, a series of clinical trials could have pointed the way to saving thousands of heart attack victims. If researchers had used a mathematical technique called meta-analysis—essentially a way of combining the results of different investigations to discover what they have in common—they would have realized the effectiveness of thrombolytic therapy (the use of anticoagulants). No one looked, and medical textbooks waited until 1988 to recommend this treatment.[23]

Physician inertia can lead to continued reliance on treatments that are inappropriate or worse. Tonsillectomies and tympanostomies (ear tubes) are two examples where that can occur. Routine chest X rays before hospital admission, begun when tuberculosis was rampant, have persisted as an ostensible screening tool for lung cancer years after that use was discredited.[24]

The reason for all these seeming aberrations from the best standard of practice has little to do with the findings of science, but a great deal to do with the culture of medicine.

THE NATURE OF CLINICAL WISDOM

A 1922 book of advice for physicians advised them to portray their office as "the sanctuary of an earnest, working scientific medical man."[25] But medical sociologist Eliot Freidson, in a landmark examination of the culture of the practicing physician published about a half-century later, observed very different behavior. Doctors acted as a consulting profession, not a scholarly one. Rather than being the "science-based . . . practicing biologist,"[26] as some put it, physicians retained a "moral commitment to intervention" on behalf of each patient, even in the absence of reliable knowledge. Their training emphasized personal intuition rather than the careful testing of assumptions and biases that characterized a scholarly profession. Modern physicians seemed at times not to have advanced very far from their eighteenth- or nineteenth-century predecessors' reliance on "empiricism," the evidence one observes firsthand. Wrote Freidson:

> The model of the clinician . . . encourage[s] individual deviation from codified knowledge on the basis of personal, first-hand observation of concrete cases. This deviation is called "judgment" or even "wisdom." . . . Since it is intimately bound up with the personal life of the knower . . . it is no wonder it has a dogmatic edge to it, resisting contradiction by embarrassing facts and contorting itself to reconcile contradictions.[27]

Freidson's characterization remains critical to understanding the gap between science and practice. Consider the fate of two initiatives sponsored by the National Institutes of Health. The first involved an attempt by the National Cancer Institute (NCI) to speed a wider community acceptance of innovative therapies. To do so, the NCI set up a Community Clinical Oncology Program featuring collaboration among academic medicine, community hospitals, and the NIH. The condition it chose to test the concept was breast cancer, a disease of terrifying importance to many women.[28]

If a woman lives to age eighty-five, there is one chance in nine that she will develop breast cancer.[29] According to the National Cancer Institute, in 1993 alone some 182,000 women struggled to cope with this disease. The treatment with the longest history of effectiveness is mastectomy, but over the past fifteen years an alternative has grown in popularity. Instead of removing a woman's entire breast (mastectomy), the surgeon excises the cancerous lump (lumpectomy), and the woman receives anticancer drugs (adjuvant chemotherapy) to kill any cancerous cells that might remain.

The NCI's cooperative program on breast cancer began in 1983, and researchers periodically returned to the communities involved to examine its impact. The results were mixed. Oncologists who participated in ongoing clinical trials "were more likely to adopt the new treatment, adopted it at a much faster rate, and were less likely to abandon the state-of-the-art treatment after initial use." Their participation also brought them referrals from other physicians. On the other hand, patients whose oncologists did not directly take part in the trial "tended to be less likely . . . to receive the consensus state-of-the-art treatment."

"Change in practice is difficult to achieve unless the physician is actively engaged in the process by which new treatments are developed and evaluated," the researchers concluded. In other words, "I don't believe it unless I personally see it"—the same retort a nineteenth-century doctor might have made.

The second NIH effort to influence everyday care was more comprehensive, spearheaded by a group with the vaguely exotic acronym OMAR. Alas, OMAR's activities do not involve spies, beautiful women, or clandestine missions to the Middle East. The more prosaic purpose of the Office of Medical Applications of Research is to bridge the gap between the nation's premier biomedical organization and community physicians.

To do that, OMAR periodically gathers top scientists, practicing doctors, and knowledgeable members of the public for a consensus development conference. For two and a half days, the group pores over the literature dealing with an important medical problem. When the conference concludes and the experts have finally agreed on the best medical practice, OMAR turns on the NIH publicity machine. An NIH press conference generates stories on television and radio and in newspapers around the country. The agency mails 20,000 to 100,000 copies of a consensus statement directly to medical professionals and others. It distributes the statements at medical meetings, arranges for publication in key journals, posts them on an electronic bulletin board, and places them in the heavily used National Library of Medicine database. Thanks to this multimedia blitz, demand for the statements more than doubled in five years.[30] Sadly, one glaring failure sours this sweet tale of success: the consensus conferences have had no measurable effect on how doctors treat patients.

RAND Corporation researchers examined the aftermath of NIH conferences dedicated to four important topics: the surgical management of breast cancer; the use of steroid receptors in breast cancer treatment; cesarean section births; and coronary artery bypass graft surgery (commonly known as "bypass" or "open-heart" surgery).

To the researchers' chagrin, the influence of these august NIH pronouncements on patient care was negligible.

"The dedicated efforts of a national agency to affect clinical practice through a consensus conference approach mostly failed to produce change at the bottom line—in the care provided by practitioners to their patients," concluded the RAND group. "Practice failed to change *even though the recommendations appeared to reflect the state of science and sound practice at the time and even though efforts to disseminate the recommendations were at least moderately successful* at reaching . . . physicians" (emphasis added).[31]

That OMAR today continues to conduct and publicize its consensus conferences in much the same way as in 1987 provides an appropriately ironic twist: just as physicians have not altered their behavior despite being shown evidence by OMAR, so too has OMAR ignored the evidence and continued in its old and comfortable ways.

Unfortunately, OMAR's persistent reliance on ineffectual methods of influencing physicians' behavior is not particularly unusual. Take the topic of continuing medical education, which is designed to keep doctors' medical knowledge current. Study after study has concluded that holding a conference is not a very good way to bring about change.[32] The scientific literature, though, is no match for the opportunity to combine business and pleasure in Vail or at Disney World or on a cruise ship. A physician with a real thirst for tax-deductible learning opportunities can subscribe to an entire magazine devoted to matching exciting travel destinations with continuing medical education courses. The authors of a 1995 article on physician education in the *Journal of the American Medical Association* lamented: "A vanishingly small [number of] . . . more effective methods [than conferences] are ever used."[33]

So how do you change physicians' behavior? It takes focused hard work, and it takes a strategy that links medical evidence directly to clinical practice. Los Angeles' Cedars-Sinai Medical Center learned that the hard way.

HERDING CATS

Cedars-Sinai knew how *not* to get doctors to change. In the late 1980s the hospital dabbled in putting out guidelines based on physician consensus. The predictable result was the kind of vague exhortations common to political party platforms and corporate mission statements. In mid-1991, the hospital's medical vice president personally recruited Scott Weingarten to try a fresh approach.

Despite his youth, Weingarten arrived with impressive credentials. For the previous two years he had worked as a primary care physician for a local health maintenance organization; therefore he had credibility as a "practicing doc." In addition to seeing patients, Weingarten also designed guidelines to help the physicians at the health plan improve their preventive care. Finally, Weingarten had academic credentials. He had earned a master's degree in public health at UCLA while simultaneously doing postgraduate clinical work. It was at UCLA that he began to learn the theoretical basis for getting physicians to change their behavior. The lessons came from a physician-researcher named John Eisenberg, a nationally respected authority on how doctors' decision making could be influenced. By the mid-1980s, doctors' decisions had become a matter of keen interest. It was not because of their effect on the quality of care; American medicine was then, as ever, self-evidently the "best." The problem was money.

Direct payments to doctors make up a small part of total health care costs. Where doctors make a difference is with their pens; of each dollar spent on health care, eighty cents begins with a physician's order. It was all well and good to talk about unneeded tests, overprescribed drugs, and hospital stays of a length more suited to vacation than recuperation. The question remained: How do you persuade doctors to do less while ensuring that the quality of care does not become worse?

In articles and a book, *Doctors' Decisions and the Costs of Medical Care,* Eisenberg argued that attempts to influence physicians would benefit from the research done by behavioral scientists. Combining that work with studies in the medical literature, Eisenberg concluded that doctors were most likely to react to new information when it was delivered by another physician in a position of clinical leadership; when it concerned quality of care as well as cost; and when there was frequent feedback. Like other adult learners, physicians quickly slipped back into old habits when reinforcement stopped.[34] (That tendency could explain the futility of most educational conferences.)

The secret to success in changing physician behavior was maintaining a clear focus. "Feedback is most likely to be successful when it addresses a single clinical problem about which physicians have reached consensus regarding standards of practice," Eisenberg wrote.

He also recommended the use of computerized databases to reduce the labor costs of reminders and feedback.[35]

Reasonable as that sounded, achieving consensus in a profession that trains practitioners to trust their own intuition was, as an often-quoted expression put it, "like herding cats." At Cedars, Weingarten confronted a very large collection of felines. The medical center employed 250 staff physicians, while another 2,000 independent community physicians held practice privileges. Weingarten seized on a clever strategy that would appeal to something all the doctors had in common. However much they varied in their treatment of patients, they all thought of themselves as logical, rational decision makers, trained in the Flexnerian ethos of respect for clinical findings. So Weingarten made a rule for himself. "It all depends on the science." If you can't back up a recommendation with scientific evidence, you don't do it.

The next problem was digging out the evidence. One reason physicians don't regularly consult the medical literature is that the task is so time consuming and confusing. Information overload is hardly a new problem. "No physician can read all of the current literature in his specialty and retain his reason," opined Duke University's Wilburt Davison in 1942.[36] "Medical Science Is Accelerating; Can Doctors Keep Up? Many Admit They Don't Learn of All New Drugs, Skills; Some Say Patients Suffer." That was the headline on a page 1 article in the *Wall Street Journal* on 30 June 1958. Still, the situation has worsened. The National Library of Medicine receives an estimated 2,500 journals.[37] The total number of randomized trials, meanwhile, is estimated at between 250,000 and one million![38] "Our textbooks are out of date, our journals are disorganized and the disparity between our reading time and our reading load is discouraging," concluded an editorial in the premier issue of *Evidence-Based Medicine,* a medical journal that appeared for the first time at the end of 1995.[39]

A modern-day Diogenes, searching for truth via modem instead of lantern, risked sinking in a swamp of citations. Contrarily, a too narrowly focused search risked missing vital studies. Searching wasn't easy even for an information age sophisticate. Weingarten had put himself through medical school by writing computer programming codes for a defense contractor. After comparing his search results with those of a medical librarian, however, he gave up and turned the responsibility over to a professional.

As articles piled up on his desk, Weingarten sorted them by means of a method adapted from the Evidence-Based Medicine Working Group at Canada's McMaster University. First, he assigned each article a letter grade based on the quality of the scientific evidence it presented in support of its conclusions. The Canadians had graded studies from A to C. Weingarten, realizing his marks would directly affect his hospital's treatment decisions, was a tougher taskmaster. he included D and E in his grading scheme. An A was for a randomized clinical trial with statistically significant results, while an E designated indirect evidence or "expert opinion." A low grade did not imply that a study was useless, but it did force doctors to confront the flimsy scientific foundation of many clinical practices they unthinkingly took for granted. "We found a lot of the information used to guide clinical decision making did not warrant a C," Weingarten said. "We wanted to make people aware that evidence existed, but also warn them [of its quality], so you could let the user beware."

The grading produced some surprises. The American Thoracic Society's guideline on when to admit a pneumonia patient to the hospital earned an E; the society's opinion was based on an opinion. A study on the same subject by the less well known University of Rochester produced a passing mark of C. Nuggets of valuable information were also mined from unlikely sources. Taking a global view of good medicine, Cedars explicitly included foreign journals. One pathway team retrieved a useful C grade study on speeding up the recovery of pneumonia patients from the *Scandinavian Journal of Infectious Disease.*

As Weingarten searched the medical literature, studies inevitably conflicted or the evidence was insufficient to answer important clinical questions. That was to be expected. The practice of medicine did not begin from scratch with the advent of clinical trials, nor should it have. Nonetheless, the sheer mass of untested practice—as much as 85 percent of what doctors did—was disconcerting. Utah researcher John Williamson, one of the first to examine the research base of medical practice, put it: "Everyone's been concerned with the cost of care, and no one's been seriously concerned about what we're buying with the money.[40] Indeed, when the American College of Physicians sought to update its guidelines on the use of magnetic resonance imaging (MRI) for brain scans, the organization found just one paper out of 285 whose evidence deserved an A grade: 15 articles got a B, 16 a C, 118 a D, and everything else an E.[41]

"This is an extraordinary finding," acknowledged the College's journal, the *Annals of Internal Medicine.* "Here we have an expensive [upward of $800 per scan], very widely-used procedure, and only 5 percent of recent reports are judged sufficient to determine its diagnostic and therapeutic efficacy. [A]nd many of those are hardly adequate."[42]

In seeking to bring scientific evidence into everyday care, the Cedars pathway teams took an approach toward physician autonomy that was similar to what LDS Hospital did with ARDS. The guidelines were based on evidence, but the individual physician could always overrule them. Still, one early pathway dramatically illustrated the pitfalls of physicians' relying on old habits. It involved the treatment of a heart defect in children known as tetralogy of Fallot.

Tetralogy of Fallot is named after E. L. A. Fallot, the French physician who first described it; it is more commonly called "blue baby" syndrome. It comprises four defects (hence *tetra,* four) in the heart and lungs. These defects rob the newborn of oxygen and hemoglobin, giving its skin a bluish tint. Surgery can eventually correct the impairments, but the complicated series of operations may not be completed until the child is four or five years old. Moreover, the surgery carries risks. Secretions and mucus can build up afterward in the lungs, leading to respiratory complications. To prevent that, a respiratory therapist at Cedars would place a vibrating apparatus on the child's back for a fifteen- to twenty-minute "chest physiotherapy" session. The procedure was repeated several times a day with the purpose of loosening secretions and stimulating coughing up. There was just one problem: the pathway team discovered that in most children physiotherapy increased the risk that the lung tissue would collapse. The evidence came directly from a randomized trial in the respected *Annals of Surgery.*[43] Even more distressing, this bad news wasn't even new. The *Annals* study had appeared in early 1982, but either no one had seen it or no one had comprehended its importance.

"It was 180 degrees different from what everyone in the room believed you should do," remembered pediatric cardiologist Burton Fink, a former chief of the Cedars medical staff who participated in the pathway team. "We found that when you challenge [practices] against data . . . maybe a bunch of stuff you thought was essential really wasn't at all."

As if the *Annals* study weren't enough, a nurse added another piece of upsetting information. Because the treatment involves vibrating the skin near a fresh surgical wound, the children getting the therapy would frequently cry out in pain. "I'm with the children," she said. "It hurts."

The tetralogy of Fallot team spent four months collecting data and translating it into a series of clear-cut recommendations Cedars doctors could follow. To make the pathway easier to access and update, the information was stored on computer. Routine physiotherapy was dropped, the number of lab tests was cut, and patients were weaned from a ventilator more quickly, reducing the chances of a hospital-caused complication such as pneumonia. Patients also were able to go home sooner.

One year after the pathway was implemented, the cost of treating a Fallot's syndrome child had plummeted by 20 to 30 percent (chest physiotherapy alone cost upward of $100 per day), but the quality of care was the same or better. Fink, a thirty-five-year veteran of the hospital, savored the victory for the new way of practice. "Sure there was skepticism, and there remains skepticism," he said. "But we've changed the mind-set. Now, we have data . . . with everybody buying into it. That will continue to change what we're doing."

Because of the fiercely competitive California marketplace, Cedars had little choice. The medical center had to reduce its costs or it risked losing the insurance contracts that bring in thousands of patients. Safely reducing costs, however, meant paying attention to every small detail of care.

The treatment of pneumonia presented a particularly inviting target.[44] Pneumonia patients typically spend seven days in the hospital receiving intravenous drugs before being switched to oral medication and then discharged. Weingarten, though, could find few clinical studies either supporting or refuting this common practice. However, some trials did suggest that low-risk pneumonia patients could be treated with oral drugs as early as the third day and then discharged one day later.

Rather than letting individual Cedars physicians pick the patients they thought would benefit, Weingarten laid out a more systematic approach. First, he would design a clinical pathway. Then, before making it official hospital policy, he would test its effect on patients. "As is the case with introducing a new drug into clinical practice," he asserted, "practice guidelines should only be introduced into patient care after evidence is available to support both the safety and efficacy of the guideline."[45]

In designing any experiment, an essential first step is defining basic terms. "Low-risk" pneumonia could be in the eye of the beholder.

To reliably measure the effect of changing pneumonia treatment, there had to be a clear and consistent understanding of which patients were safe candidates for the new therapy.

A panel of Cedars physicians first examined medical records. They found that a third of the pneumonia patients had symptoms that qualified. Just to be sure, the doctors looked at the outcome of care for these patients to see whether the "low-risk" guideline excluded people who subsequently suffered a life-threatening complication or died. The guideline passed the test. In fact, had the guideline been in place in the past, the quality of care would have stayed the same for 98 percent of the low-risk pneumonia patients.

For more than a decade, researchers had been calling fruitlessly for practice guidelines to be used in treating pneumonia. Weingarten, determined to get his guideline adopted for everyday treatment, decided to rigorously monitor its results. If a quicker discharge caused patients to be readmitted to the hospital or to need sharply more medical care outside the hospital, the guideline would be justified neither medically nor economically. Just to be cautious, Weingarten used medical records and a patient survey to examine what happened to patients up to thirty days after they left the hospital. Because the average discharged patient was nearly seventy years old, he even checked death records against patients' Social Security numbers.

Weingarten dubbed this the "Ann Landers method." In one column Ann asked readers to write and tell her what happened after they took her suggestions. Did the upscale businesswoman marry her auto mechanic lover? Were they still happily together? "Ann Landers is looking for outcomes validation," Weingarten explained. "With a guideline, you should have that same degree of inquisitiveness. Did it improve patient care or did it worsen patient care? You want to know."

Of course, first someone had to take the advice. Cedars set up a computerized system to alert nurse case managers when a pneumonia patient was admitted who fit the pathway criteria. The case manager, in turn, reminded the treating doctor. Physicians overrode the guideline for low-risk pneumonia about a quarter of the time (a rate typical for other Cedars guidelines as well). Some simply disliked outside advice, but most had a good reason.[46]

"You want physicians to be thinking about their individual patients," stressed Weingarten, who still sees patients one day a week at the hospital's urgent care center. "Often, [doctors] recognized a clinical nuance or a social circumstance that the guideline couldn't possibly address."

After nearly two years of testing, pneumonia patients were going home sooner but remained satisfied with their care and ready to recommend the hospital to their friends. Clinically, meanwhile, "the overall outcome of care was favorable compared to previously published values." (A survey of a comparable group of patients was used as a comparison.)

"Very few of these patients would have benefited from a longer duration of hospital stay," wrote Weingarten. "Use of our guideline could significantly reduce health care costs."[47]

Other Cedars improvement projects touched more sensitive nerves. As at virtually every hospital, the process of systematically examining treatment uncovered some care that did not live up to what the scientific evidence demanded. Cedars, which saw itself as "one of the finest teaching hospitals in the country" was forced to deal with the inexplicably low rate of DVT prophylaxis.

DVT stands for deep-vein thrombosis, or clotting of the blood within the deep-lying veins; "prophylaxis" means prevention. Patients who undergo knee surgery or a hip replacement, common procedures in the elderly, are at particularly high risk for this painful and sometimes dangerous complication. If clots become extensive, they can break loose and travel to the heart or lungs, a rare development but possibly fatal. Surgeons can prevent DVT with a timely dose of the blood thinner Coumadin or use of a special compression device. Unfortunately, one in five knee and hip surgery patients at Cedars was receiving a type of preventive therapy that a 1991 study had specifically identified as ineffective. One in four got no DVT prophylaxis at all—which may still have been better than the national rate.[48] The chairman of a hospital committee that monitored medical privileges quickly responded with an ultimatum. Orthopedic surgeons were told to either improve DVT prophylaxis or face disciplinary action. Within a year, the DVT prophylaxis rate shot up to 91 percent, on its way to 95 percent. The change may have saved one or two lives a year, Weingarten estimates.

An even more delicate problem involved the hospital's kidney transplant program. A successful transplant capability brings prestige and money. Cedars boasted of its "reputation for excellence and leadership in transplantation surgery." A quiet investigation by the hospital's board of directors, however, found that the kidney program's costs were high, but its outcomes were no better than average. What was needed was not a clinical pathway but a complete redesign of the process of care. Marianne Deignan, director of Cedars's resource management department, was tapped to help oversee the effort.

When Deignan began to analyze data the hospital collected on its kidney transplant patients, she saw large variations in care. Although each transplant patient was operated on by a full-time staff surgeon, a private nephrologist from the community took over once the patient left the operating room. Each nephrologist liked to do things a little differently, and the numbers reflected it.

The hospital faced a dilemma. The wide variation in care had to be reduced, but the community nephrologists needed to be appeased. After all, staff surgeons weren't the ones who admitted paying patients. After lengthy discussions, an inspired compromise was reached. To make care more consistent, a special renal transplant team composed of full-time staff physicians took charge of treatment. However, the community nephrologists would accompany the staff doctors as they made their rounds and would be invited to make "suggestions" about the care of their patients. This solution preserved the sacred physician-patient relationship, was respectful to the community nephrologists, and not incidentally, allowed the specialist to continue to bill for services provided in the hospital.

One year later, quality of care had improved: the number of transplanted kidneys that were rejected by patients fell to zero. The cost of care plunged as the average time each patient stayed in the hospital dropped from thirteen days to five. And the variation virtually disappeared. Happy hospital marketers, meanwhile, helped increase the number of patients by a third, from thirty-five patients a year to fifty.

PUTTING EVIDENCE INTO PRACTICE

Confronted by evidence that lemon juice prevented outbreaks of scurvy among ships' crews, the eighteenth-century British Navy took fifty years to respond. In our era of genetically engineered drugs and computerized medical devices, we look backward with condescension at such inexplicable slowness to reap the benefits of scientific research. Yet how much has really changed?

"Development [in medicine] has been limited by the rate of discovery," noted one commentator in the *British Medical Journal,* "but now it's limited by the rate of implementation."[49]

Practice guidelines represent a serious attempt to take the human tendency to act on pattern recognition—the kind of "autopilot" syndrome that can lead to medical errors—and turn it into a positive force for the improvement of care.[50] A well-designed guideline provides a template that is a starting point for improvement, not a definitive formula. Certainly not all guidelines meet the test of codifying best practice. Some are designed with an eye on the bottom line and threaten the flexibility that doctors need to serve each individual patient. Some good guidelines are implemented with a rigidity that threatens innovation. But the alternative to care that is guided by the evidence is care that relies on each doctor's memory.[51] Or perhaps care that conforms to whatever the patient's insurance company believes is best. "It comes down to using the scientific method," says Scott Weingarten. "You use information to drive decision making."

In a clear signal that guidelines are gaining acceptance as a legitimate means of protecting and enhancing the professionalism of physicians, the American Medical Association is giving its stamp of approval to guidelines based on solid scientific evidence. The AMA's House of Delegates, though long suspicious of any hint of infringement of physicians' freedom, approved the initiative in December 1996. On the one hand, the AMA imprimatur is designed to encourage doctors to pay closer attention to guidelines whose recommendations come out of the scientific literature. Just as important, however, the withholding of AMA approval is meant to send a public message of disapproval to health plans and hospitals whose guidelines cannot withstand a rigorous scientific review.[52]

One fact is unassailable. Doctors and hospitals sorely need help. Knowledge is very clearly *not* the same as action. This book has given example after example of how guidelines can improve care, and the clinical literature regularly suggests new opportunities. There are even signs that the mainstream physician community is starting to open its eyes to the high cost in patient lives of relying on each doctor's instant and unaided recollection of the entire body of medical knowledge. In the 8 January 1997 *JAMA,* researchers once again reported glaring deficiencies in heart attack care. When asked whether they believe that beta-blocker drug therapy "definitely improves survival" for heart attack victims, physicians generally said it does, and they were right: it increases survival by 20 to 40 percent. Yet only about a fifth of the elderly patients with heart attacks received the therapy in one state whose data were extensively analyzed.[53] An accompanying editorial praised clinical practice guidelines, particularly when they pop up on a computer screen at the time of treatment, as one way to "alert clinicians about the existence of innovation."[54]

Separately, the federal Agency for Health Care Policy and Research is spending nearly $5 million to fund research in software for computerized decision support in medicine. The areas of study as of early 1997 ranged from the prevention of drug errors to the treatment of depression to the management of bone marrow transplant patients after their discharge from the hospital.

"If we asked the question of whether physicians have based their practice on scientific principles, it is clear that the profession has been sorely lacking," says Kenneth I. Shine, president of the Institute of Medicine, a part of the National Academy of Sciences. "When we see threefold and fourfold differences in the use of procedures and interventions in various parts of the country, and no evidence that either the population or the outcomes differ, how can we argue that the use of those technologies is based on science?"[55]

In 1994 the *British Medical Journal* phrased the challenge to physicians this way: "to promote the uptake of innovations that have been shown to be effective, to delay the spread of those that have not yet been shown to be effective and to prevent the uptake of ineffective innovations."[56] It is past time for physicians to take up that challenge.

PART 2

Changing the Paradigm of Medical Practice

CHAPTER SEVEN

Trust Me, I'm a Doctor

There is nothing more difficult to plan, more doubtful of success, nor more dangerous to manage than the creation of a new order of things. . . .Whenever his enemies have occasion to attack the innovator they do so with the passion of partisans.
—Niccoló Machiavelli, *The Prince,* about 1513

When the Crimean War broke out in 1854, Florence Nightingale quickly volunteered to lead a group of her fellow nurses to the front. There, as "the Lady of the Lamp," she became famous for her nighttime rounds to comfort the wounded soldiers lying in British military hospitals. What is much less well known about Nightingale is her role as an ardent and early advocate of information-based medicine.

Appalled by the unsanitary conditions she witnessed overseas, Nightingale carefully gathered statistics to buttress her case about the high mortality rate in military hospitals. Her appeal to Parliament relied as much on hard data as on well-orchestrated emotionalism. Educated by her father in mathematics, history, philosophy and five foreign languages, Nightingale came to regard statistics "as the source of a keen aesthetic pleasure," wrote one biographer.[1] Another quotes her as saying: "To understand God's thoughts, we must study statistics, for those are the measure of His purpose."[2]

After the war, Nightingale tried to transfer her campaign for better care to the civilian world. "There is a growing conviction that in all hospitals, even in those which are best conducted, there is a great and unnecessary waste of life," she wrote.[3] Elected to the British Statistical Society in 1858, Nightingale penned a *Proposal for Improved Statistics of Surgical Operations,* which included a plan for reporting the results of care at all British hospitals in a uniform and comparable manner. But while Nightingale the nurse was a hero, Nightingale the statistician encountered little success. She was what we today would call a "paradigm pioneer," urging her society to look at medical care in a way that it had never looked at it before.

The word paradigm comes from the Greek *paradeigma,* meaning "pattern" or "example." It refers to the unconscious framework that shapes our perception of the world—"what water is to a fish."[4] It provides both the mental framework for how we solve problems and the context for what we can see as a problem in the first place.[5] A paradigm filters our worldview under the guise of common sense, tradition, or dogma.[6] Warner Brothers chief Harry Warner, asked in 1927 about the future of motion pictures using sound, responded with the dismissive tone of the expert completely oblivious to the possibility that a paradigm can change. Said Warner: "Who the hell wants to hear actors talk?"

In medicine, the old paradigm says that physicians are craftsman-scientists whose trained judgment is what allows them to respond appropriately to each patient's needs. Scientists were once thought to be immune from the biases and blind spots that distort the perceptions of others. Then along came Thomas Kuhn, a Harvard-trained theoretical physicist turned science historian. In a landmark 1962 book, *The Structure of Scientific Revolutions,* Kuhn punctured the reassuring belief that scientific progress is an orderly affair. He showed that scientists, like ordinary mortals, tend to ignore evidence that contradicts what they already believe. Altering a scientific paradigm is traumatic and disruptive, necessitating "the community's rejection of one time-honored scientific theory in favor of another incompatible with it." It occurs only when the defenders of the old ways of thought can "no longer evade anomalies that subvert the existing tradition."[7]

Years before the present-day push for evidence-based medicine, guidelines and computerized expert systems, a handful of individuals tried mightily to subvert the old paradigm of medical practice and substitute a new way of thinking that emphasized systematic use of information. They failed, but their stories carry important lessons about today's battles to transform health care.

In this country, a puckish turn-of-the-century Boston surgeon named Ernest Amory Codman tried to shock the medical community into incorporating information on patient outcomes as a regular part of care. Like Nightingale, Codman possessed the self-confidence of a revolutionary from a comfortably affluent background.[8] Both Nightingale and Codman also displayed an early love of detail. At twenty, Nightingale's hobby was reading public health reports; the young Codman started a logbook of his hunting trips that recorded the ratio of birds shot to shells expended.[9] Both showed a flair for attracting public attention. But where Nightingale was a proper Victorian, Codman was a self-described atheist who enjoyed using exaggeration and humor to deliberately provoke his peers.

Codman joined the staff of the Massachusetts General Hospital, a Harvard teaching facility, in 1895, after schooling at Harvard College and Harvard Medical School. Despite this conventional background, he was never one to be satisfied with the status quo. While still a medical student, he wrote down on small cards the condition of each patient before and after receiving anesthesia. Being "put to sleep" was still a crude procedure. A classmate, Harvey Cushing, watched in horror as his first anesthetized patient vomited and died while Cushing was trying to learn proper techniques. The attending surgeon shrugged off the fatality as not uncommon, but Cushing became depressed. Codman and Cushing decided to have a contest to see who could obtain the better patient outcomes, with the winner getting dinner. As a result of that bet, the two men created the first formal anesthesia records, including a graph that plotted the patient's pulse and respiration every five minutes. (It's unclear who won their wager.)[10]

Codman remained obsessed with systematic improvement of patient outcomes. Most surgeons of the time claimed success if their patients left the hospital alive; Codman said they should monitor the patient's health for a year afterward, and he proposed what he called the "End Result Idea." This was "merely the common-sense notion that every hospital should follow *every* patient it treats long enough to determine whether or not the treatment has been successful, and then to inquire, 'if not, why not?' with a view to preventing similar failures in the future."[11]

Codman's timing seemed fortuitous. The famous Flexner Report had just been released. As the movement to "standardize" medical education gained momentum, Codman's system of what we would call performance measurement seemed a way to bring similar standardization to patient treatment. Moreover, Codman belonged to an influential group of progressive surgeons across the country who were dissatisfied with the paucity of reliable scientific information for improving practice.[12] In 1912 that group formed the American College of Surgeons. Its first president, Philadelphia surgeon Edward Martin, immediately appointed two committees: the first to do organizational work and the second, chaired by Codman, to examine hospital standardization.[13] The End Result Idea seemed poised to change the practice of medicine.

Codman was very much a part of the medical establishment of

his era. A man of broad scientific and clinical interests, he pioneered the diagnostic use of X rays and developed an important procedure for treating lesions of the shoulder. He also lived at a time when science and business were eager to learn from each other. America was being transformed from an agrarian society into an industrial one. The harnessing of steam power and other advances in the physical sciences had led to the industrial revolution and to a fundamental alteration in the economic structure of manufacturing. It was the era of John D. Rockefeller's big oil, Andrew Carnegie's big steel, and Henry Ford's Model T assembly line. Advances in medical science were bringing similarly sweeping changes to hospitals. The advent of surgical sterility and the "twilight of safe sleep," as anesthesia was advertised, made surgery safe enough for the middle class. The hospital immediately began shedding its old role as warehouse for the poor and started to evolve into a more sophisticated "physician's workshop" for curing disease.

In the business world, an industrial engineer named Frederick W. Taylor conducted the first careful time and motion studies of factory workers. "Taylor Societies," dedicated to industrial efficiency and "scientific management," sprang up all around the country. In the medical world, New York city physicians interested in these concepts sponsored a joint meeting between the industrial management experts of the New York Taylor Society and the Harvard Medical Society.[14]

To Codman, hospitals were also in business to make a product: patients who were cured. Yet while "a factory . . . takes pains to assure itself that the product is a good one . . . the hospital does not." He called on the businessmen trustees on hospital boards to support measurement of patient outcomes as a kind of "inventory of the goods delivered."[15] It was a very different concept from that of the hospital as physician workshop, where the implicit "product" was satisfied doctors.

For a time, Massachusetts General gave Codman's ideas a try. "The most important achievement of recent years has been the establishment of the 'follow-up' system urged by Dr. E. A. Codman . . . ," read the 1913 annual report of the hospital's general executive committee. "There has been no way of being sure that the medical and surgical work of the institution is as good as the present state of knowledge and the resources of the hospital, personal and financial, permit."[16]

Codman also started his own small hospital. Each medical and surgical patient got an end result card that included symptoms, the doctor's diagnosis, the treatment plan, any complications that resulted before the patient left the hospital, the correct diagnosis at discharge, and the results of care a year later. Codman eventually published at his own expense a volume showing the "end results" for all the patients his hospital treated during a five-year period.

Even today it is astonishing to read the kinds of information Codman made public. It was hardly the material of your ordinary annual report. It included a listing of the deaths due to actions "partially controllable" by better surgical management (such as "lack of technical knowledge") and deaths that, for various reasons, were beyond the surgeon's control.

Meanwhile, the regents of the American College of Surgeons in 1913 unanimously accepted the recommendations made by Codman's standardization committee for "efficiency" in hospitals. The College even sent a copy of the report to the American Medical Association, the Canadian Medical Association, and every hospital in North America.[17] Never before—or since—had the idea of judging the success of hospitals and physicians by the direct results of patient care received such powerful professional support. And yet measuring patient outcomes did not evolve into a standard feature of American medicine. In fact, the existence of Codman's system was forgotten, as was Codman (except by a few researchers), until a revival of interest in the 1980s. It is instructive to examine why this revolution that seemed poised for success ultimately failed.

One major problem was money. Professional rhetoric was not matched by a concomitant financial commitment. The Flexner Report's call for reform of medical education was subsequently backed by millions of dollars from the Carnegie and Rockefeller Foundations. By comparison, Codman's proposal to have all 2,700 hospitals in the United States measure the end results of their care attracted a grand total of $500 in funding from the College of Surgeons. The surgeons' priority was the much more limited goal of developing a standardized patient record.[18] At the time, many doctors were suspicious of sharing the records of "their" patients with the hospital and other physicians, and some physicians doubted the need for a written record at all. The Carnegie Foundation donated a modest $30,000 to the College for quality improvement, but those funds were earmarked for developing "minimum standards" of hospital quality.[19]

An even thornier problem was the threat Codman's ideas posed to the existing power structure of medicine. His proposals for public performance reports would have opened up medicine to the scrutiny of outsiders, a development many saw as an attack on their professionalism. Codman urged hospitals and individual surgeons to disclose both their successes and their failures to each other (for peer review) and to the public (so patients could choose the best qualified specialist). The reaction from colleagues was decidedly unenthusiastic. Sighed Codman:

> I am called eccentric for saying in public: that hospitals, if they wish to be sure of improvement, must find out what their results are, must analyze their results, to find their strong and weak points, must compare their results with those of other hospitals [and] must care for what cases they can care for well, and avoid attempting to care for cases which they are not qualified to care for well . . . must welcome publicity not only for their successes, but for their errors.

He added optimistically: "Such opinions will not be eccentric a few years hence."[20]

It's entirely possible that Codman did not realize the magnitude of the challenge his system presented. The truth was that the average hospital could barely meet minimum standards. In October 1919 the results of the first large-scale inspection of hospitals with at least one hundred beds were given to the regents of the American College of Surgeons, who were meeting at New York City's Waldorf-Astoria Hotel. Of 692 hospitals surveyed, only 89 passed. Those that failed to meet these minimum standards included some of the nation's most prominent institutions. Afraid that this list of individual scores would fall into the hands of the press, the surgeons took the pages down to the furnace in the hotel's basement. There, at midnight, they burned them.[21]

The Waldorf-Astoria incident dramatized the catastrophic potential of publicizing the end results of care. It was one thing for "scientific" physicians to denounce "unscientific" medical schools, as the Flexner Report did. But at a time when "scientific" physicians and hospitals were still fighting for public acceptance, publishing standardized outcomes information could impose a devastating degree of scrutiny.

Nor was there any outside pressure for accountability. In the early part of the century, malpractice suits against doctors were rare to nonexistent. Costs were not an issue, and not-for-profit hospitals were immune from liability for patient injuries as "charitable institutions."[22] As Codman quickly perceived, the absence of any tangible reward to doctors and hospitals for quality improvement was critical. "For whose *interest* is it to have the hospital efficient?" he asked. "Strangely enough, the answer is: No one . . . There is a difference between interest and duty. You do your duty if the work comes to you, but you do not go out of your way to get the work unless it is for your interest."[23]

There was a final factor working against Codman that can easily be overlooked in retrospect. In Codman's time, even a significant improvement in the quality of medical treatment paled in comparison with public health concerns. This was still the era of deadly infectious diseases that physicians were powerless to either prevent or treat. The death toll was staggering. In 1916 polio struck nearly 29,000 Americans, killing 6,000 and crippling thousands more. In 1918–19 the "Spanish" flu, which actually began in China, killed an almost inconceivable thirty *million* people worldwide, or more than 1 percent of the world's population. In this country, there were shortages of coffins as some 550,000 Americans died. This was on top of the just-concluded world war that had killed another ten million.[24]

Codman's old medical school classmate, Harvey Cushing, followed the prevailing paradigm of medical practice and had a long and brilliant career. He became known as the "father of brain surgery," wrote a Pulitzer Prize–winning biography of the revered surgeon William Osler, and was honored after his death by a portrait on a stamp. Codman, by contrast, had to dip into his own pocket to publish an account of his work on the End Result Idea. His surgery practice suffered as colleagues shunned him, and he was forced to borrow against his insurance policy to make ends meet. After Codman's death, there was no picture on a stamp. Instead, he was erased from some of the history books. The 1950 annual report of Massachusetts General Hospital traced the institution's workings over the previous half-century. After noting that "the 1913 report contained some very significant items," the historical review conspicuously omitted the most prominent accomplishment named in 1913—Codman's follow-up system.[25]

Codman's fate did not stop others from pushing for systematic improvement of medical care, but it contained a prescient warning about the forces within the medical profession working against change.

THE DOCTOR BUSINESS

In 1956 the *Wall Street Journal* sent a reporter for the first time to cover the annual meeting of the American Medical Association. It was an acknowledgment of the changing character of the medical profession. Before the war, a third of all depression-era physicians eked out a living on less than $2,500 a year. Nearly one in five earned less than $1,500.[26] After the war, the situation changed dramatically. There was a severe doctor shortage, so even the many physicians who kept their fees at a modest level saw incomes rise as they worked increasingly long days. Meanwhile, thanks to the growth of health insurance, more people could afford to see doctors or use the hospital. Blue Cross served two and a half times more subscribers in 1956 than in 1946. One of every ten Americans spent time in the hospital in 1945; by 1955 the figure had jumped to one in eight.[27]

The profession did not quickly forget the years of hardship. A little-noted 1955 AMA report found that "most" of the doctors it interviewed "display a consistent preoccupation with their economic insecurity. They think about money a lot—about how to increase their incomes, about the cost of running their offices, about what their colleagues in other specialties make, about what plumbers make for house calls and what a liquor dealer's net is compared to their own."[28]

Still, a page 1 *Journal* article, "Medic Merchants," reported that none of the three hundred speeches and medical treatises being presented at the 1956 AMA meeting dealt overtly with economics. It continued:

> Many a doctor still doesn't like to talk about such an earthy topic as money in connection with his profession. But a peek behind the average doctor's professional mask reveals a fellow with just about as many economic problems as any other small businessman.
>
> "The doctor is essentially a small businessman," says Dr. Frank G. Dickinson [Ph.D.], head of the AMA's bureau of medical economic research. "He is selling his services, so is as much in business as is anyone else who sells a commodity."[29]

Unfortunately, there was a great temptation to sell merchandise the customer didn't really need. Doctors were subjected to only the gentlest external control. As a result, some of the medical community's small businessmen behaved with the same lack of restraint as the big businessmen who ran steel or oil companies in the old robber baron days. The consequences of this behavior for the doctor's patients were not only financial, however; patients often paid for medical excesses with their health. Treatment-caused injuries (whose alarming growth was chronicled in chapter 3) frequently resulted from treatment that was inappropriate in the first place. It is a tawdry story that helps put our present system of regulating medical practice into context, but it is not a story that the leaders of the medical community ever publicize today. It is more convenient to hark back to a counterfeit golden age of professional self-control.

The halcyon 1950s were placid only in retrospect. In truth it was a time when the AMA was trying to persuade doctors to give up the all too common practice of taking kickbacks from laboratories, pharmacies, and makers of eyeglasses. Forty-three percent of patients thought their doctor charged too much, according to a 1956 AMA poll, while a 1959 cartoon in the *New Yorker* satirized the greed of a middle-aged physician making a house call to an elderly matron. As she glares from her bed, the doctor opens his little black bag and wads of paper money pop out. "Pshaw! I grabbed the wrong bag," the doctor exclaims.[30] (Interestingly, a 1993 AMA poll, taken right before the boom years for managed care, found that 69 percent of the public thought doctors were too interested in making money.)

In the 1950s, the American College of Surgeons remained locked in a decades-long struggle against "fee splitting," in which a surgeon rewarded the referring doctor by kicking back part of the patient's payment. The College was also trying to curb "ghost surgery," where, unknown to the anesthetized patient, his chosen surgeon secretly subcontracted the operation to a different doctor. The first surgeon charged the patient a fee, paid the "ghost" a lower one (some "ghosts" joked of belonging to the Twenty-five Dollar Club) and then pocketed the difference.

The headline of a 30 October 1953 article in *Collier's* advised "Why Some Doctors Should Be in Jail." "The M.D.'s Are off Their Pedestal," said a February 1954 piece in *Fortune*. That same month, *Harpers Magazine* warned its readers of the danger of the "commercial" surgeon who was "usually a good salesman."[31] Paul Hawley, the College's president, dared speak openly to *U.S. News and World Report* about these types of abuses. Outraged delegates to the AMA's 1953 annual meeting introduced eleven separate resolutions—condemning Hawley, of course.[32]

If tonsillectomies were an early surgical fad, "female surgery" was now all the rage. "Hysterectomy: Therapeutic Necessity or Surgical Racket?" demanded University of Michigan gynecologist Norman Miller in 1946.[33] "Unnecessary Ovariectomies," scolded Los Angeles gynecologist James Doyle in a 1952 article on misuse of ovary removal.[34] Doyle also followed Miller's work with his own research that reviewed twenty-five times as many procedures. His "Unnecessary Hysterectomies" still found that about four in ten were inappropriate.[35]

Doyle's study presented a horrifying picture of casualness involving a procedure that takes away a woman's ability to bear children: 160 of the women, many in their twenties and thirties, received no preoperative diagnosis. Some 185 hysterectomy recipients were diagnosed with only a single symptom called "pain." Another 86 women had hysterectomies after they complained to their doctors of a backache!

"An appalling number of the patients aged twenty to twenty-nine who were subjected to hysterectomy had no disease whatsoever (30 percent)," wrote the usually dispassionate Doyle after reviewing postoperative pathology reports. "In women aged thirty to thirty-nine, 18 percent had no lesions. In women forty to forty-nine, 9 percent had a uterus that was normal."

Some surgeons responded that they were only doing what patients wanted. "Were the women subject to these unnecessary operations in better health and happier and well content to have been operated upon or were they not?" asked one. "If they were, I suspect the operations were not unnecessary." Another surgeon cited the placebo effect. "Often time patients prefer to be operated upon; they get well quicker if an operation is done which is not really necessary."[36]

It was in this atmosphere that physician and epidemiologist Paul Lembcke tried to take up the fight for systematic quality measurement and improvement where Codman had left off. The "medical audit" was Lembcke's method to ensure that patients received the most appropriate and effective care. Lembcke was one of a new breed of physicians who combined clinical and public health training. After attending medical school in his hometown of Rochester, New York, he joined the state department of health and showed an immediate knack for tackling tough issues.[37] There was a nationwide epidemic of diarrhea among newborns, and one-quarter to two-thirds of the infected babies were dying. Lembcke discovered that hospital administrators were not seeking assistance from the local health department in addressing infection outbreaks because they feared bad publicity. "Don't cover up!" Lembcke urged in a 1943 article in *Modern Hospital*.[38]

A few years later Lembcke decided to examine whether postgraduate medical education made a difference in the outcome of patient care. To his surprise, he found there was no accurate method of comparing the results achieved by different hospitals. Lembcke responded by developing standardized measures of individual diseases and conditions that came to constitute the medical audit.[39]

The phrase was a deliberate tribute to Codman, who had urged hospital trustees to audit end result reports "as they do financial accounts." Without such an audit, wrote Codman, trustees "rely on what the staff is said to be able to do, not what it actually does do, to the patients."[40] Although cognizant of Codman's eventual failure, Lembcke was nonetheless willing to try once again to make hospital standardization more than a "watered-down program" of "minimal standards."[41]

His medical audit arranged information into disease classifications (such as major female pelvic surgery), verified the statements made in the clinical record, and independently established the accuracy of laboratory and other test results. Next the audit compared the verifiable facts from each hospital with outside standards of good care, such as the appropriate indicators of a surgical operation. The final step was comparing the audited hospital's score with the average score of a group of hospitals "of acknowledged merit"—what we would today call benchmarking. In addition, Lembcke recommended comparing how frequently different surgeries were performed in different communities—essentially, an investigation into the kind of "small-area variation" that Wennberg and Gittelsohn later carried out in New England.

Lembcke first applied these methods to examine appendectomies in twenty-three hospital service areas. He had spent enough time in the trenches to know the tricks of the trade. For example, there was a tendency for surgeons to describe the removal of a patient's normal, nondiseased organ "with euphemisms or anatomic terms that could be construed to disguise this fact." Or a surgeon who waited until after the operation to write up his preoperative observations "perhaps inadvertently made the preoperative diagnosis correspond to the postoperative diagnosis or even the pathology report."[42]

Lembcke's 1952 article on appendectomies found "considerably more operations . . . done than are necessary."[43] The popular press had already guessed as much: *Harpers* dubbed the problem "chronic remunerative appendicitis."[44] Lembcke went on, however, to articulate a standard for appraising the quality of medical care that was decades ahead of its time. He wrote: "Measurements of quality should be expressed in terms that are uniform and objective, and that permit meaningful comparisons between communities, institutions, groups and time periods, and with a general standard [of care]."

As chapter 3's discussion of medical errors showed, the traditional medical culture focused on the doctor's actions rather than what happened to the patient. As the old saw put it, "The operation was a success but the patient died." Lembcke, though, dared to look at medical treatment through the patient's eyes. He wrote: "The best measure of quality is not how well or how frequently a medical service is given, but how closely the result approaches the fundamental objectives of prolonging life, relieving distress, restoring function and preventing disability."[45]

Unlike Codman, Lembcke was soft-spoken and well liked by those he worked with. Unfortunately, that work was cut short; Lembcke died of a brain tumor on 1 December 1964 at age fifty-six. Some hospitals did launch medical audits, just as a few tried to implement Codman's ideas. But medical auditing was difficult. Without any widespread intellectual support or the financial incentive to tough it out, hospitals and doctors gave up. The latest attempt at institutionalizing a new paradigm of American medicine fizzled.

Unlike Codman's work, Lembcke's did not totally disappear. The W. K. Kellogg Foundation eventually recommended his audit methodology to a physician-researcher at the Southwestern Michigan Hospital council who was also interested in hospital standardization. The researcher, Vergil Slee, was extolling the virtues of using a new tool that few people really understood. That tool was the computer.

THE OPTIMIST

> It is human nature to shrink from too close self-examination . . . when a convenient belief persists that no matter how we behave personally, there always can be some vicarious substitute for self government, with its painful necessity for thought.
> —William Howard Hay, M.D., about 1900

In 1952, the year Lembcke's article on excess appendectomies appeared, a computer assisted for the first time in the news coverage of a national election. The UNIVAC I (UNIVersal Automatic Computer) on loan to CBS News correctly predicted the eventual landslide presidential victory of Republican Dwight Eisenhower less than forty-five minutes after the polls closed. However, CBS's political analysts, confident in their own experience, refused to air the results and ordered the computer reprogrammed. Thanks to this human intervention, the computer (incorrectly) predicted a close contest between Eisenhower and Democratic nominee Adlai Stevenson.[46]

About the same time America was deciding it liked Ike, the American College of Surgeons was relinquishing its unique role as guardian of hospital standardization. Because of the doctor shortage, there were fewer surgeons available to perform surveys. Worse, the shortage also meant that hospitals being surveyed had a tougher time meeting the minimum standards. When a hospital failed it led to embarrassment, political fallout for the College, and the need for an additional visit. Wearying of the drain on money and time, the College helped form a new Joint Commission on Accreditation of Hospitals (JCAH). The board included the surgeons, the American College of Physicians (representing internists), the AMA, the Canadian Medical Association, and the American Hospital Association. (The Canadians dropped out in 1959. In 1987 the JCAH become the Joint Commission on Accreditation of Healthcare Organizations, or JCAHO.)

Still, after thirty-four years, the College of Surgeons was not ready to completely abandon its interest in standardization. Hospital revenues now exceeded the revenues of steel companies, but the way hospitals handled information remained primitive. In a bid to jump to the cutting edge of technology, the surgeons joined the Kellogg Foundation in backing the work of Vergil Slee, a University of Michigan professor who promised to put hospital records onto a computer.

If Codman was a skeptic and Lembcke a realist, Slee was an optimist, a paradigm revolutionary convinced that revolutions could be bloodless affairs if one only convinced oneself that they weren't really going to change much. "The medical profession has long sought an effective, practicable and inexpensive method by which medical staffs of hospitals can evaluate the quality of patient care," said a scientific exhibit put together for the 1955 AMA annual meeting by Slee, Robert Hoffmann, a statistician colleague at Michigan, and physician Robert Myers, assistant director of the College of Surgeons.[47] That sentiment might have been more persuasive if this hadn't been the same AMA assembly that heard about physicians' desperate efforts to keep pace economically with liquor store owners.

For a short while, Slee's upbeat outlook seemed justified. He persuaded a group of Michigan hospitals to collect standardized information, code it onto computer punch cards, and then send the cards to the University of Michigan School of Public Health for processing and analysis. Unlike LDS Hospital's Homer Warner, whose work in Salt Lake City was discussed in chapter 4, Slee was not personally involved in patient care. Still, Slee proposed to do nothing less ambitious than build a comprehensive, computerized, national database on the clinical quality of patient care—*and* make the results available to the public.

The implications of the blandly named Professional Activity Study (PAS) were explosive. In 1954, speaking as if the system were reality, Slee painted the following picture:

> A friend came to us one day and said, "One of the members of my family has to be hospitalized. How can I tell what hospital to put him in?"
>
> We answered, "Professional services statistics are designed to give the answers to questions like that. We'll just see which hospital is the safest to go into, or in which you may expect the most dramatic results of treatment. . . . Let's see which hospital reports the greatest percentage of recoveries on discharge."[48]

In Slee's vision, hospitals using the PAS system would examine the results of care for their patients and compare the results with those of other hospitals—much like the benchmark "hospitals of acknowledged merit" described by Lembcke. The medical staff could also use the system to analyze the performance of its own physicians, making possible Codman's goal of assigning each patient to the best qualified doctor.

As appealing as this prospect was (at least to patients), the effort required to make the PAS system function smoothly was considerable. It involved tedious hand coding of procedures, transferring those codes to punched computer cards, and giving careful attention to every medical record. Moreover, the results of a PAS pilot study in the early 1950s were not likely to make physicians clamor for its widespread use. Given the abuses of the time, Slee's system inevitably cast medicine in an embarrassing light. In the pilot study, about a third of the surgeons who performed ten or more appendectomies a year were consistently wrong in their diagnosis; in fact, they diagnosed acute appendicitis correctly less than a third of the time.[49] Just three of seventy-nine physicians ordered chest X rays for every patient they diagnosed with pneumonia, while ten doctors ordered them for fewer than half their patients. And the range of hospitalized diabetics who never even had their blood sugar tested ranged from 5 to 55 percent!

To be sure, serious quality-of-care problems over the years were not limited to hospitals. As far back as the 1930s, medical leaders acknowledged that "little is known about the quality of medical care . . . rendered by private practitioners" in their offices.[50] In the mid-1950s the Rockefeller Foundation commissioned internist Osler Peterson to observe "family doctors" in North Carolina whose education and training resembled national norms. Despite being observed by internists as they saw patients, 45 percent of the doctors failed to meet a set of minimal standards. For instance, when giving patients a physical exam, "physicians were observed attempting to [hear] the heart or lungs through several layers of [patient] clothing, or dropping the stethoscope chest piece down through the open neck of the clothing in this attempt," reported Peterson. "Similarly, several physicians failed to recognize the impossibility of feeling a soft, rounded liver edge through several layers of heavy clothing.[51]

To Slee, problems were the proverbial opportunities in disguise. "Medical staffs now can . . . use [these] facts to help them guide the practice in the hospital," he wrote sunnily.[52] The way doctors and hospitals really behaved, however, was captured in the report of a blue-ribbon commission appointed by Michigan's governor to examine hospital quality and cost. The commission report provides a candid contemporary snapshot of health care circa 1958.

"Many hospitals are not properly using many of the techniques of quality control that have been devised," the commission concluded. "Boards of trustees seem to be reluctant to assert themselves in the area of quality of care, even though they have the legal obligation to do so; but without the board's leadership, the medical staff may be reluctant to impinge upon the freedom of individual staff members." Medicine's failure to keep up with the latest therapies, discussed in chapter 6, was already apparent three decades ago in "the lag between advances in medical science and their application by all physicians and hospitals to the care of patients."[53]

The commission added a warning that would not be fully appreciated until years later: "Direct control of quality by doctors and hospitals is not likely to reach full expression without external inducements."[54] In other words, doctors, like anyone else, were not going to change until they had to. There is no more sobering illustration of that truth than the little-known story of the National Halothane Study.

WHO LIVES, WHO DIES, WHO CARES

The National Halothane Study began in the mid-1960s as a classic clinical investigation. Halothane, a common general anesthetic, was strongly suspected of causing fatal postoperative damage to the kidneys, a condition known as massive hepatic necrosis. Because the drug was widely used, the National Academy of Sciences, the Public Health Service, and national professional societies cooperated in organizing an urgent review of patient records that was unprecedented in its scope.

Researchers went to extraordinary lengths to ensure that the information was statistically meaningful. A research team examined both the overall surgical death rate and deaths from hepatic necrosis at thirty-four hospitals during the years 1959 through 1962. Researchers extracted data from more than 856,000 patient records, paying particular attention to about 10,000 surgeries where hepatic necrosis was a complication.

The good news in the researchers' 1968 report was that halothane, "rather than being a dangerous anesthetic, demonstrated a record of safety."[55] Contrary to impressions, halothane was actually associated with *fewer* deaths on average. But the bad news threatened to overshadow the good. The halothane team had discovered large differences in the surgical death rates at the participating hospitals. Only one explanation could be offered with certainty: halothane use was not the reason.

"Raw" mortality rates at different hospitals can vary considerably without there being a genuine difference in care. So it was not altogether surprising that researchers found as much as a twenty-four-fold disparity between hospitals in the percentage of patients who died within six weeks of surgery. What was unexpected, however, was the magnitude of the gap that remained even after the raw figures were adjusted to take into account factors such as patient age, physical status, and the seriousness of the operation. The "standardized" mortality rates for six common operations, such as gallbladder removal and hysterectomy, varied more than sevenfold, ranging from seven patients per thousand at the low end of the scale to as high as fifty patients per thousand at the high end.

In several hospitals, over 200 patients died who would have lived had the hospital's mortality rate been at the expected level. There was a total of 1,750 "excess" deaths at the hospitals with medium and high death rates.[56] Since there were only 17,000 surgical deaths in all, a difference of 1,750 lives was substantial.

Nothing on this scale had ever before been documented. Was the reason an inadequate adjustment for the physiological variation in patients? Might a hospital's high surgical death rate be due to differences in the decision about which patients to send to surgery? Some hospitals might operate as a last resort on sick patients who otherwise would die of "medical" conditions such as pneumonia. If the patient died anyway, it became a surgery-related death. Or did the numbers really point to substantial differences in the end result of care?

National Halothane Study statisticians Lincoln Moses and Frederick Mosteller said that they were not even going to attempt to answer such "important and delicate questions."[57] For one thing, they weren't certain where to begin. It wasn't obvious which institutions should be studied, or what kinds of factors should be examined, they wrote in the 12 February 1968 issue of the *Journal of the American Medical Association.* In what seems to be an expression of priorities shaped by the dominant paradigm of a different era, the men expressed the most concern about the effect a public outcry might have on doctors and hospitals. It would be "too easy to set in motion what could, in fairness, only be called a circus," they advised.

What to do instead? "We are not persuaded that 'strenuous efforts to correct the situation' are necessarily called for," they wrote, but "someone" (they put the word in quotation marks) should take action.

> Indications of [problems of] such importance based on so much data should not be swept under the rug—and we do not suggest that they should. We feel that at a minimum, "someone" should recognize that there may be a problem here and not a trivial one. Further, "someone" should try to ascertain which institutions, though inexplicable by our data, are readily understood as "naturally" having high death rates because of, say, poverty of their clientele or other compelling and well-understood reasons.[58] Finally, we feel that "someone," after finding a remaining set of hospitals whose death-rate experience can-

not be dismissed, should cause these to be thought about. *Quiet, unofficial, cooperatively oriented inquiries into opportunities for studying the problems should be sought.* [Emphasis added]

Were "strenuous efforts" not called for? The numbers work out this way: If there were 1,750 "excess" deaths in four years at thirty-four hospitals, that translates into about 308,000 "excess" deaths among the nation's roughly six thousand community hospitals.[59] Divide that result by four, round it off conservatively, and you get 75,000 "excess" deaths every year. Moreover, those 75,000 deaths were based on just *six* common surgical conditions. They do not include excess deaths from other surgeries or from nonsurgical treatment.

In 1968, as in the era of Codman, Lembcke, and Slee, the only force pushing for an answer to the questions raised by the halothane study was the professionalism of the medical community. Apart from a couple of cities in California, the impact of what was then called "prepaid group care"—we'd call it "managed care"—was negligible. There were no consumer groups making loud accusations. Ralph Nader would not form the Public Citizen Health Research Group until 1971. As for the news media, their coverage of science and medicine still consisted largely of a dutiful chronicle of clinical advances. The malpractice lawyers were just starting to flex their muscles, and doctors remained almost untouchable by politicians, particularly on matters of clinical quality of care.

In sum, the medical profession was free to conduct, or not conduct, its own discreet inquiry into whether 75,000 patients each year were dying unnecessarily. Moreover, the National Halothane Study had appeared in the AMA's professional journal, making it practically a poster child for self-regulation. Coincidentally, the study appeared about the same time a federation of seventy-five voluntary and professional societies called the National Health Forum announced that "Quality in Health Care" would be the theme of its annual meeting. The meeting promised to "assess standards and procedures for assuring quality in health-care services and consider proposals for strengthening these standards and procedures."[60]

Despite all the high-minded declarations, nothing happened. The original halothane study was designed to examine a specific clinical question. Neither the federal government, organized medicine, nor charitable foundations appropriated one extra dime to examine the quality of the health care system as a whole.

A physician, a sociologist, and a biostatistician at Stanford University believed they could find answers to the questions raised by the halothane report. At the urging of Stanford anesthesiologist John Bunker—chairman of the National Halothane Study and later the mentor of variations pioneer John Wennberg—federal agencies gave leftover funds from the original study to Stanford's Center for Health care research. The center got $500,000 to conduct follow-up research on the excess deaths, or a little under $7 for each fatality.

Eight years after the original halothane results appeared, the Stanford team published its Institutional Differences Study. The researchers had examined the treatment of 8,600 patients undergoing fifteen types of surgery at seventeen hospitals. The data were carefully adjusted to take into account as many factors as possible that were unrelated to the actual care patients received. In some cases observers even went into the operating room to make certain the information was accurate. However, because the study did not carry the prestige of its predecessor and was not published in a clinical journal, few people ever read the dramatic findings.

First, the Stanford group concluded that hospitals' performance could be compared using outcomes. Lembcke and Slee's vision of comparing hospitals was scientifically validated.

The second conclusion was even more important: there were real and significant variations among hospitals in the outcomes of patient care. After all the adjustments, a threefold difference remained between the best and worst hospitals. The excess deaths uncovered by the National Halothane Study were neither a fluke nor an error. Although the magnitude of excess deaths might be open to dispute, "substantial variation in outcome among hospitals does exist, independently of differences in patient mix," the Stanford team concluded.[61]

The Stanford study was "quiet, unofficial, and cooperative," precisely as Moses and Mosteller had wished. "Someone" had done something—but no one paid any attention.[62] The research documenting that the wrong choice of hospital could triple a surgical patient's chance of dying was not used to improve the care of a single person. It had even less effect than the exhortations of Ernest Amory Codman a half century before; Codman, after all, was a practicing surgeon who could at least affect the care of his own patients. The Stanford researchers didn't even affect the Stanford hospital.

I asked biostatistician Byron Brown, a member of the study team and now chair of Stanford Medical Center's Department of Health Research and Policy, about the study's negligible influence. Brown made it clear that he never intended to be a paradigm revolutionary.

> I grew up in a small town. You know there are differences in the competence from one doctor to another. We all know there are differences in [auto] mechanics, and there are differences in doctors. That was common sense then, it's common sense now.
>
> We didn't attempt to make any splash with [the study]. I don't think we even tried to get it into the *New England Journal*. I avoid talking to reporters as much as possible, including you.[63]

LOOKING OUT OF THE FISHBOWL

In Codman's day, "scientific" physicians and hospitals were still nervous about exposing their flaws to a public that didn't yet fully believe in their virtues. Those worries were only a faint memory by the time Lembcke, Slee, and the National Halothane Study appeared on the scene. Yet if having a precarious grip on power makes one cautious about change, being entrenched in power only reinforces that tendency. "The better you are at your paradigm," notes Joel Arthur Barker, author of *Future Edge*, a book about paradigm shifts, "the more you have invested in it, and the more you have to lose by changing paradigms."[64]

Paul Sanazaro, a physician pioneer in medical quality research, remembers visiting "probably over 1,000 hospitals," as a part-time surveyor for the Joint Commission during the 1950s and 1960s. He recalls little commitment to systematic improvement of patient outcomes. When he suggested using Professional Activity Study data to one medical association, the staff responded, "If you take it out of the boxes, you can use it." The printouts that no one really understood or cared to understand were neatly stacked in a closet.[65]

As for the medical community's reaction to halothane, John Bunker described a situation not unlike the metaphor this chapter began with: that of the fish unable to see outside its fishbowl. "Doctors ask, 'What's the relevance of this to my daily work?' In the early age [of medicine], it was a question of what we call clinical freedom. Doctors were able to hide behind that for a long time. Now I think times have changed."[66]

CHAPTER EIGHT

The Doctor's Car and the Car Companies' Doctors

There is a tide in the affairs of men,
Which taken at the flood, leads on to fortune;
Omitted, all the voyage of their life
Is bound in shallows and in miseries.
—William Shakespeare, *Julius Caesar*

At the end of World War II, Ford Motor Company and Chrysler Corporation were approached about buying Germany's Volkswagen. They dismissed the idea out of hand. Sneered one Ford executive about the VW Beetle: "You call that a car?"[1]

Paradigm shifts are revolutions, but the signs of a brewing insurrection can easily be overlooked. A public wearied by years of economic travail and war was in no mood after World War II to talk about lowered expectations, be it in cars or any other aspect of life. "More" was better.

America's love affair with the auto was obvious. Automobiles offered a seductive blend of freedom, privacy, and the opportunity to show off material success. By the early 1950s, more than 60 percent of Americans owned a car, and they clamored for relief from clogged roads. Congress responded by passing the 1956 Highway Act, opening the way for a radical change in the national landscape.

Postwar medicine was also popular. In 1946 Congress passed the Hill-Burton Hospital Survey and Construction Act, which eventually pumped $700 million into hospital expansion. The nation added or renovated 170,000 hospital beds in only ten years, changing the map of the United States health care system as radically as federal highways changed the road map.[2] Medical progress provided an important measure of freedom as well, even if not quite so obviously as a bright red convertible. New drugs and vaccines gradually freed the nation from deadly plagues. And just as the auto industry promised exciting improvements every model year, important medical discoveries seemed to arrive at dependable intervals. On television, viewers saw the fictional Dr. Wayne Hudson pioneer a different treatment each week on *Dr. Hudson's Secret Journal.*

Tonsillectomies and tail fins symbolized progress. Driving a new car showed that an individual had "made it"; building a new hospital demonstrated the same for a community. The auto companies offered power steering to ease the stress for anxious women drivers; doctors proffered Valium. Automakers seized on fads like push-button gear shifts; doctors and hospitals tried out gastric freezing. Carmakers built souped-up engines; hospitals built bigger and better emergency rooms.

In California, industrialist Henry J. Kaiser tried his luck at autos and health care simultaneously. He bankrolled the expansion of the Oakland-based Kaiser Permanente Health Plan, originally set up to serve his company's workers, and also poured millions into Kaiser-Frazer autos. The health plan prospered. The car company and its little-remembered "Henry J" model sank into oblivion after just a few years.

For all the financial success and prestige enjoyed by both the automobile and health care industries, however, there were signs that the good times would not roll on forever.

"THE SKY WAS THE LIMIT"

> Health, as a vast societal enterprise, is too important to be solely the concern of the providers of services.
>
> —William L. Kissick, M.D.

A man who headed a large New York City hospital in the 1950s and 1960s spoke candidly, in return for anonymity, about how his hospital used to operate:

> We were always concerned about quality within the institution, but nobody cared about geographic variation and nobody cared about appropriateness. Not that we didn't know in a piece of our mind that was an issue. But we felt we were pretty good. . . .
>
> It didn't really start becoming a problem until Medicare, Medicaid, because all of a sudden, issues like length of stay and . . . doing inappropriate procedures and the whole issue of the national expense on health care started then. Before then, who cared?
>
> When Medicare and Medicaid first passed, there was no limit on reimbursement. I remember sitting in our planning rooms and saying, "Hey, they've just passed a national bill without an upper limit

> on the per diem [daily rate a hospital charged]." I predicted that in two years they'd wake up and find it was out of control. So I said, "Let's go now and spend as much money as we can, and get the rate up as high as we can, so at the point that they close it, we'll be on top."
>
> We were in the voluntary [not-for-profit] sector, but we weren't stupid. It wasn't just us: everybody realized the sky was the limit. [President Richard] Nixon woke up one morning and said, "They're out of control"—and they were out of control.

Indeed they were. The Medicare program for the elderly and the Medicaid program for the poor took effect on 1 July 1966. The cost of a day in the hospital increased by an average 7 percent annually between 1963 and 1966, climbed 13 percent per year from 1966 to 1969, and then accelerated nearly 16 percent annually from 1969 to 1970—the year Nixon imposed national wage-price controls. Between 1965 and 1969 the net income of nonprofit hospitals shot up 76 percent.[3]

President Lyndon Johnson had struck a deal with the American Medical Association in order to get the powerful group's promise not to tie up Medicare and Medicaid legislation in Congress. Johnson agreed that the government would pay doctors treating the elderly whatever fee was "usual, customary, and reasonable," a level of reimbursement significantly more generous than that of private insurers.[4] (Medicaid fees were set by states.) Despite doctors' denunciations of "socialized medicine," the new system encouraged profit maximization. Before Medicare, many doctors essentially conducted their business according to the principles of Karl Marx, the father of communism: "From each according to his abilities, to each according to his needs." Physicians charged higher fees to patients who could afford to pay and smaller or no fees to those who could not. Medicare, though, promised to pay whatever fee was "usual." The penniless senior citizen was instantly upgraded from charity case to full-fare customer. Although physicians' earnings in 1965 were already five times the median average income,[5] the rate of increase in their fees promptly doubled.[6] Doctors weren't stupid, either.

On the other hand, the cost of care was no longer a private matter between doctor and patient. Just as physicians had feared, a powerful outside force now evinced a keen interest in examining what care doctors delivered for their money. As the federal share of national health expenditures jumped from 25 percent in fiscal 1965 to nearly

40 percent five years later, the Medicare trust fund plunged into the red and Congress held its first public hearings on medical misdeeds.

Just a few years earlier, the automakers had been in the same position. Accustomed to basking in public praise, the industry was put on the defensive by the publication of Ralph Nader's *Unsafe at Any Speed: The Designed-in Dangers of the American Automobile*. Unlimited autonomy gave way to unprecedented government regulation of everything from auto safety features to, eventually, gas mileage and tire standards. In 1969 the health care industry started down this same path. A system with virtually no external checks or balances was about to get outside scrutiny of what it did and how much it charged. There would be no turning back.

Financial scams were an easy first target. At Senate hearings in 1969, investigators trotted out tales of an abused public trust. Senators castigated "ruthless providers of health services" who charged Medicare an average of two to four times as much as they charged commercial insurers for the same surgical procedures.[7] One general practitioner had billed Medicare $58,000 for home visits to forty-nine patients, leading Senate Finance Committee chairman Russell Long (D-La.) to quip: "Who says you can't get a doctor to make a house call anymore?"

Just days later, the White House staged its own press conference at which President Nixon stressed his "personal concern" about the state of the health care system. At the same time, he unveiled recommendations from the Department of Health, Education, and Welfare (HEW) for cutting medical costs and improving quality. "We face a massive crisis in this area . . . in the next two or three years unless something is done about it immediately," Nixon declared.[8] The HEW report called for "drastic measures" that would "challenge . . . the private sector to begin the process of revolutionary change in the medical care system."

Doctors and hospitals were as surprised to find themselves on the defensive as auto executives had been. The abuses of the past were becoming intolerable—if not to the profession, then to society. Just as the excesses of the pharmaceutical industry prompted a strengthening of the Food and Drug Administration's powers, the excesses of doctors and hospitals provoked a political backlash whose effects are still being felt. John G. Veneman of HEW made an extraordinary pronouncement, the more so because it came from an official in a conservative Republican administration: "In the past, decisions on health care delivery were largely professional ones," declared Veneman. "Now, the decisions will be largely political."[9]

The politicians dared challenge the profession so boldly only because they had public opinion on their side. In a 1970 survey of heads of families, three-quarters agreed with the statement: "There is a crisis in health care in the United States." The extent of the change in the public's attitude can be seen by looking at the news coverage provided by *Fortune,* a quintessential Establishment magazine read by corporate managers. A 1954 *Fortune* critique of doctors' behavior portrayed greed that led to inappropriate surgery as an aberration. The magazine gave passing mention to cases of outright incompetence, but in the indulgent tone used to discuss schoolboy pranks. "The physician, after all, is organized into a guild whose rules require mutual back scratching and forbid face clawing," the magazine advised. "The physician cannot say aloud that a hospital has weak departments or that a medical school has inadequate equipment. . . . [But] so long as they do not violate guild rules and name names, they will even talk about the occasional incompetence and rascality in their profession.[10]

The deference to doctors was completely gone from the January 1970 *Fortune.* There was no hint of amusement in an editorial that pronounced "much of U.S. medical care, particularly the everyday business of preventing and treating routine illnesses . . . inferior in quality, wastefully dispensed and inequitably financed. . . . [M]ost Americans are badly served by the obsolete, over-strained medical system that has grown up about them helter-skelter . . . the time has come for radical change."[11]

The public backlash against the auto companies had been so strong in part because Nader showed that Detroit knew about safety problems but did nothing to fix them. In the mid-1960s, a spate of exposés began to make that same point about the leaders of medicine. In 1966, for instance, Martin Gross's *The Doctors* estimated that two million unnecessary operations were performed annually. Surgeon "Lawrence Williams," writing under a pseudonym, produced a candid book-length exploration titled *Unnecessary Surgery* in 1971. Dr. Alex Gerber's *The Gerber Report* presented an acerbic laundry list of medical misconduct. In *A Surgeon's World,* Dr. William Nolen, a respected elder statesman, shamefacedly admitted turning a blind eye to collegial lapses in competence and ethics. Sociologist Marcia Millman's *The Unkindest Cut,* a brutally honest account of the goings-on in one unnamed hospital, caused a national sensation. Newspaper and magazine articles and television news reports added to the pressure.

Congressional investigators moved on from probing financial shenanigans to examining clinical misconduct. In 1974 a House subcommittee held the first hearings on inappropriate surgery and concluded that the number of unneeded procedures had grown about 20 percent since Gross's 1966 book appeared. Gradually the federal government chipped away at the medical community's immunity to outside oversight. The original Medicare law required hospitals to set up utilization review committees to ensure that the elderly received effective and appropriate care. Half of all hospitals never bothered reviewing any admissions at all.[12] As health costs increased, however, congressional scrutiny became more persistent. In the early 1970s, Medicare had set up EMCROs (experimental medical care review organizations) to peer over doctors' shoulders. Those turned into PSROs (professional standards review organizations), which looked a little more closely, and eventually PROs (peer review organizations), which looked more closely still.

Oversight, however, was no substitute for the "revolutionary change" the Nixon administration had promised. Here, despite the catchy rhetoric, the Republicans had a problem: no one was quite sure what a reshaped health system should look like. The man the administration eventually turned to for guidance in reshaping one of the largest pieces of the United States economy was a pediatric neurologist who specialized in treating children with polio. Paul Ellwood Jr. also had a second specialty: prescribing therapy for the paralysis afflicting the American health care system.

CAPITALIST TOOL

Paul Ellwood always knew he wanted to do more than provide patient care. As an intern at Stanford University Medical School in the 1950s, Ellwood made unusual use of some free moments: he read *Concept of the Corporation,* Peter Drucker's classic management study about the organizational structure of General Motors. "Gee whiz, that's health care," Ellwood thought. From then on, he began applying a mental business model to the problems of the health care system.

Ellwood grew up in Oakland, California, where industrialist Henry Kaiser's Kaiser Permanente plan flourished as a "prepaid group practice." In a prepaid practice, all the patient's medical needs were met by one group of doctors in return for the annual insurance premium. "Wellness" care (such as prevention and rehabilitation) and "sickness" care were covered equally. Drawing on that experience, Ellwood decided that a more rational health care system would combine the efficiency of prepaid groups with the adherence to quality standards Drucker wrote about. To keep down costs, the prepaid groups would compete for customers. To encourage good care, the plans would be evaluated based on who took the best care of the patient's complete health needs.

There were formidable barriers to turning this vision into reality. Not the least of them was that the AMA and many fee for service doctors had long regarded prepaid group practices as falling somewhere between socialism and communism. Ellwood, undeterred, became a public policy entrepreneur, unabashedly peddling what amounted to a paradigm revolution to whatever center of political power could help him carry it off.[13] His natural first stop was the health insurance industry, but the prospect of alienating large numbers of physicians gave the insurers cold feet. Next Ellwood approached congressional Democrats, certain they would be interested in this progressive approach. The Democrats responded that the real solution was national health insurance. That left Ellwood with a single option: Nixon was the one.

Domestic policy was not the Nixon administration's strong suit. By mid-1969, however, the administration had no choice but to take a stand on health care.[14] Massachusetts senator Edward Kennedy, invoking the legacy of his slain brother, Robert, was vowing to push national health insurance through the Democratically controlled Congress. The Nixon administration, caught flat-footed, scrambled to find an alternative. So it was that on 5 February 1970, HEW undersecretary Veneman and assistant secretary Lewis Butler came to visit Ellwood in his suite at Washington's Dupont Plaza Hotel. As long-haired teenagers gathered in the nearby park to smoke marijuana and protest the Vietnam War, the president's men listened intently to Ellwood's plan to recast prepaid group practices as a model of cost-effective yet compassionate capitalism.

Doctors in prepaid groups hospitalized their patients less often than fee for service physicians, who were paid more to do more, but studies showed the quality of care was comparable. Still, a reform plan whose centerpiece consisted of promising to "do less" for patients was political suicide. So Ellwood cleverly asserted that prepaid groups would actually "do more" for people by letting them visit their doctors at no charge for preventive treatment. To emphasize this purpose and downplay the controversial financing mechanism, Ellwood gave prepaid group practices a new label. He called them "health maintenance organizations," or HMOs.

The high-level political visitors seemed impressed, but Ellwood could not be certain he had carried the day. As soon as the men left his hotel room, the stress overwhelmed him. He went straight to the bathroom and threw up.

He needn't have worried. Like Ellwood (and Nixon), Veneman and Butler were Californians who had firsthand experience with prepaid care. They didn't fear Reds under hospital beds.[15] On 18 February 1971, the president announced a "national health strategy" whose cornerstone was the HMO. It was an extraordinary action when one considers that at the time a mere thirty-three HMOs served the entire country. In any event, one thing was perfectly clear: no one was going to accuse Richard Nixon of being soft on communism. The same cold warrior credentials that later enabled this president to establish diplomatic relations with the "Red" Chinese made Nixon the perfect advocate of prepaid care. In December 1973 Congress passed the Health Maintenance Organization Act, conferring government financing and support on HMOs that met certain federal standards. Although the HMO Act's full effects would take years to be felt, its impact was truly revolutionary. It set the stage for a fundamental change in the structure and incentives of medical practice.

The next step in the paradigm shift was to get private industry to notice its power.

WHO LIVES, WHO DIES, WHO PAYS

In January 1903 the magazine *Horseless Age* published a special eighty-six-page issue praising the contribution of physicians to the fledgling auto industry. Many doctors were avid motorists, welcoming the horseless carriage for their personal use and for its contribution to speedier and more economical house calls. (Unlike a horse, a car didn't need to be fed and cared for.) In 1904 automakers Jonathan Maxwell and Benjamin Briscoe decided to produce a special "doctor's car" that featured special high wheels for better clearance on mud-filled side roads. Several other automakers followed suit; one auto advertisement later claimed the car was "dependable as the doctor himself."[16]

Maxwell Motor Company was bought out by Walter P. Chrysler in the early 1920s and renamed the Chrysler Corporation. Time passed until in March 1982 Chrysler again offered a "doctor's car"—of sorts. The auto company told six thousand doctors and dentists it would give them a rebate of $500 to $2,000 on Chrysler cars in return for the clinicians' cutting their fees to company workers by 10 percent. Unfortunately, house calls were history, and a mere four hundred doctors and dentists took advantage of the discount deal.[17]

What made the Chrysler offer remarkable was not the money involved, but the calculation behind it. The cost of health care services had become so important that Chrysler was treating physicians not as individual car customers, but as suppliers to the company. In essence, the rebate offer amounted to a kind of barter deal: you cut your prices, and I'll cut mine.

At the time of the Chrysler offer, the nation was in the midst of economic turmoil. In 1982 America was emerging from its worst slump since the Great Depression. The overthrow of the shah of Iran in 1979 had set off a replay of the traumatic 1973 oil crisis. Simultaneous double-digit inflation and double-digit unemployment mocked economic theorists. Prices soared, gas rationing set in, and auto sales slumped to a twenty-year low. Chrysler, the domestic auto company with the worst gas guzzlers, hemorrhaged red ink. The company lost $1.7 billion in 1979, surviving only because of controversial federal loan guarantees of $1.5 billion approved in 1980—that, and the skills of the company's brash new chairman and chief executive officer, Lee Iacocca.

Iacocca began his auto career began at Ford, where he rose swiftly to the presidency. In 1978 he was abruptly fired by Ford chairman Henry Ford II himself, but resurrection arrived a year later, when Iacocca was recruited for the top spot by a desperate Chrysler. In a whirlwind of activity, he stanched the financial bleeding, lobbied for the loan guarantees, and spearheaded an advertising blitz in which he personally pitched Chrysler cars to consumers. That done, he soon discovered that Chrysler's costs for health care were rising faster than any other company expense. In fact, Chrysler's largest single vendor was Michigan's Blue Cross and Blue Shield plan. And though General Motors had the highest health costs per worker among the auto companies, Chrysler's sales volume was so low that each of its cars carried a disproportionate share of the medical costs for its active workers, laid-off workers, and retirees.

Iacocca telephoned Joseph Califano Jr., an old friend who had been secretary of HEW under President Jimmy Carter, with a bold offer: a seat on Chrysler's board of directors and a chance to confront rising medical costs head-on. Califano recalled a dinner meeting where the two discussed the details.

> Iacocca was aghast at Chrysler's health care costs. "They'll break this goddamn company if we don't do something about them."
>
> I agreed. I had tried unsuccessfully to alert American businesses to the dangers of rising health care costs when I was HEW Secretary. But it was like dropping a grain of sand on a beach. I had no impact. No one heard.
>
> Iacocca was getting me excited about the prospect of joining the Chrysler board. "Look," Iacocca said, "I'll set up a committee. . . . You say you want to do something about health care costs. You chair the committee, the health care committee of the board."
>
> I was hooked. No other corporate board had such a committee. . . .
>
> We started work almost immediately. What we found was appalling waste and inefficiency that exceeded my worst concerns about the health care system as Secretary of HEW.[18]

During the boom times of the early 1960s, Santa Claus had replaced Scrooge in corporate personnel departments. Like other large unionized companies, Chrysler paid every penny of its workers' medical costs. And like every other company, Chrysler received a federal tax deduction for these expenses. Every few years the company would add more goodies, such as coverage of prescription drugs or eyeglasses. Chrysler wasn't alone in this approach. Nationwide, about one in five workers paid for their own health insurance in 1963. By 1980 only one in twelve did.[19] A visitor driving down Detroit's East Jefferson Street to the United Auto Workers (UAW) headquarters in the early 1980s counted more hospitals and medical offices than gas stations.

At the same time the auto companies were encouraging workers to treat doctor and hospital visits like an all you can eat buffet, they were also agreeing to pay doctors the kind of "usual and customary" fees that nearly bankrupted Medicare. Califano, who had been a young White House aide when President Johnson cut his deal with the AMA, was horrified. Doctors were being given "the power to write their own checks on the Chrysler bank account," he complained.[20]

But the balance of power between private industry and the medical community was changing, just as had happened with the federal government. Once more, the reason was financial. When Congress passed Medicare and Medicaid in 1965, employer contributions for health insurance amounted to less than a tenth of pretax profits. A federally sponsored National Conference on Medical Costs held in 1967 had no corporate purchasers of health care on its advisory committee.[21] But from 1977 to 1983, as hospital inpatient expenses doubled every five years, corporate America started to wake up.[22] By the end of that period, employer expenses for health benefits equaled half of pretax profits. Just as soaring Medicare and Medicaid costs had prompted the politicians to slap controls on hospitals and doctors, private industry, too, reacted to the assault on its bottom line.[23] One key tool was the Employee Retirement Income Security Act (ERISA), passed in 1974. ERISA regulated pensions, but it also gave corporations that self-insured nearly unlimited freedom to design their health benefits plans.

About the same time that ERISA became law, the political involvement of the business community in health care issues was also changing. A group of large national companies formed the Washington Business Group on Health to focus the energy of corporate America on the health care delivery system. Locally, business could use ERISA to take control away from the health insurers, who depended on doctors' goodwill. Nationally, business could use organizations such as the Washington Business Group to increase policy clout. Revolution was in the air.

Unlike the government, Chrysler couldn't regulate or legislate its way out of its big medical bills. On the other hand, it could pick and choose which hospitals and doctors it would give its business to. In a decision that completely broke from the past, Chrysler's board-level health care committee—Califano, UAW president Douglas Fraser, and Jerome Holland, former head of the American Red Cross—voted to evaluate both the cost and the quality of medical providers. Chrysler would deal only with hospitals and doctors who operated efficiently *and* provided appropriate care.

Doctors and hospitals warned Chrysler that its tough stance would hurt workers. Califano and colleagues were uncowed. "We rejected the myth that aggressive cost controls would reduce the quality of care," wrote Califano in a later book titled *America's Health Care Revolution: Who Lives? Who Dies? Who Pays?* "Unnecessary hospitalization is an increased risk. Unnecessary surgery is an inexcusable risk.

So are unnecessary X-rays, blood tests or transfusions, biopsies and other lab tests. One of the first conclusions we reached was that cost controls and efficient health care delivery were essential to assuring our employees care of the highest quality."[24]

Consumer advocates agreed. "Bad medicine is what's costing us a lot of money, not good medicine," asserted Charles Inlander, president of the People's Medical Society. "If you cut out unnecessary medicine, there would be no cost crisis."[25]

With half a billion dollars in medical costs at stake, Chrysler embraced the concepts of medical auditing and computerized analysis that Lembcke and Slee had tried to persuade hospitals and doctors to adopt years before. Prodded by Chrysler, Blue Cross and Blue Shield of Michigan hired Boston's Health Data Institute to subject thirty months of Chrysler's medical expenses to a computerized review. The study involved over 67,000 separate hospital admissions and more than $217 million in charges. It uncovered widespread overutilization, inefficiency, waste, and fraud. For example, two-thirds of the hospitalizations of Chrysler workers for lower back pain were unnecessary; in three of eight hospitals audited, not a single one of the admissions for back pain was needed.

With union backing, Chrysler approached local hospitals to discuss needless hospital stays. The dental plan was altered to make employees more cost conscious. The company even began offering workers the chance to join an HMO. Health care costs for 1984 came in at $58 million under budget.

The money Chrysler saved was important, but the principles established by Chrysler's actions had a longer-lasting impact: private corporations had the right to review clinical information related to the overall medical treatment of its workers and to hold doctors and hospitals accountable for meeting standards of good practice. "The gospel lesson," wrote Califano, "is that hard-negotiating buyers, who treat health care like the other products they purchase, can change the system."[26]

Those "hard-negotiating buyers" did not have to be major corporations. They could be average consumers. But what companies like Chrysler and the general public both needed first was reliable information. Chrysler had its bills analyzed by an expensive consultant. In order for society at large to begin to move to the paradigm of medical accountability, the public needed more and better information about clinical care.

WHO LIVES, WHO DIES, WHO KNOWS

In the early 1970s, Ralph Nader's Public Citizen Health Research Group decided to publish a consumers' guide to health care. The activists stayed close to home, targeting the Washington, D.C., suburban area of Prince Georges County, Maryland. And by today's standards, the information the group sought was tame. Even Nader's Raiders lacked the temerity to ask about the outcome of care. Instead, Public Citizen requested information on fees, office hours, hospital privileges, and the doctors' attitudes toward prescribing certain drugs that were then controversial. This was still enough to set off an immediate confrontation with Maryland's state medical society.

Maryland law explicitly prohibited "information that would point out differences between doctors." Similar laws, based on the AMA's code of ethics, were on the books in thirty-two states, ostensibly to block misleading advertising. Any doctor who answered the survey risked expulsion, the state society declared. Only one-quarter of the doctors surveyed dared to respond.

On 17 January 1974, Public Citizen responded with a sharply worded press release and a lawsuit. Said the group:

> That this country tolerates the very worst along with the very best quality of medical care, the poorly trained doctor along with the well-trained, those who overcharge along with those who charge reasonable fees, can best be explained by the total lack of information consumers have about doctors. . . .
>
> If public access to information concerning differences in credentials, fees, accessibility and the like is regarded [as] illegal and unethical, what likelihood is there that information about differences in doctor quality will be judged the right of patients to know?[27]

Separately, Public Citizen asked a federal district court to enjoin the medical society from disciplining doctors who answered its questions, arguing that the Maryland law violated the First Amendment. Before the case could go to trial, the society settled out of court.[28] The magazine *Consumer Reports* followed that victory with an article telling people all over the country how they could undertake similar surveys in their own states. A key barrier protecting the medical community from outside scrutiny had broken down.

A much more famous federal court action about the same time also involved release of information. In 1974 a unanimous Supreme

Court ordered President Richard Nixon to give hundreds of tapes that had been secretly recorded in the privacy of the Oval Office to prosecutors investigating the Watergate scandal. Not long afterward, Nixon became the first president in American history to resign.

The Watergate affair marked a turning point in American life. "Freedom of information" laws, "open meetings" acts, and other statutes and regulations removed traditional barriers hiding government information from the public. Legal changes aside, changes in public expectations about accountability ultimately reverberated through the cloistered world of medicine. If presidents could not claim immunity from prying questions by outsiders, then how could physicians or hospitals? On a more practical level, increased accountability meant that government information on physicians and hospitals was not automatically secure from prying eyes.

Sure enough, the first published comparison of hospital mortality rates was triggered by the troubles of a public hospital, Long Island's Nassau County Medical Center. Pressured by questions about alleged problems in open-heart surgery, the medical center released its mortality figures to *Newsday* reporter David Zinman. Zinman then persuaded a private local hospital that had an excellent reputation to release its figures as a point of comparison. Next he persuaded most other Long Island hospitals doing the surgery that they would look bad if they didn't also make their results public. A story in the 30 June 1973 *Newsday* subsequently revealed that Nassau County Medical Center had nearly triple the death rate for open-heart bypass surgery as the second-worst Long Island hospital and nine times the rate of the best one.[29]

Others in the news media also began to discover comparative clinical information. *Chicago Tribune* science writer Ronald Kotulak used freedom of information laws to write about the death rates at Chicago-area hospitals from both open-heart surgery and cancer.[30] The *Baltimore Sun* used state data on mortality rates to compare costs and quality of hospitals statewide.

These efforts were only a prelude to the most influential public release of health quality information, that of the Health Care Financing Administration's mortality rates for Medicare patients. No less than the advent of HMOs, federal oversight, or corporate monitoring of health care, the publicity surrounding the HCFA mortality rate information marked the beginning of a new era. Although the initial information was flawed, and mostly ignored, it established a precedent that is rapidly being built upon today.

In the mid-1980s policymakers were worried that Medicare's transition from "cost plus" reimbursement for hospitals to a "fixed price" system would prompt hospitals to discharge patients before they received all needed treatment. To protect the elderly, HCFA compiled mortality rates for groups of procedures at selected hospitals. The calculations were crude, but officials intended the list only as a "tip sheet" for Medicare peer review organizations. HCFA flagged hospitals that were above or below a kind of arbitrary norm. Then it was up to the peer reviewers to examine patient medical records to determine if there really was a problem.

Unfortunately for HCFA, *New York Times* reporter Joel Brinkley found out that the list existed. His story prompted hundreds of requests for a copy of the document, and to the great surprise of HCFA bureaucrats, federal attorneys ruled that the federal Freedom of Information Act required the government to hand it over. The list ended up as a page 1 story in the 12 March 1986 *Times* and the lead item in countless other newspapers and television news broadcasts.[31] The bureaucrats and the medical community immediately predicted the worst.

"This was never meant to be used by consumers," lamented acting HCFA director Henry Desmaris, while fearful hospital executives called the release "dumb" and "utter folly." But the cat was out of the bag. The American Association of Retired Persons argued, "It is better to err on the side of providing more information to consumers."

HCFA showed 142 hospitals with death rates higher than average and 127 with lower than average rates. The agency warned that its information was tentative. As if to emphasize the point, the institution with the highest death rate turned out to be a hospice in Nevada.

Technical flaws aside, the news that comparative information on clinical quality could be—would be!—released to the public with real hospital names attached sent shock waves through the medical community. Physicians and hospitals had been unable to either prevent or prepare for an event they bitterly opposed. Legitimate concerns were mixed in with bizarre objections. One downstate Illinois hospital complained about HCFA's using a patient's age as a factor in adjusting for the underlying death risk. The hospital noted that the Medicare patients who died there the previous year were generally older than their average life expectancy. Under those circumstances, the hospital couldn't understand the fuss.[32]

The permanent HCFA administrator who took office a couple of months after the first release of information proceeded to make a virtue out of necessity. If Ralph Nader and his allies favored consumerism from a liberal perspective, the conservative Reagan administration would champion data release as a critical part of a free market. "At HCFA, we believe consumers should have the information they need to make intelligent choices for their health and well-being," said William Roper, a soft-spoken Alabama pediatrician.[33] Roper pointedly emphasized that he had the full political support of his boss, Health and Human Services secretary, and fellow physician, Otis Bowen.

Roper improved the methodology and expanded the list to include all hospitals. Although the medical community remained unhappy, Roper became famous for his often-repeated admonition: "Don't let the perfect be the enemy of the good." The government, said Roper, should be part of "an advocacy effort to inform the public." Roper was also keenly aware of the precedent HCFA's action set. "We believe this will have an important spillover effect," he said.[34]

Roper tirelessly lobbied the leaders of the hospital and physician community to support his quality measurement agenda. Quality measurement and management started to become socially acceptable. The journal *Inquiry* devoted its spring 1988 issue to "the challenge of quality." There was even a long section on Ernest Amory Codman. And the *New England Journal of Medicine* proclaimed the arrival of "the Era of Assessment and Accountability." This was nothing short of a revolution, wrote editor Arnold Relman in a much-quoted editorial that frankly acknowledged the role played by economic necessity: "We can no longer afford to provide health care without knowing more about its successes and failures."[35]

And then . . . the revolution temporarily petered out. In November 1988 George Bush was elected president, and Bill Roper left HCFA the next year for a domestic policy position at the White House. Changing paradigms is hard work; although medical leaders may have been charmed by Roper, the rank and file continued to regard quality measurement and accountability with the same suspicion as in Codman's day. Roper himself had attributed HCFA's success to the "golden rule"—he who has the gold rules.[36] When the pressure from HCFA eased and an improving economy loosened tight corporate medical budgets, the interest in "assessment and accountability" waned.

Back in 1973, Paul Ellwood and coauthor Michael Herbert had

written in the *Harvard Business Review* that "the health maintenance organization (HMO) offers corporations a means of getting a better health care product to the consumer at a better price than the conventional form of health care delivery." The two men pointed out that corporate purchasers could utilize their "vast purchasing power" in HMO contracts.[37] But it would take a few years before the force of that argument hit home and accountability came to stay. Meanwhile, the old paradigm still had some life left in it. "When the [political and financial] pressure's on, people do [quality measurement]," sighed John Ball, former president of the American College of Physicians "As soon as the pressure's off, they don't."[38]

Nonetheless, a turning point had been reached. The performance of doctors and hospitals would now be subjected to outside scrutiny and evaluation by the government, private industry, and the public. Sometimes that would be uncomfortable. Like the automakers, doctors and hospital administrators now worried about picking up the morning newspaper and reading an unflattering performance review. Being held accountable for performance can churn up such basic human emotions as fear, shame, guilt, blame, and anger. Not only that, it changes behavior.

PART 3

Holding Medicine Accountable for Results

CHAPTER NINE

A New York State of Mind

> We talk about the interests of the medical profession, the interests of the hospitals, the interests of the nursing homes; but above all else, the whole of the health care system exists for one person, and that's the individual who needs it.
> —David Axelrod, M.D., 1990

It is almost 7:00 P.M. at Winthrop-University Hospital in Mineola, New York, when William Scott and Scott Schubach enter the empty offices of the cardiac surgery department and flip on the light in a narrow conference room. The two men began operating on their first patients of the day some twelve hours before. Now, their surgical garb exchanged for coats and ties, they are looking over the medical charts and diagnostic scans of the men and women who will be their surgery patients tomorrow. When the review is completed, one last ritual awaits before the two men can go home. Together, Scott and Schubach visit the rooms of each of the patients whose hearts they have operated on in the past few days and those they will operate on starting twelve hours from now.

The two surgeons radiate understated confidence. Schubach, clean-cut, trim, and in his early thirties, grew up in Long Island, the suburban New York City area where Winthrop-University is located. He was practicing at New Hampshire's Dartmouth-Hitchcock Medical Center when he was wooed back to his native region by Scott, Winthrop-University's chief of cardiac surgery. Schubach's senior by about a decade, Scott has tousled brown-and-silver hair and a salt-and-pepper mustache. The diplomas in his office reflect blue-chip credentials: medical school at Harvard, training in cardiac surgery at Stanford, and a teaching position at Yale–New Haven Hospital. But as Scott chats with patients in the thick accent of his native Wilkes-Barre, Pennsylvania, he exhibits no trace of the self-importance that sometimes affects senior surgeons at academic institutions.

The first room where Scott and Schubach stop is occupied by a sixty-eight-year-old retired engineer for a medical products company. As might be expected, the patient shows a keen interest in the technical details of his imminent surgery. Scott swings easily into a discussion of the clinical specifications of the artificial heart valve he plans to implant the next day. When the patient asks warily whether the preferred model comes in a variety of sizes, Scott assures him there are plenty of choices on the shelf in case a last-minute substitution is needed. The man's adult son, noting the lateness of the hour, jokes nervously to dispel the unspoken worry that hangs in the air.

"You going home early tonight or what?" the son asks.

"Absolutely," replies Scott genially.

"Can I send anything over to the house [to help you sleep]?" shoots back the son, to laughter.

Other patients seek reassurance in other ways. Down the hall from the engineer, a woman in her forties—a rarity on a cardiac floor—recalls that both her grandfathers died young of massive heart attacks. Her bypass surgery is aimed at avoiding that fate. A few doors from her, an African American man of fifty-eight anxiously voices his need to shed the disability brought on by his persistent chest pain and get back to full-time work at the nearby aerospace company.

Whatever the patient's mood, Scott and Schubach spend an unhurried few minutes responding to questions both spoken and unspoken. They soothe, they reassure, they explain. Then, when it is time to leave, one of the surgeons always looks the patient in the eye and offers a personal promise: "We'll take good care of you tomorrow."

It is a poignant moment, one that speaks to the soul of the patient-physician bond. What makes the pledge particularly interesting in New York State is that bypass surgery patients do not have to take a surgeon's promise wholly on faith. A public scorecard shows the success rate of each hospital and almost every surgeon, allowing potential bypass patients to check out the "win-loss" record much as they would for a baseball or football team. Actually, the bypass scorecard is more precise than the sports standings. A sports team's win-loss record doesn't reflect whether the opponents it faced were strong or weak. By contrast, New York's bypass surgery scorecard is "risk adjusted" to take into account the difficulty of success—the extent to which the patient's illness before surgery created a risk of death.

Using this risk adjustment, the New York State Department of Health calculates the success rate for bypasses (formally known as coronary artery bypass grafts, or CABG) for every hospital and for every surgeon at the hospital who performs a certain minimum number of procedures. The mortality rate, and how it compares with the state average, is printed in a brief booklet released to the news media and made available without charge to consumers. Some patients prefer, as always, to trust the choice of hospital and surgeon completely to their cardiologists. Others, though confident about their cardiologists, also do a little checking on their own. One of the Winthrop-University patients confides, "I was reading it just last week."

It is doubtful that any potential patient who read the pamphlet just a couple of years earlier would have picked Winthrop-University for this life and death procedure. The hospital's heart program finished a discouraging twenty-sixth out of the thirty similar programs in the state, and the individual surgeons at Winthrop-University generally ranked just as poorly. Within the hospital, the subpar results were not a total surprise. The hospital's own cardiologists were discreetly referring some complicated cases to surgeons at competing hospitals, and the Winthrop-University administration had launched a national search for a new chief of cardiac surgery. The publicity, though, ratcheted up the pressure for quick action. To persuade Bill Scott to leave Yale–New Haven Hospital, Winthrop-University's chief executive promised him patients, political support, and deep pockets. The important thing was to "fix the problem."

In the popular imagination the surgeon is a lone hero, the warrior whose cool-headedness in the heat of battle allows him to single-handedly create order out of chaos in the fight against sickness and disease. Yet the most successful surgeons, like successful generals, abhor unpredictability. Rather than conquering chaos, they seek to minimize it through painstaking preparation. They are obsessed with anticipating potential problems and figuring out how to avoid or react to them. The maxim of *Poor Richard's Almanac,* "a little neglect may breed great mischief," is ingrained in their every action. They believe:

> For want of a nail, the shoe was lost.
> For want of a shoe, the horse was lost.
> For want of a horse, the rider was lost.

Bill Scott was the kind of man who checked every nail in every horseshoe before he ventured out for a ride. Every patient was subjected to a meticulous examination. There was no such thing as "routine" heart surgery. Cardiologist Anthony Gambino made an analogy. "You bring your car in and it needs to be fixed," said Gambino. "Certain mechanics will look through in five minutes and . . . change [a] part, but you've still got that same 'click.' Other mechanics who investigate the problem more in depth make sure they cover all the bases. Bill covers all the bases, and he expects everyone else around him to do the same."

"He's really very strict," agreed Richard Steingart, the hospital's chief of cardiology. "By going into the surgery with an understanding of exactly what the operation is that's going to be done, you minimize the number of surprises when the patient is [cut] open and defenseless. You want to make sure you don't get fooled."

Not every surgeon goes to the same trouble. Perhaps the problem is that what was once a miracle procedure has become routine. Bypass surgery was introduced into widespread use in the mid-1960s. It became so popular so quickly that it was part of everyday practice well before clinical trials could evaluate it.[1] By the mid-1980s, it had become one of the most common of all surgical procedures. Still, "routine" is not the same as "simple," and even a run-of-the-mill bypass provides ample drama.

The patient undergoing a coronary artery bypass lies heavily sedated on the operating room table, tubes and hoses protruding from both sides. The open chest cavity is framed by thick clamps holding apart the two halves of the chest wall. Inside that cavity, exposed and vulnerable, sits the heart, its color more a mix of red and purple than the bright red of a Valentine's Day card. To the patient's left, a piano-sized heart-lung machine stands ready to take on for a few minutes the job that this fist-sized organ does for a lifetime. The machine will remove the blood, cleanse it of carbon dioxide, infuse it with oxygen, and then pump it back through the patient's body once again. When the patient is ready, the surgeon carefully pours a special cardioplegic solution directly onto the heart's surface. (In one hospital they hold the fluid in a heart-shaped purple plastic container.) Like water dousing a candle flame, the fluid snuffs out the regular thump-lump beating of the heart. It goes silent, and the electrodes monitoring its every movement send a flat-line picture to nearby cathode-ray terminals. At that moment, a race against time begins.

A heart-lung machine mimics the functions of a real heart, but it cannot quite duplicate them. The trick is to rely on the device for as little time as possible. As the patient's own heart lies still and surgical technicians call out readings from the machine, the heart surgeon begins to stitch a pathway to life. He methodically sews a healthy artery extracted from the patient's chest wall onto each side of a clogged coronary vessel running through the heart. When this mending is completed, the arterial blood that barely squirmed through the blocked coronary passage before surgery will bypass the obstruction and travel freely along the detour. Depending on how many arteries are clogged, the surgeon may repeat this procedure up to four times before restarting the heart.

In the harsh lights of the operating room, this stopping and starting of a human heart is a technical accomplishment: on; off; on again. Yet something mysterious occurs that no monitor or gauge can record. While the patient's conscious mind passes the time in a deeply drugged sleep, a part of the brain nonetheless records this terrifying dress rehearsal for death. In subconscious mourning for themselves, some bypass patients suffer profound depression in the weeks following their operation.

Of course, in the surgery's immediate aftermath, simply waking up to life renewed is a feeling sweet enough to sweep some patients into a kind of euphoria. At Winthrop-University, surgeons Scott and Schubach visibly relax as they visit the room of a patient who is preparing to spend his last night in the hospital before discharge the next morning. Art Segal is going home.

Segal is a gregarious, thin man in his mid-fifties. He holds forth in a room filled with get-well cards from family and friends. His surgery is over, memorialized by assorted scars and by a souvenir heart-shaped red pillow bearing the Winthrop-University name. He is elated. "You don't want to have this [procedure] done, but if you have to, this place is great," Segal pronounces. He points to Scott. "He does three surgeries, he's in here making visiting hours . . . and you'd think he'd go, 'Uhhh!' But the guy's as fresh as like he's not doing anything!" A pause, then the punch line. "The only problem is, he's twenty-seven, and he looks. . . ."

Segal's condition on arrival at Winthrop-University was no laughing matter. A local cardiologist had found blockages in all four of his coronary arteries, with one key vessel more than 90 percent shut. "If I can get you Dr. Scott, that should be your first choice," Segal recalls his cardiologist saying. Winthrop-University promptly arranged for a private ambulance to bring Segal in. Still, Scott didn't rush Segal into the operating room. Instead, the surgeon ordered a detailed physical workup, which discovered another ticking time bomb. It wasn't only Segal's coronary arteries that were clogged. His carotid artery, the main carrier of blood to the brain, was also nearly closed. For Scott this new finding waved a yellow caution flag. If he operated on Segal, the difference between a natural heartbeat and the artificial pumping of the heart-lung machine used during bypass surgery could prove catastrophic.

"The patient's heartbeat on bypass is not the same as beating on its own," Scott explains. "It's not the same pulsital flow, it's not the same distribution of blood flow. It doesn't exactly have the same characteristics. Certainly, it doesn't have the same [high] pressure. . . . If you have a carotid problem, the incident of stroke is somewhat higher during the bypass. Stroke during bypass could leave you with real trouble. You could wake up with a significant neurologic deficit [severe brain damage] or you could die." Art Segal is an active man who is only in his fifties. Says Scott, "I think a stroke [can be] worse than dying."

Scott invited a neurosurgeon into the operating room to clear the blocked carotid before he began the bypass. As a result, Art Segal did not have a stroke. Nor, of course, did he die. A tone of unmistakable pride creeps into Scott's voice as he relates this story."We spend a lot of time making sure the patients are ready for [the] operation," he says. "We spend a lot of time taking care of patients postoperatively. One of the things that lets our program get a little bit of an edge is we spend a lot of time thinking about each patient."

When Scott took over the Winthrop-University program, his first goal had to be improved patient survival. He methodically reviewed the charts of the twenty-five patients who had died the year before, making careful notes about the course of care. Then he sat down and talked about each patient death with the surgeon involved."I got a lot of excuses: it was the patient's fault, it was the nurse's fault, it was the scheduling's fault. It was God's fault. It was never their fault. . . . At the end of the conversation, I told each of them it was *their* fault, because it was *their* patient. That put things in perspective."

As with many tasks where the margin of error is small, there is a well-documented link in heart surgery between how frequently the procedure is performed and the likelihood that the patient will survive—the "practice makes perfect" principle. Because of that, New York State has strictly regulated the number of hospitals that can do the procedure. Other states, such as Illinois, have rules regarding surgical minimums but leave enforcement to the honor code. And still other states allow hospitals to perform whatever procedures they wish.

Some years ago an Intersociety Commission for Heart Disease Resources, composed of prominent surgeons and other medical society representatives, issued guidelines advising hospitals what personnel and minimum caseloads were necessary to do the bypass procedure properly. Professional self-control proved no match for the enthusiasm generated by a procedure that was new, promised potentially enormous patient benefit, and was lucrative for both hospital and surgeon. In 1969, just two years after the technique was formally described in the medical literature, only 5 percent of the 480 hospitals performing bypasses met those standards. By the mid-1970s, most still didn't.[2] By 1995, just two-thirds of the 1,023 United States hospitals performing open-heart surgery met the recommended minimum volume.[3]

In recent years the Society of Thoracic Surgeons has assembled detailed clinical information on outcomes of the procedure. However, the society prohibits public release of figures on individual doctors or hospitals, or even comparisons among states or regions of the country. There is one exception: surgeons who want to disclose their personal results—even if just for marketing purposes—can do so. "This whole system was designed for the individual surgeon for his own use," the head of the society's data committee explained to the *Chicago Tribune* in 1993.[4]

At Winthrop-University Hospital, Scott was not as forbearing as the professional societies have been. He quickly informed a couple of heart surgeons that their personal caseloads were too low. Each heart surgeon had to be the "primary" surgeon on a minimum of fifty open-heart procedures a year and either the primary or secondary surgeon on a total of at least one hundred cases. Shortly afterward, two surgeons stopped doing the procedure and a third signaled that he was ready to stop. One of those doctors also filed a lawsuit against Scott, an outcome he shrugs off as a cost of doing business.[5]

"Organized medicine has always been reluctant to police itself with teeth, except for obvious people on the fringe [such as drunks]," Scott says.

Scott's next step was to beef up the entire surgical team. The individual surgeon's skills are a key component, but only one component, of successful surgery. Like a football coach trying to turn around a losing franchise, Scott began investing in the heart program's future. He bought new equipment, such as an echocardiograph to image patients' hearts before surgery, and upgraded older equipment, such as the perfusion machines to keep patients breathing during bypass. He recruited new players in the "free agent" market, luring physicians' assistants, nurses, and medical technologists who specialized in the specific and delicate choreography of the open-heart procedure. He brought in a new cadre of "assistant coaches," installing individuals who shared his approach to surgical care as directors of the cardiac surgery operating room, the cardiac surgery intensive care unit, the perfusion service, and cardiac anesthesiology.

All these changes were accompanied by a revamped "playbook." The best equipment and the most skilled quarterback cannot compensate for a team that is confused. A revealing study of intensive care units at thirteen sophisticated hospitals across the country illustrates the critical role played by well-coordinated care. All the ICUs had similar technical capabilities, but there was a frightening difference in mortality rates. Patients at the best ICU had a 41 percent greater chance of surviving than would have been predicted, given how sick they were before treatment, while patients at the worst hospital had a 58 percent greater chance of dying than would be expected. What caused this yawning gap was not technology, but "the interaction and communication between physicians and nurses."[6]

At Winthrop-University, Scott stressed teamwork. For example, the cardiac unit's system of handling lab results was streamlined to make sure surgeons received certain vital information before surgery. And after surgery, the patients were monitored around the clock by specially trained nurses. Scott, meanwhile, kept checking the "game film," looking at patients' charts, looking for ways to improve.

The hard work paid off as Winthrop-University rose steadily in the standings. After a year, the state health department ranked the hospital fifteenth, in the middle of the pack. Within another year, Winthrop-University first in Long Island. In the cardiac surgery department, copies of a newspaper article on the hospital's new status were passed from hand to hand and posted triumphantly on bulletin boards. The hospital's program has stayed near the top, and Scott and Schubach make no secret of their belief that this success reflects the constant attention to a hundred small things every day.

"The patients have a better chance of surviving," Schubach says. "It's not just random. Whether it's that we put the stitches in differently or whether [it's because] we're there at eight o'clock at night talking to patients and reviewing all the information, . . . these changes in numbers have happened for a reason. The system has changed."

New York State's decision to publish a cardiac report card "was a remarkably enlightened act," adds Scott. "I think the concept is something we as physicians should have done many years ago. . . . Outcomes analysis [like the state report] has forced us all to deal with the wide spectrum of results and of quality of care in this country. [It] has forced organized medicine to deal with problems from within." Schubach concludes, "The statistics make . . . people accountable for their actions."

It was the kind of accountability that would have pleased Nightingale, Codman, Lembcke, and Slee. It did not, however, please most surgeons in New York. Giving up secrecy in favor of public disclosure of outcomes information was not their idea. In New York, however, when the state health department talks, doctors and hospitals have little choice but to listen.

DON'T ASK, DON'T TELL

> When people's ill, they comes to I,
> I physics, bleeds and sweats 'em;
> Sometimes they live, sometimes they die.
> What's that to I? I lets 'em.
> —Satirical verse punning on the name of British physician
> John Coakley Lettsom, 1744–1815

In 1988 a studious biostatistician named Edward Hannan received a deceptively simple assignment. Hannan's boss was David Axelrod, commissioner of the New York State Department of Health. New York has a unique database on hospital admissions. In reviewing information from it, Axelrod had become concerned about the persistently large differences in the bypass death rates at different state hospitals. The state health department keeps a strict regulatory grip on everything to do with medical quality. Hannan's mission was to find out to what extent the differences in death rates were related to the types of patients treated and how far they reflected the quality of patient care.

To do that, Hannan set out to design what he called a "statistical model that predicts the normative probability of death for each patient, based solely on the presence of preoperative risk factors."[7] Put plainly, Hannan's model was going to give the presurgical odds that a heart bypass patient would leave the hospital alive.

Hannan was not the only one interested in this topic at the time. Researchers in neighboring New Jersey were investigating the same question, but they were trying to develop a research tool.[8] Hannan needed something that could be used to improve everyday hospital treatment by assessing the quality of patient care. To ensure that the final product was clinically credible, he turned to the state's Cardiac Advisory Committee and asked its members to compile a list of the important indicators that predicted whether a bypass patient would survive. Not surprisingly, the list quickly stretched to a length that appeared utterly impractical. But Hannan wasn't through. He took the list and put each item through a stringent series of mathematical tests. Known as "regression analysis," the technique was designed to tease out which of the proposed indicators were essential in predicting death and to decide how to weigh the significance of each factor against the others.

Take a simple example of cause and effect. Suppose doctors agreed that heart bypass patients over eighty years old had an increased likelihood of dying from surgery. Although that might seem obvious, the obvious might not hold up under closer scrutiny. Maybe eighty-year-old patients with no earlier heart attacks fared as well as sixty-year-olds; perhaps eighty-year-olds with a previous heart attack were really the ones at higher risk.

Moreover, patients rarely vary in just one clinical sign. One eighty-year-old may have diabetes and be overweight; another could be overweight without diabetes; a third could have diabetes, have her weight under control, but smoke. Which is more important: age or smoking? Weight or diabetes? Relying on the doctor's intuition and experience to predict the influence of each of these variables is a hopeless task. Regression analysis balances all the multiple influences in a consistent way and then produces a probability of death for each patient based on that patient's specific clinical signs.

Unlike the Health Care Financing Administration, when it assembled the hospital mortality rates discussed in the previous chapter, Hannan had the luxury of crafting a customized system that focused on one very specific clinical event. Moreover, since the federal government was responsible for every hospital in the nation, it was forced to rely on a computerized analysis of medical claims forms. Hannan could tap into clinical data reported by the doctors and nurses directly involved in the procedure.

By mid-1990, a New York surgeon could type a list of clinical signs into a program called "prob mort," press a couple of keys, and play God. "Prob mort" stood for "probability of mortality." The number that appeared on the screen represented the chances, give or take a small margin of error, that the average patient with these same signs and symptoms would not leave the hospital alive.

At Winthrop-University Hospital, for example, Art Segal's initial "prob mort" was a mere 2 percent. Despite his severe coronary blockages, he was only in his fifties. Then the complications began. Segal's heart stopped several times while he was undergoing further diagnostic work. Next the blocked carotid artery was discovered. By the time of Segal's operation, the odds of surgical success had changed from a slam dunk to something worrisomely like a coin toss. "Prob mort," said the emotionless computer, was 52.7 percent.

An elegant mathematical model is only as reliable as the information going into it. To encourage conscientiousness in gathering and reporting information, the state health department informed the hospitals' directors of cardiac surgery that each would be held personally responsible for providing good data. To emphasize the point, the department sent in inspectors at the beginning of the program to compare the information on the cardiac surgery reporting system with actual medical records.

Hospitals could have declined to participate in the cardiac project. No rule required them to spend the considerable amount of time, energy, and money it took to collect the information. In practice, however, the health department controlled what hospitals could charge and what services they could offer. (That long-standing system was phased out at the end of 1996.) The department also inspects for violations of safety and quality rules and metes out punishment to transgressors. Like a prison inmate accepting the warden's "invitation" for lunch, every hospital with a heart program "volunteered" to go along with what the state wanted.

After collecting and analyzing six months of data, the health department produced a list of hospitals whose performance was significantly better or worse than predicted. Then the department collected all the medical records of bypass patients who died at these "best" or "worst" facilities. A case-by-case physician review of each patient's chart validated the measurement system. The disparity in outcomes was due to the care, not the type of patients treated. At the worst hospitals, the number of deaths where there were questions about care ranged from 18 to 64 percent. At the very best hospital, the figure was just 10 percent.[9]

Finally, in December 1990 the state let the public in on the results. Nearly three decades after the National Halothane Study and fifteen years after the Stanford Institutional Differences Study, the truth about the wide range of outcomes in medical care was finally major news.[10]

The relation between a hospital's mortality rate and its quality of care "has rarely been tested in studies that adjust [the] mortality rate for [patient] severity of illness," Hannan wrote later. Now "indications are that this relationship . . . may be strong."[11] "Indications," indeed. Even when initial condition was taken into account, a patient undergoing heart surgery was 4.4 times as likely to die at the lowest-performing hospital in New York State as at the best-performing one.[12] Moreover, when the state dug a little deeper, the cause of the differences seemed clear: low-volume surgeons, like those whose privileges Bill Scott had revoked at Winthrop-University.

Among heart surgeons performing at least one hundred procedures a year, the risk-adjusted death rate ranged from zero to 11 percent. For those doing fewer than one hundred operations, by contrast, the death rates of individual surgeons ran as high as 82 percent for a doctor doing only nine cases.[13] By comparison, the average statewide death rate, adjusted for patient risk, was just 3.7 percent.[14]

Hannan's July 1989 article in the *Journal of the American Medical Association* prompted an immediate demand for names. A Freedom of Information Act (FOIA) request from *Newsday* reporter David Zinman, the journalist who published the first comparative information on heart surgery mortality rates back in 1973, finally pried loose the doctor statistics with the names masked. The result, published in March 1991, resembled an old joke: "Here are the latest baseball scores: 10 to 3, 4 to 1, and in a squeaker, 1–0." *Newsday* went to court to get the physicians' identities.

"In talks I had with David Axelrod, he was supportive of my getting this information and making it public, but he felt it wouldn't be politically correct for him to say it, because he would lose credibility with the medical establishment," Zinman recalled in an interview.[15] "But he encouraged me to file an FOIA and follow it with a [law]suit."

To Zinman's pleased surprise, his editors agreed to take on the state. Meanwhile, state lawyers ignored pleas from the health department to argue against data release on technical grounds (some experts felt the numbers were not yet statistically significant). Instead, they argued that the public wasn't smart enough to understand the information. "The data [will] be misunderstood and misused by the public, resulting in significant adverse impact upon the physicians identified by the data, with little public benefit," the health department asserted in its legal brief.[16]

State Supreme Court justice Harold J. Hughes ruled in favor of *Newsday*. "Following the department's position to its logical end, it appears that if members of the public were more intelligent, it would be in the public interest to disclose this information, he wrote in an October 1991 opinion."[17] On 18 December 1991, *Newsday* published the first doctor-specific performance information ever made public.[18] An angry Cardiac Advisory Committee promptly recommended that the state stop collecting information on individual doctors altogether, but it reluctantly changed its mind under pressure from Axelrod. In a second vote, the committee approved releasing individual rankings using a three-year rolling record of surgeons who performed at least two hundred operations during that period. The health department's rationale for reversing itself was simple: its members knew that releasing the results would save lives.

THE DIFFERENT FACES OF TRUTH

Two views of the same events:

The first perspective: A hospital misuses information to end the career of a blameless physician. At a meeting on the topic of quality improvement, a respected cardiac surgeon from New England emotionally denounced the New York State rankings for "ruining institutions." Asked privately to substantiate that assertion, the surgeon related an anecdote. He told how a mentor and friend was asked by Strong Memorial Hospital, an affiliate of the University of Rochester, to stop doing bypass surgery. The wronged doctor was a "legendary teacher," the New England surgeon said indignantly.

The second perspective: A hospital responds to information and makes tough decisions in order to improve patient care. Robert Panzer is associate medical director for quality improvement at the University of Rochester Medical Center, which includes Strong Memorial. Strong's heart surgery program was ranked as one of the worst in the state in the health department's initial 1990 report. At a workshop sponsored by the Healthcare Forum, a trade group, Panzer candidly explained what happened next. "Not the thing you want to wake up and see [in the newspaper], but it gets your attention rather quickly. . . . The clinicians in the [cardiac] area . . . had some soul-searching discussions."

Although Strong Memorial prides itself on its commitment to

continuous quality improvement, the hospital never suspected problems in its cardiac unit. But as a skeptical team of physicians dug through patient records, some disturbing patterns began to emerge. If a patient already on a medical floor required emergency heart surgery, the hospital raced to find the first available surgeon. That seemingly logical response, however, contained a hidden flaw. By definition, the hospital's busiest heart surgeons were the ones who had the most cases. That volume, in turn, made these busy surgeons the ones most likely to obtain good results in complex cases. Yet precisely because the high-volume surgeons were busy, they were rarely available to handle emergencies. It was a catch-22: the emergency patients whose condition demanded the highest level of skill were most likely to be operated on by the lower-volume surgeons whose skills were not the best.

There was one more important twist. Because these more "difficult" emergency patients had a higher probability of death to begin with, the informal quality assurance system of peer review failed. No individual surgeon had made an egregious error. It was only after the state database sounded an alert that the hospital reexamined every patient death. Taken aback by what it found, Strong Memorial changed its triage system.

"We act as if all physicians and all parts of the system are equally capable for all patients, and I don't think that's so," said Panzer. "[Instead], we found need for [surgeons'] retirement." Without the objective data from the state, he adds, "it's very hard for people to be open [about colleagues]."[19]

"I SAY IT'S SPINACH, AND I SAY TO HELL WITH IT"

> One of the most time-consuming things is to have an enemy.
> —E. B. White

It is a few days before the Fourth of July weekend, and officials from the New York State Department of Health are facing a roomful of heart surgeons, cardiologists, and cardiac nurses who have gathered in the ballroom of a hotel on the outskirts of La Guardia airport.

Since saving lives is the point of heart surgery, state officials should be getting a hero's reception. The risk-adjusted death rate for bypass patients has dropped by an eye-catching 40 percent since the cardiac reporting program began. That translates into hundreds of lives saved. New York boasts the lowest reported CABG mortality rate in the nation.

Other factors also argue for harmony. Commissioner David Axelrod's relationship with the state's medical community was increasingly marked by acrimony and confrontation. Axelrod, however, has been succeeded by Mark Chassin, a third-generation New York physician.[20] Chassin is no shrinking violet. Ambitious and driven, he holds an undergraduate degree, an M.D., a master's degree in public policy, and a doctorate in public health from UCLA. He is also a widely published researcher in the area of quality of care. But Chassin has also spent twelve years as a practicing emergency room physician, so he is ready to hold out an olive branch to the doctors "in the trenches." To the vast majority of physicians trying to do their best, he offers cooperation in a journey of continuous quality improvement. "The health department ought to be helping institutions to look at each other's processes of care," Chassin declared in his June 1992 inaugural address. "The goal [is] not to punish, but to share best practices among institutions so that everybody's quality is improved."

Unfortunately, the surgeons and cardiologists at this 1994 meeting are refusing to follow the upbeat script. A large number believe neither that the patient's risk of death is measured accurately by the health department nor that the outcome of care has improved because of it. Moreover, despite steps the state has taken to tone down sensationalist reporting, many surgeons are still angry that their names appear in the paper every year. The accumulated resentment prompts a steady barrage of hostile questions. The conciliatory answers from Chassin and his colleagues, whether based on statistical analysis or on testimonials from working surgeons who have used the data to improve care, have no effect on the audience's mood. Although Chassin may want continuous improvement, what he gets is fear and loathing. The assembled clinicians' attitude most closely mirrors that of the little boy being urged to eat his vegetables in a famous *New Yorker* cartoon. Responds the child: "I say it's spinach, and I say to hell with it."

On its face, this is a puzzling response. If a researcher discovered a drug or device that reduced bypass deaths by 40 percent, surgeons would loudly demand immediate regulatory approval. Moreover, the state's cardiac surgery reporting system (CSRS) has been subjected to repeated scientific peer review. "CSRS became the first profiling system with sufficient clinical detail to generate credible comparisons of providers' outcomes," wrote New York University Medical Center researchers Jesse Green and Neil Wintfeld in a *New England Journal of Medicine* commentary. "For this reason, CSRS has been recognized by many states and purchasers of care as the gold standard among systems of its kind."[21]

Yet the ill feeling remains. Opponents insist that the performance reports have backfired. Good surgeons are allegedly avoiding operations on sick patients out of fear that a bad result could lead to professionally devastating publicity. V. A. "Manny" Subramanian, chief of cardiovascular and thoracic surgery at Manhattan's Lenox Hill Hospital, gives voice to a common theme. "Sick patients are not getting taken care of," charges Subramanian, whose hospital is on the wealthy Upper East Side. "It happens every day."

Not surprisingly, Ed Hannan sees things differently. As a Ph.D. in applied mathematics, he tries to employ logic. Whenever surgeons raise an objection to the prediction methodology, the objection is mathematically tested, says Hannan, who is now a consultant to the health department and a professor in the State University of New York's School of Public Health. If some clinical factor is found improve the predictive ability of the algorithm (formula), it is added. Otherwise it is left out. Over time, the algorithm has grown to forty risk factors for each patient. As for the belief that surgeons are penalized for treating sicker patients, the system overpredicts the risk of death for those who are most severely ill, precisely to discourage doctors from turning them away.[22] Hannan won't back off: "I think lives have been saved," he declares.

As logical as the health department's reasoning may be, it omits a key variable than can't be punched into a calculator. Public perceptions count. State officials once held high hopes that their "gold standard" would be widely adopted, thereby making possible accurate national comparisons of bypass surgery. Instead, not one state has adopted New York's methodology. The doubts spread by opponents of the measure have even infected the state's most powerful newspaper, the nationally respected *New York Times.* Warned the *Times* in a 1995 editorial: "Doctors can reach the top of a report card because they turned away hard cases." Similarly, the state legislature quickly punctured a health department trial balloon to link the outcome of care to payment. Medical lobbyists got the state legislature to expressly ban even an experiment with that approach.[23]

The state health department was trounced so thoroughly in the public relations battle that Albert Siu, a physician and frustrated

Chassin deputy, decided that making public the performance scores of individual surgeons had been a mistake. Siu (after leaving office) told a meeting of health researchers that the department ended up spending too much of its energy fending off surgeons' attacks on the validity of the individual data.[24]

Yet for all the criticism of New York's effort, the undeniable trend is to increasingly hold hospitals and individual physicians accountable for the results of patient care. In that context, what happened in New York holds lessons for the entire country. Has the New York report card saved lives, as proponents say, or has it backfired and hurt patients, as critics claim? Or is there some rhetorical truth on both sides?

A hint of the likely answer comes from quality improvement legend Joseph Juran, founder of the Juran Institute. "With licensed professionals, they have a monopoly and resist change," said Juran. "The last reason they'll give is, 'This is a threat to my monopoly, to my status.' They'll give more plausible reasons. You have to look beyond that."[25] Except that, oddly, no one ever did.

BEARING FALSE WITNESS

> The great enemy of the truth is very often not the lie—deliberate, contrived and dishonest—but the myth—persistent, persuasive and unrealistic.
>
> —John F. Kennedy, 1962

The allegation that sick patients are being turned away so that doctors will look better on their state report cards is a plausible one. This is, after all, a world where airlines fiddle with flight schedules to boost their on-time record and colleges scheme to look good in magazine rankings. "Gaming" results also has a long history in medicine. William and Charles Mayo grumbled about surgeons whose reporting of their surgical successes seemed based on a careful definition of which cases to include in the analysis. In eighteenth-century Scotland, one of the first recorded attempts to gather accurate hospital mortality statistics was frustrated because the reporting institutions repeatedly tinkered with the true numbers.

The first step to take in investigating an allegation is to ask for evidence from the person making it. At the New York State Department of Health seminar, I repeatedly asked dissident surgeons for an "off the record" assessment: Had they ever turned away a patient or known, firsthand, anybody who had? In each case the answer was no. In fact, each surgeon assured me he personally did such a good job that it was his ethical obligation to tackle the tough cases.

Others who allege dire consequences appear equally removed from firsthand evidence. The Medical Society of the State of New York (MSSNY) has a history of opposing the collection of detailed information on physicians' activities.[26] In 1993 the staff of the American Medical Association asked MSSNY for its evaluation of the cardiac reporting system. Here, from an AMA document, was the response:

> MSSNY continues to be "very concerned with the inappropriate dissemination of [physician-specific health care] data." *Although MSSNY has not collected any scientific data* regarding the impact of NYSDH data releases on the quality, access and cost of care, *its perception is that some physicians within the state may have become more selective in treating high-risk patients.* [MSSNY] . . . "looks forward to the time when the statistics have proven to be dependable and meaningful and can be reported fairly and responsibly." [Quotation marks in the original; emphasis added]

In other words, in the absence of real data, the society passed along its "perception" that patients were being harmed and that the data were undependable, meaningless, and unfairly reported.[27] Meanwhile, the state medical society did warn that "patients may suffer *psychologically* [emphasis added] if they have to get treated by a surgeon with a higher than average mortality rate."[28]

My analysis of news stories about patients allegedly turned away found distortions and exaggerations. The most prominent such article, a 1992 opinion piece in the *New York Times,* has metamorphosed in the retelling into a news story—something quite different from one person's opinion. The author, Mindy Byer, told a frightening story of how her very sick mother was nearly unable to find a heart surgeon. The reason, said Mindy, was because doctors were afraid they would look bad in the state report if Mrs. Byer died.[29] Fortunately, the seventy-six-year-old Mrs. Byer was eventually accepted for surgery at a Manhattan hospital, where a skilled surgeon saved her life. "If we weren't vocal, my mother would have died and nobody would have known anything about it," Mindy said.

The moral of the story is supposed to be that the state data system is dangerous. An interview with Mindy, however, yielded detail that made that conclusion a lot more ambiguous.[30]

To begin with, Mrs. Byer needed valve surgery, and the state data include only bypasses. Surgeons surely would have known that. Even so, one Long Island hospital immediately accepted Mrs. Byer. Unfortunately, the bed was filled by an emergency patient before she could be transferred. That's when the alleged problems began: another Long Island hospital said it had no open cardiac bed, but a medical resident confided to Mindy that the real reason was that the hospital wanted to treat low-risk patients to help out its performance rating. Was the resident correct, or was this just one more opinion? It's impossible to tell. Surgeons at two other hospitals told Mindy they thought her mother was too sick to survive the rigors of surgery. At a third hospital, however, a surgeon agreed to accept Mrs. Byer. Happily, she survived her surgery. Acknowledged Mindy, "If they thought they were going to lose her at [the other hospitals], it probably worked out better in the end."

So was Mrs. Byer the near victim of a surgical backlash against the state performance report, or did the story illustrate only a legitimate difference of medical opinion about when surgery is appropriate? New York State has one of the lowest levels of inappropriate bypass surgery in the nation.[31] Does Mrs. Byer's surviving her operation mean that the doctors who were reluctant to operate were wrong? Or does it mean that hindsight is always twenty-twenty and that Mrs. Byer was fortunate to have vocal children? The answers are not obvious.

The story of Mrs. Byer was retold by her son, Alan, a few months later in an 11 May 1992 *Newsday* article. *Newsday* also quoted another patient who had needed a bypass and valve surgery and was turned down by a local hospital, only to go to another hospital and do well. The newspaper quoted several surgeons asserting that they "knew" of patients being turned away, but "none of the cardiac surgeons interviewed said that they themselves turned away cases."[32]

The third media report about a hospital turning away heart surgery patients raises some interesting questions. A spokesman for North Shore University Hospital in Manhasset, Long Island, told *American Medical News* that the hospital turned away twenty-three high-risk patients in order to improve its bypass outcomes for that year. Because it did so, asserted the spokesman, North Shore's risk-adjusted mortality rate dropped from 5.15 percent in 1989–90 to 3.25 percent in 1991.[33] The North Shore spokesman portrayed the hospital's actions to *American Medical News* as "a form of health care rationing." This shocking public admission by a hospital deserves closer examination.

North Shore University is within an easy drive of several other institutions with open-heart programs. If the hospital was a "last resort"—the spokesman's words—then the rejected patients and their doctors either gave up on needed surgery when North Shore wouldn't do it or found that no other hospital would accept them. Alternatively, perhaps the rejected patients underwent surgery elsewhere, only to suffer complications or even death because no other hospital was as capable as North Shore.

However, there is no evidence that North Shore tracked what happened to the patients it rejected before making these serious allegations. And in any event, if the effect of being turned away at North Shore University was really so dire for these twenty-three individuals, is the state to blame? After all, there are laws requiring doctors to provide care in life and death situations, no matter what. Is North Shore really saying that it cared more for its report card score than it did about having "rationed" lifesaving care to these people? Or was the hospital perhaps engaging in a piece of rhetorical overkill that was encouraged by surgeons who shared the prejudices that lay behind it?

Arthur Levin, director of New York City's Center for Medical Affairs, is one who scoffs at the contention that patients with bad hearts are having trouble finding good surgeons. "I think it's a straw man," Levin says. "If some doctors turn away patients who don't do well [operating] on those patients, that's a public benefit."As it happens, Levin's assessment seems to be supported by the New York cardiac rankings for 1990 through 1992. During that period, North Shore University Hospital was the only hospital in Long Island with a death rate higher than expected. The hospital's chief of cardiac surgery also had results that were significantly worse than average.[34]

Until now, however, no one has linked those rankings to these anecdotes. Moreover, turning away sick patients is such outrageous behavior—if it happens—that one would think critics of the cardiac program would have rushed to document it. Yet no such studies have been published in the medical literature more than six years after the first physician "report card" appeared.

Some critics cite a 1996 *Circulation* piece that reported an increase in the number of New York residents going to the Cleveland Clinic for bypass surgery.[35] This article allegedly documents an access problem for New Yorkers with cardiac problems. The study, however, covers a five-year period; the New York data for hospitals were public for only three years of that time, and the information on named individual surgeons was public for just two of those five years. More to the point, even if the outmigration is true (and a paper presented to the 1996 American College of Cardiology meeting reached the opposite conclusion), it's hard to argue that patients' health—as opposed to physicians' wealth or egos—is harmed when New York residents pass over a local hospital in favor of the Cleveland Clinic's nationally respected cardiac surgery team. The team performs more open-heart procedures than any other institution in the country.[36]

To be sure, there is some evidence that New York surgeons tried to "game" the system in other ways. The reported prevalence of chronic obstructive pulmonary disease (COPD) among bypass patients soared at one hospital from 1.8 percent to 52.98 percent after the public reports began.[37] At another hospital the percentage of bypass patients reported to have angina rocketed from 1.9 percent to 20.8 percent. And the differences among patients treated by different doctors also widened with suspicious rapidity. Among all New York surgeons, noted a report in the *New England Journal of Medicine,* the reported prevalence of pulmonary disease ranged from 1.4 to 60.6 percent, while different surgeons' reported rates of unstable angina ranged from 0.7 to 61.4 percent.

Yet there is more than a little irony if the game playing really occurred. If critics truly believe that the rankings penalize surgeons who treat the sickest patients, then they should make their patients appear *less* sick, not *more* sick. The gaming represents a perverse vote of confidence in the rankings. In any event, the gaming still accounted for only four percentage points of the state's extraordinary reduction in the cardiac surgery death rate.[38]

Moreover, if one is judging a program by anecdotes, then the other side of the coin is to ask whether the stories of success—like those of a Winthrop-University Hospital—are truly representative. I believe they are. Consider: of the thirty-one hospitals performing heart bypass surgery in New York State, six *publicly* admitted that the performance report prompted new quality improvement initiatives. A seventh hospital suspended its heart surgery program completely until it could correct problems.[39] Is the system perfect? No. Should it be used blindly? No. Has it detected real problems in care and motivated improvement? Yes.

Finally, let's look at individual surgeons, such as the "legendary teacher" forced away from bypass surgery by Strong Memorial in Rochester. According to state records this surgeon, nearing retirement age, operated on just thirty-five patients in 1989–90. The state-recommended minimum is fifty surgeries. (The data do not reflect operations in which a doctor was the assistant.) This surgeon's risk-adjusted mortality rate of 10 percent was well above the state average. I wonder whether this man's admiring former student examined what happened to the surgeon's patients before voicing his public criticism of the New York program or whether he relied entirely on his former teacher's feelings of indignation.

In early 1996 Hannan, Chassin, and Barbara DeBuono, health commissioner under the Republican administration that replaced Democrat Mario Cuomo in early 1995, cooperated on an article that addressed the issue of the physicians whose jobs were affected by the state reports. Instead of emotional anecdote, they cited data:

> Between 1989 and 1992, 27 low-volume surgeons stopped performing CABG in New York State. In each of those four years, *the low-volume surgeons who discontinued CABG had risk-adjusted death rates in their final year of practice that were 2.5 to 5 times the state average* and more than twice the average rate for all low-volume surgeons. In all, their combined risk-adjusted operative mortality rate between 1989 and 1992 was 11.9 percent, as compared with a statewide average of 3.1 percent. [Emphasis added][40]

When it comes to the surgeons and hospitals who have gained and lost as a result of the state performance reports, O. Wayne Isom, chairman of the division of cardiothoracic surgery at the highly rated New York Hospital–Cornell Medical Center, draws an analogy with playing poker during his youth in the small town of Idalou, Texas. Says Isom: "The winners tell jokes, while the losers say, 'Deal the cards, damn it.' "[41]

CHANGE WHEN YOU HAVE TO

> One of the greatest pains to human nature is the pain of a new idea. It . . . makes you think that after all, your favorite notions may be wrong, your firmest beliefs ill-founded.
>
> —Walter Bagehot

Many cardiac surgeons don't like "report cards." Two of the nation's most prominent cardiologists (the medical specialty that sends its patients to be operated on by cardiac surgeons) do. Eric J. Topol and Robert M. Califf put it this way in an article in the *Annals of Internal Medicine:* "Initially, most practitioners react defensively to the concept that medical outcomes should be measured and made available to physician peer review organizations, insurers, patients and the public. . . . [But] overall, appropriate implementation of scorecards could ultimately lead to a substantial improvement in the quality of U.S. cardiovascular medicine."[42]

Whether a statewide effort is needed or whether having each individual hospital focus on improvement is sufficient is open to question. That clinical information needs to be collected and used effectively to improve care—and that hospitals and surgeons need to be motivated to do it—is not.[43] In New York, the state health department, which tried from the start not to upset surgeons, ended up losing the battle to shape public perceptions about how useful its mortality information really was. Only in 1995 did the state start providing reporters with positive anecdotes in the press packet filled with statistics. There was, for instance, the story of Albany's St. Peter's Hospital, which in 1991 and 1992 had a 30 percent death rate among forty-two patients who received high-risk grafts. In response to the poor showing in the state's report cared, the hospital launched a quality improvement campaign. In 1993 it had no deaths among thirty-six patients who received high-risk grafts.

The result of this public relations initiative? A *New York Times* story that mentioned the state's assertion of lives saved but focused mostly on a young surgeon at St. Peter's whose reputation appeared unfairly hurt. His poor ranking seemed due to systemwide problems at the hospital, not any personal failing.[44] Once again the patients whose lives were saved—the Art Segals of the world—remained faceless statistics. The focus, yet again, was on the livelihood of doctors, and only on a doctor who appeared to have been hurt unfairly (a very safe approach from a legal point of view).

The legendary political schemer Niccolò Machiavelli understood the importance of carefully choosing friends and enemies alike. "The innovator makes enemies of all those who prospered under the old order," he wrote, "and only lukewarm support is forthcoming from those who would prosper under the new." Performance reports take away professional control, leaving surgeons and hospitals subject to a public scrutiny they never anticipated and often deeply resent.

"In the past, if a procedure was done right and the proper process was followed, then it was OK even if the patient died," Hannan told *Hospitals and Health Networks.* Commented the magazine, "Previously, no one presumed to question surgeons' methods, because their work was still unique enough that there was little basis for comparison. Things have changed."[45]

CHAPTER TEN

The Empire Strikes Back

Follow the money.
—Deep Throat, in Robert Woodward and Carl Bernstein, *All the President's Men*

Pause for a moment to pay tribute to the company benefits manager. His colleagues, the number crunchers, operations experts, and marketing wizards, are all paid in the coin of glory or disgrace. Benefits managers are rarely either praised or pilloried; mostly they just go unnoticed. "Our people are our most important asset," the company's chairman ritualistically proclaims, but the reality remains that no one from the personnel cum "human resources" department is ever likely to climb to the top of the organizational ladder.

Obscurity, however, should not be confused with powerlessness. In a nation where health insurance is still largely tied to the workplace, benefits managers wield considerable clout. Those at America's largest corporations oversee the health care needs of spreading armies of workers, retirees, and their families. Giant General Motors writes checks to nearly every hospital in the country and to five out of six doctors. In smaller cities and towns, benefits managers hold the power of economic life and death over doctors and hospitals.

Still, the managerial culture stands awkwardly apart from the culture of medicine. Physicians can draw on a rich history celebrated in literature, music, and art. There are no bards of benefits management and no odes to employee open enrollment season. Some scholars claim that the first group benefit was offered by the burial societies of ancient Rome (a tentative link, perhaps, to early physicians). The first reference to benefits funds cited by the *Oxford English Dictionary* does not occur until 1875, however, and the evolution of the modern benefits management position dates back only to the 1940s.

In contrast to medicine's obeisance to the individual artisan, the benefits manager is by definition an organization man. Not to put too fine a point on it, he is a bureaucrat. Although this word has turned into an epithet, "bureaucrat" began life as a badge of honor. The bureaucrat was a modernist, a progressive. While others followed an individual patron to whom personal loyalty was owed, the bureaucrat rejected this feudal model of organizational structure and pledged allegiance to an objective and explicit set of rules.[1] While others indulged in mythmaking, the bureaucrat was a rationalist. Generations of doctors cherished an ancient Greek oath or glorified the serpent on a staff symbol of the pagan god of healing. The bureaucratic mind remained unaffected. Facts, not emotion, made the difference.

Sociologist Max Weber, who codified the culture of bureaucracy in the late nineteenth century, wrote: "Bureaucratic administration means fundamentally the exercise of control on the basis of knowledge."[2] The would-be bureaucratizers of medicine, however, faced formidable barriers to acquiring the knowledge they sought. Physicians spent years in training learning to unravel the unseen workings of the body. Those painstakingly acquired insights would not and could not readily be shared with someone who had never held the sobering responsibility for the life of another human being. Moreover, the very mysteriousness of medical knowledge conferred extraordinary power. Patients, standing in awe of their doctors, frequently feel better even if the only medication the doctor provides is a sugar pill and sincere assurances that all will be well. (In some experiments, the "placebo effect" has been as much as 70 percent effective.)[3] Even the boldest bureaucratic rationalist hesitated when confronted by such potent magic.

It was only when the fight for control shifted from the clinical arena, which doctors fiercely claimed as their birthright, to a financial setting, where the corporate bureaucrats reigned supreme, that physicians gave ground. The victory over "socialized medicine" left physicians vulnerable to the depredations of capitalists far sharper of tooth and claw than any government paper pusher. In other industrialized countries, which almost all have national health insurance, governments control the "global budget" available for health care but typically leave doctors alone to make treatment decisions. Of course there is no "global" budget for all of United States medicine. Instead, there are tens of thousands of different organizations whose small "global" budgets for medical expenses add up to the nearly trillion dollar national health care bill. Benefits bureaucrats oversee this money, whether for the government (administering Medicare and Medicaid) or for private sector health programs. With money comes power.

For years, however, benefits managers hesitated. Even Chrysler's challenge to its hospitals and doctors came not from the benefits department, but from Joseph Califano, a member of the board of directors committee specifically set up by the company's chairman to deal with medical costs. How could the average benefits bureaucrat turn into the "hard-negotiating buyer" Califano envisioned? A solution to the bureaucrats' befuddlement was suggested by an intense health care evangelist from Minneapolis named Walter McClure. McClure called his approach "Buy Right."[4]

When Walt McClure gazed out over the health care landscape, he saw not bad doctors, but bad incentives. This analytic view of medicine came naturally. Trained as a physicist, McClure gave up his job at a government physics lab in 1969 to join the InterStudy think tank founded by Paul Ellwood, the proponent of HMOs. After a few years at InterStudy, however, McClure grew restless. The theory of HMO competition bore little resemblance to the reality. Instead of competing on quality and efficiency, HMOs were competing like fee for service plans: "You find out what your competitor is doing, price just a little lower, and add benefits so people will shift."[5] McClure also believed that physicians were deceiving themselves about their ability to practice cost-effective medicine in an unrestricted fee for service system whose incentives encouraged excess. It was, he said, similar to the way early Christians genuinely believed "they could abstain from the carnal pleasures."

McClure founded his own group, the Center for Policy Studies, and preached a gospel of capitalistic redemption. Those who purchased medical care needed to "buy right"; that is, reward high-quality, low-cost doctors and hospitals for the desired behavior by bring them more patients and more income. Let others worry about intellectual paradigms. McClure, the practical physicist, wanted to connect physicians' reimbursement to patients' health. "When doctors say the health care system is doing well, they mean doctors are doing well. . . . That's not crass on their part. They can't separate the welfare of doctors from the welfare of patients."

One response was to constantly stare over doctors' shoulders and second-guess them. This was called "utilization review" (UR), a drab description of the delicate job of pushing doctors to spend less money on each patient without really hurting anyone. The "review" typically meant requiring physicians to dial a toll-free phone number and ask a nurse or clerk for permission to hospitalize a patient or to keep the patient hospitalized past a certain time. Doctors hated UR, but it was a perfectly logical response to a system created by the doctors themselves. If each individual physician insisted on total autonomy in the treatment of each individual patient, then the only way to control the doctor's decisions was to review them one at a time. In 1983, just 14 percent of big companies included UR in their health plans. By 1988, 95 percent did.[6] The Mayo Clinic, with patients from all over the country, reported dealing with some one thousand different UR programs in 1988 versus just one in 1984.[7] To many, it seemed an odd way to improve economic efficiency.

McClure argued for a different approach, one that carefully reordered the economic incentives of the entire system rather than reviewing decisions one by one. "In the health-care system, we say doctors are bad and greedy, instead of [saying that] the incentives punish them for doing the right thing," he said. The same held true for hospitals. Yet "if a hospital were to reduce prices, screen admissions, control ancillary services [such as laboratory tests and X rays] and shorten length of stay, it would not gain a single patient or attract a single physician by its efficient behavior; it would simply lose revenue. . . . In contrast, if the hospital were to raise prices, encourage admissions and ancillary use and increase length of stay, it would not lose a single patient or physician; it would gain substantial revenue. There is little wonder, then, why providers gravitate to inefficient and elaborate practice styles."[8]

In order to funnel patients to the efficient and high-quality doctors and hospitals, however, one needed first to identify them. But where could one obtain reliable performance information? Here McClure was fortunate. A 1975 Supreme Court ruling had held that the traditional "learned professions" of law and medicine were subject to antitrust law. As chapter 8 described, attempts to compare physicians in even a rudimentary way met with immediate opposition from state medical societies or ran afoul of state laws sponsored by those societies and the American Medical Association. The Supreme Court decision, however, meant that professional societies could no longer prohibit advertising and other forms of open competition among their members. In the years following that ruling, additional court decisions and regulatory findings gave corporations the green light to contract with groups of physicians.[9]

When physicians exercised monopoly power, the lack of information about qualitative differences between them allowed everyone to claim the high price due the "best" doctors. But when doctors had to compete among themselves for patients, what was a strength got flipped by a kind of economic jujitsu into a weakness. If quality was equal, then medical treatment could be bought like corn or wheat or any other commodity—solely based on price.

Doctors and hospitals were trapped. They disliked the micromanagement of utilization review, but they even more virulently opposed a government-financed health care system. The only remaining alternative, a competitive marketplace for medical services, demanded that they disclose information on the quality as well as price of care.

The earliest calls for measuring and managing the quality of medical care had come from idealists within medicine: nurse Florence Nightingale, surgeon Ernest Amory Codman, internist Paul Lembcke, and others. Now, though, the demand for information came not from idealists but from the people who paid the bills. Sticking to the old paradigm—"just trust us"—threatened to bring highly unpleasant consequences. As McClure succinctly put it: "You scare the providers that the purchasers are either going to buy right—or they're going to buy cheap."[10]

Scare the providers enough, and they might even agree to have their performance measured and results disclosed to the public.

FOR ALL PRACTICAL PURPOSES

> While a factory . . . takes pains to assure itself that the product is a good one . . . the hospital does not.
>
> —Amory Codman

Less than seventy-two hours before Mark Baas was scheduled to undergo open-heart surgery, the Allentown, Pennsylvania, resident stumbled upon some information that caused him to abruptly change his plans. The information was contained in a simple booklet showing the bypass success rate of individual surgeons and hospitals in Pennsylvania. Unlike the similar report on bypass surgery put out by New York State, this one was designed to be easily usable by consumers. The rankings were simple. A minus sign next to a name meant that more patients died than would be expected given their risk of death before surgery; a diamond meant the mortality rate was within the expected range; and a plus signified that a doctor or hospital performed better than expected. There was also information on cost.

Baas was understandably upset to see a minus sign next to the names of both his hospital and his surgeon. Although his cardiologist assured him that "I would let [the surgeon] operate on my own mother," the forty-year-old stacker crane operator decided to check out a different hospital not much farther away. This hospital had a diamond rating for its surgical program and a plus rating for one of its surgeons.

Rather than just switching hospitals, Baas quizzed doctors at the second institution about their higher score. The surgeons spoke of being trained by the military during the Vietnam War to take total responsibility for patients. They talked about high morale among nurses and about the nurses' attention to a hundred details of care. Baas was persuaded. His surgery at the second hospital took place without incident. And because the surgery was triggered by a mild heart attack a few weeks earlier, Baas decided to do some prudent postsurgical planning for the future. "I got on the mailing list for the new report," he said, "in case I have a second heart attack."[11]

Baas's story is the kind that brings a pleased smile to the face of Ernest Sessa, executive director of the Pennsylvania Health Care Cost Containment Council, the state agency that issued the consumer booklet on bypasses. Unlike the New York State Department of Health, the council's sole mandate is to curb costs while improving the quality of care. It unabashedly believes that the best way to do that is to give the public and businesses the kind of information they need to "buy right."

The decision to embrace informed purchasing as a way to change doctors' decisions arose out of a sense of frustration felt by state business leaders in the early 1980s. Two years of working cooperatively with physicians and hospitals to design a voluntary system to collect and disclose information on health care costs and quality had gone nowhere. The Pennsylvania Business Roundtable, representing the state's largest corporations, said it was ready to support regulatory price controls similar to those in the neighboring states of Maryland, New Jersey, and New York. At about that same time, several local business coalitions interested in Walt McClure's "Buy Right" program announced that they were fed up too. They were ready to buy health care from the lowest bidder unless they received solid information demonstrating that a higher cost was justified.

A task force hastily assembled by Pennsylvania's governor decided to opt for a marketplace approach rather than regulatory controls. The state's powerful physician and hospital associations reluctantly made the same choice and endorsed public performance standards. The providers were backed into a corner. As the national weekly *Medical World News* reported:

> Hospitals and physicians were "very afraid" that without outcomes assessment "medical care decisions would be based on cost alone," says Dr. Robert Tyson, a retired surgeon who was president of the Pennsylvania Medical Society. . . .
>
> How do state physicians feel about having their "batting averages" printed in newspapers? "If the data are complete and accurate, I think we can live with outcome assessment," says Dr. Tyson. "As doctors have learned about the program, they have supported it. They understand the reasons for assessment—and the alternatives."[12]

The act setting up the Pennsylvania Health Care Cost Containment Council became law on 8 July 1986. It was part of the same activist approach toward medical cost containment that was sweeping the nation. As late as the mid-1970s, ignorance about the components of rising medical costs was so nearly total that there was not even published information on the annual number of surgeries performed nationwide.[13] A decade later, some eighteen states were requiring hospitals to provide a wealth of comparative information.[14]

What made the Pennsylvania agency unique, however, was the sophistication of the data it gathered on the quality of care. The council's logo read, "Pennsylvania's Declaration of Health Care Information," complete with a small drawing of the Liberty Bell. Though hokey, the analogy was not far from the truth. The council's legal mandate represented a revolutionary assertion of the public's right to know about the most important aspect of care: its effect on patients. The state law requires the council to include measures of medical quality along with cost data in all reports, unless no appropriate quality indicator is available. Even more boldly, Pennsylvania became the first state to legally require a public report on individual doctors.

The political clout of a legislative mandate and unabashed focus on economics clearly differentiated the Pennsylvania effort from New York's. The New York State health department saw itself as operating within the traditional paradigm of professional self-improvement. It spent a great deal of time cajoling cooperation from surgeons and hospitals. Moreover, because of the state's tight regulatory controls, cost comparisons were less urgent. In Pennsylvania, however, cost and quality were linked from the start. The question was value: How can we get our money's worth out of the medical dollar? Nondoctors had a legal right to information that could help answer that question. Doctors and hospitals could either cooperate to improve the data or sit on the sidelines and watch the data get published anyway.

The council was dominated by those who bought or used medical care. Its twenty-one members showed little tolerance for esoteric debate. Early on, some doctors objected to reporting the "treatment effectiveness" of hospitals, asserting that they would be penalized for bad outcomes when the problem was that the patient was very sick to begin with. A labor representative pounded on the table and smashed through the technical detail. "We're spending all this money on these hospitals," he declared, "and you're telling me that what goes on with patients has nothing to do with what you do in there?" The discussion moved on to the next topic.

The council's technical advisory committee took a similar attitude, even though it was largely composed of doctors. When a hospital suggested that a certain bypass death should not be counted because the patient was almost dead before surgery, the committee replied that the hospital shouldn't be operating on dead people—and the fatality remained part of the state's calculations.

The appointment of Sessa as the council's executive director set the tone. Neither a public health expert nor a researcher, Sessa brought with him the political survival skills and contacts of a lifelong bureaucrat. Born in Philadelphia, Sessa attended a Jesuit college in the city before grabbing the opportunity for a management trainee position with a large insurance company. Jobs were scarce in 1957, and plans for law school were put on what turned out to be permanent hold. Sessa built a solid track record in a variety of benefits jobs, both public and private. He capped his career with a thirteen-year stint as administrator of the Benefits Trust Fund established for state workers.

The fund's governing council was composed of union and management representatives, and both sides agreed on the need to curb health care inflation. "We all bought into the fact that quality was really what counted," said Sessa. "If you got quality, cost would fall into line." Sessa threw himself into the effort to pass the legislation that established the cost containment council. In February 1987 Sessa and an assistant became its first full-time employees.

Sessa's friends warned him that the council would be sued by an angry hospital or doctor, but no lawsuits ever came. Sessa insisted that his staff pay attention to every detail. As the council waded through a paperwork swamp containing information on 154 types of hospital admissions for 175 hospitals, each of the hundreds of thousands of records was painstakingly checked for accuracy. Only then did it become part of the public database.

One of the council's early reports used the kind of small-area analysis of medical practice variation pioneered by Dartmouth's John Wennberg nearly twenty years before. After dividing the state into eight regions, the council showed that citizens living in the northeastern part of the state were 25 percent more likely to have surgery than the average Pennsylvania resident. The next highest region, northwestern Pennsylvania, was only 2 percent above the average. Slapping tight limits on medical prices didn't make much sense if the volume of surgery was out of control. Noted Sessa, "The most important question that small-area analysis allows us to ask is this: 'In a community with large variations, are we getting the best value for our health-care dollar?' "[15] (Present council reports on specific conditions, such as cesarean sections, include geographic variation data next to information on variations in cost and length of hospital stay.)

However important varying rates of surgery might be, it was hardly the stuff of coffee-break conversation. What finally enabled the cost containment council to capture the public's attention was a report that everyone could understand. It was a report that let the public see the clear difference between the new paradigm of public accountability for the results of care and the old paradigm of private, professional self-regulation.

In many ways Philadelphia is the hometown of American medicine. Pennsylvania Hospital was chartered there on 11 May 1751 as the nation's first hospital. The first American medical school opened its doors in 1756 at the College of Philadelphia, later known as the University of Pennsylvania.[16] Crucial financial and political support for the hospital came from a state assemblyman named Benjamin Franklin. Franklin also helped select an excerpt from the biblical story of the Good Samaritan for the hospital's official seal ("Take Care of Him and I Will Repay Thee"), and before more pressing issues consumed his time, he served as head of the hospital board. The British occupied Pennsylvania Hospital for nearly a year during the American Revolution, then left without paying for supplies. Perhaps they reasoned, as the thrifty Franklin might have put it, that "a penny saved is a penny earned."

Philadelphia remains a national center of medical education, with five medical schools crowding within the city limits. When the hospitals associated with those five schools cooperated to compare their heart bypass programs, the results were of interest around the country, but they created the biggest stir close to home.

On 14 August 1991, the *Journal of the American Medical Association* published the first detailed examination of hospital outcomes to appear in a major medical journal since the National Halothane Study of 1959.[17] The magnitude of the differences in the results of care stunned Philadelphians. For the first eighteen months of the two-and-a-half year study, unnamed "Hospital D" had a mortality rate about half that of the other four teaching institutions. During the next twelve months, Hospital D experienced a modest increase in its mortality rate, while the mortality rate dropped sharply at Hospital A. The rates at the other three hospitals stayed roughly constant.[18] Even more compelling, "there were threefold differences in surgeon-specific mortality rates," wrote Sankey Williams, David Nash, and Neil Goldfarb, the Philadelphia-based authors of the *JAMA* article. When some surgeons changed hospitals, the mortality rates changed too, although the researchers cautioned there was only "inconclusive evidence for an association with surgeons' clinical skills."

An innocuous-looking table on an inside page proved to be the most provocative part of the article. There the researchers listed the expected and actual mortality rates of thirteen individual heart surgeons who had operated on a certain minimum number of people. Each surgeon's rate was adjusted for what the patient's chart indicated was the risk of death before the operation. From a patient's point of view, there was just one problem: in keeping with standard research protocols, the doctors' names were masked, just as the hospital names had been. An angry public felt manipulated.

A *Philadelphia Daily News* editorial titled "Which Hospital Is Which? That's Bypassed in Bypass Report," cut to the heart of the matter:

> Anonymity was a condition of the study, the authors explain. . . .
>
> This makes sense to detached observers everywhere.
>
> Yet it can't help but further the suspicion (however unfounded) that doctors have more loyalty to their colleagues than to their patients.
>
> Or that the truth is so damaging it has to be hidden.
>
> It's hard to imagine that many members of the local medical com-

munity are ignorant of just where those hospitals and surgeons placed. Why should they know something the poor joker on the gurney doesn't?

If a hospital's survival rates resemble those on Omaha Beach, surely the patients have a right to know.[19]

Study coauthor Nash acknowledged later that the editorial writer had a point. Doctors were able to figure out which surgeon was which, but patients weren't. Said Nash, "Everyone in Philadelphia in the business identified the surgeons perfectly." However, many doctors, unlike the newspaper editorial writer, felt outraged that the surgeons had been embarrassed in front of their peers. Few doctors really believed in this thing called risk adjustment. "Nobody had published work like this," said Nash, who is still at Thomas Jefferson University Hospital, one of the five centers profiled. "There are people who still don't talk to me because of that piece."[20]

Only three years earlier, the *New England Journal of Medicine* had editorially endorsed the revolutionary new "era of assessment and accountability," as recounted in chapter 8. When the time came to personally man the barricades, however, the editors scurried to hide behind their lawyers. As Nash remembers it, the table listing surgeons' individual patient outcomes was too controversial, even with the doctors' names omitted. "They said, 'This is libelous. We can't publish it.' " *JAMA,* owned by the AMA, was braver. In the end, of course, no one sued.

Just seven days after the *JAMA* article appeared, the state cost containment council released its *Hospital Effectiveness Report* examining care at Philadelphia hospitals in 1990. The council reported the mortality rate and major complications for fifty-seven medical and surgical conditions, including bypass surgery. Purely by happenstance, the public was treated to a comparison of medical guild internal oversight and bureaucratic oversight.

As pure research, the *JAMA* study masked hospital identities on the outcome of care and only implicitly mentioned cost. The state cost containment council report, by contrast, reflected the council's legislative mandate to shake up the local health care system. Its numbers had actual hospital names attached to hard figures on both cost and quality. The Hospital of the University of Pennsylvania charged $80,285 for a preoperative diagnostic angiogram and a bypass; Presbyterian Hospital charged $40,929. At the university hospital five people died in 122 procedures; about three deaths were expected. At

Presbyterian, four people died in 232 operations, and about six and a half deaths (statistically speaking) were expected. (The university objected that the state did not adequately account for the severity of illness of its patients.)

The contrast between the *JAMA* article and the council report was unmistakable. When a hospital group warned about information "simplified for a mass audience," an editorial in the *Philadelphia Inquirer* responded: "All across Philadelphia, hospital officials are, well, *jumpy*. They've had their first thorough going-over by a state agency that presumed to lift the veil of secrecy surrounding their business. And, like anyone suddenly exposed to unaccustomed public glare, they are flinching."[21]

Although the publicity helped the council, its effect was short-lived. By the end of 1992, amid a budget dispute between the Democratic legislature and the Republican governor, the council's vital signs were fading rapidly. Its coffers contained just enough cash to meet one final payroll for its thirty workers (down from forty the year before). With the clock running down, the council issued its first report that linked the names of individual physicians to the results of care. This consumer guide—the same one that stacker crane operator Mark Baas eventually picked up—finally revived the council's political pulse.

The booklet examined the cost and outcome of heart bypass operations performed by 170 cardiac surgeons at thirty-five hospitals. Here was information that any patient could immediately grasp. The public flooded the council's office with more than ten thousand phone calls and letters requesting the council's report. Pennsylvania's politicians got the message and renewed the council's mandate to the year 2003.

"When the council first began to publish hospital performance data, there was a great outcry from the medical community," wrote Sessa in a review of his group's activities. "One would have imagined that the world was about to end. . . . [But] life goes on. Hospitals have not gone out of business. Reputations have not been destroyed. What has happened is that over time, a relatively cooperative relationship has developed—a process strengthened by the spotlight of public attention and awareness of hospital and physician performance."[22]

Sessa "carries a big stick, but he speaks softly," commented J. Marvin Bentley, an economist at Pennsylvania State University at Harrisburg. "It's such a balancing act. He has some sympathy with the organizations he reports on, but not so much that he gets snookered by them."

The story is told of a math professor who defined the phrase "for all practical purposes" to a roomful of students this way: If a boy and a girl walk toward each other, and with each step cut the distance between them in half, they will never actually touch—at least not according to mathematical theory. But within a few short strides, added the professor, the two will be close enough "for all practical purposes."

In Pennsylvania, the cost containment council always remembered that its practical purpose was to improve care and control costs. At least one major Pennsylvania company used the council's data to "buy right" and try to achieve that goal.

HEALTHY, WEALTHY, AND CHOCOLATE

On a day when the wind is right, the thick, unmistakable aroma of chocolate hangs heavy over the south-central Pennsylvania town of Hershey. The municipality takes its name from Milton Snavely Hershey, born shortly before the Civil War to a poor Mennonite farm couple who lived in the region. Milton Hershey parlayed a teenage apprenticeship to a confectioner into a corporate empire. In addition to locating his chocolate company's headquarters and factory in the eponymous town, Hershey established the M. S. Hershey Foundation; the Milton Hershey School, which first served orphans, then expanded to include vocational training; and the Milton S. Hershey Medical Center, part of the Pennsylvania State University system.

In the middle of 1992, a health care consultant named Ted Ackroyd brought bad news to the management of Hershey Foods Corporation. Ackroyd was an economist and researcher specializing in medical outcomes. He was hired by Hershey as part of an unusual effort to tackle the problem of soaring medical bills. Hershey Foods' health care expenses were rising 15 to 18 percent annually, meaning they would double in less than five years. As managers of a manufacturing company, Hershey executives believed in the teaching of "continuous quality improvement," that is, that higher quality meant lower costs. Their belief was so firm that Hershey decided to handpick a network of doctors and hospitals that considered both the quality and the price of the care—much as Chrysler had done a decade earlier. But Hershey was seeking far more sophisticated information than Chrysler had. It was interested not only in the appropriateness of treatment but in the outcome of care for a whole list of procedures. Ackroyd's job was to assemble the data that Hershey managers needed to decide who to invite into its network.

No local hospital had more riding on that decision than Hershey Medical Center. The medical center and Hershey Foods had close ties. For one thing, the hospital was right next door. One could almost toss a package of Reese's Pieces from a factory gate to the medical center's front steps. More to the point, the medical center was virtually a company creation. In March 1963 Samuel Hinkle, then president and chairman of both Hershey Foods and the Hershey Foundation, telephoned Penn State president Eric Walker to inquire if the university was interested in starting a medical school. "There's not a nickel" of state funds available to do that, said Walker. Hinkle then asked how much money it would take. Responded Walker, "Oh, about $50 million." "What would you say if we told you we had $50 million to start with?" "That would be different."[23]

Given that history, consultant Ackroyd wasn't looking forward to his task. After evaluating hospitals, he had to tell the Hershey Foods managers that Hershey Medical Center did not look good. Going strictly by the numbers, Hershey the hospital did not qualify for inclusion in the primary care network of Hershey the candy company.

Ackroyd clearly remembers the response to his bombshell: in his presence, no one reacted at all. No one brought up the hospital's history, and no one mentioned that the food company's chairman, Richard Zimmerman, was also the chairman of the board of the university that operated the hospital. Though some of the Hershey Foods managers had suspected the hospital might not make the cut, they were still stunned to hear the news. Regrouping, they quickly decided the first thing to do was inform Zimmerman. Yet rather than trying to reverse the decision of his underlings, Zimmerman too was restrained. "Let's be sure we're being fair," he said. To satisfy himself, Zimmerman asked careful questions about the data and the analysis. Then he made a tough call of his own: to Dr. C. McCollister Evarts, the hospital's chief executive officer.

In the business community as elsewhere, bold and principled words can conceal timid and opportunistic deeds. Vows by employers to buy health care based on "quality" have often been nothing more than window dressing. In 1985, for example, a group of large employers organized by the Midwest Business Group on Health garnered national publicity in their search for "high-quality" doctors and hospitals in a Rockford, Illinois, a mid-sized city west of Chicago. When the smoke and mirrors cleared, "they didn't really end up evaluating the hospitals," a former business group staff member acknowledged later. "They were looking for a discount."[24] More recently, the medical director of a Northeast HMO (who also has a doctorate in economics), recounted this conversation with the benefits manager of a large company that was a potential client. "Every once in a while in the middle of the conversation, he'd say the three words, 'cheap, cheap, cheap.' And it wasn't necessarily related to the conversation. We were there talking about quality, and he kept reminding us that his interest was 'cheap, cheap, cheap.' It was half in jest, but [at the same time] not in jest."

The concept that a nonphysician could make cost and quality judgments about medical care is one it has taken benefits managers some time to accept. After all, one of the earliest and most important academic studies of health economics concluded that its special nature made it an exception to normal market forces.[25] Stanford University economist Kenneth Arrow, who made this assertion in 1963, later shared the 1972 Nobel Prize for his contributions to general welfare economics. A young economist named Mark Pauly, now a professor of health care systems at Philadelphia's Wharton School of Business, wrote a Ph.D. dissertation that disagreed with Arrow and had it published during the 1970s.[26] The impact, though, was modest.

Several factors combined to enable Hershey Foods to break out of the mind-set—the paradigm—of most of its peers. Call it a mixture of idealism, pragmatism, and opportunity.

The idealism part was genuine. Hershey initially pursued the "high quality-low cost" strategy because executives were reluctant to take the knee-jerk steps of cutting benefits or raising premiums to reduce the company's health care bill. That reluctance was partly due to fear of a confrontation with a local workforce that was about half unionized, but it was also because founder Milton Hershey had instilled a strong tradition of paternalism throughout the company. Asked what his religion was, Hershey is said to have replied, "the Golden Rule": Do unto others as you would have them do unto you. Company managers periodically make a pilgrimage to the Milton Hershey School to talk with the underprivileged children who live there in a deliberate effort to "keep our priorities straight." The Hershey chief executive officer in the late 1970s and early 1980s was himself a graduate of the Hershey School, placed there as a child by his widowed father. The Hershey Trust, which operates the school, is still the company's majority shareholder.

The pragmatic motivation for Hershey Foods' quality initiative was also partly cultural. The parsimonious Pennsylvania Dutch management particularly disliked wasting money on unnecessary medical care. In an analysis of claims data, Hershey Foods discovered (like Chrysler and many others) that one out of seven medical procedures performed on Hershey employees was unnecessary. The audit found waste amounting to some $448 per worker, or $2.7 million for the central Pennsylvania workforce.

Finally, there was a much larger financial issue. On 21 December 1990, the Financial Accounting Standards Board announced new accounting rules pertaining to the future benefits that companies promised to their retirees. FASB, though nominally a private group, functions as the financial umpire of corporate America. Its rulings may sometimes be unpopular, but they still determine how everyone plays the game. FASB's Financial Accounting Statement 106 required companies to calculate the effect of inflation on promised benefits such as medical coverage and long-term care and then set aside a financial reserve to keep those promises to the future. The reserve reduced earnings. FAS 106 directly affected corporate balance sheets, profits, and by implication the selling price of the company's stock. Suddenly health care costs became very interesting to the most senior levels of management.

With FAS 106 scheduled to take effect in 1993, the "free lunch" approach to handing out ever-richer health benefits, born during the Second World War, was about to officially end. "For some, [FAS 106] . . . will have a devastating impact on earnings," read one consulting firm's analysis of the new rules. "But there is a silver lining to the cloud: Before FASB began work on the rules for post-retirement benefit accounting, most employers had no idea how large their liabilities had grown. Now, at least they are aware of the problem and can take steps to manage it."[27]

The cost of medical benefits had become "a CEO issue," summarized Sharon Lambly, Hershey Foods' vice president of human resources. At Hershey, the management response was straightforward. Said Lambly: "We think that if you drive quality, you lower price."

The final ingredient that enabled the Hershey program to be effective was opportunity. The town of Hershey has fewer than twelve thousand residents. Hershey Foods, with a workforce drawn from the town and the surrounding countryside, employs some six thousand people and provides health insurance for roughly fifteen thousand, including workers and their families. Size equals clout.

Of course, community hospitals that treated a small number of Hershey workers still might have refused a request to give Hershey data on their care. That's where the Pennsylvania Health Care Cost Containment Council came in. Every state hospital was already measuring and reporting information on quality. As a result, the door was open for a pioneering effort in "value" purchasing that considered both quality and cost.

Hershey's scoring system for potential participants in its new network assigned 30 percent of the points based on price and 70 percent based on the hospital's score on quality indicators. For instance, hospitals had to be accredited by the Joint Commission and offer a full range of services, with special emphasis on outpatient services. The staff working in certain key areas, such as the emergency room, needed to be board certified.

The Hershey team also assessed the actual performance of twenty-three hospitals in a nine-county area by using the Pennsylvania health council data.[28] Hershey examined some fifty-five diagnostic categories of illness that together accounted for more than a third of the conditions that sent company employees to the hospital. The information included quality indicators that no individual worker would think of asking for, much less get: both the death rate (mortality) and the rate of complications, including items such as infection after surgery.

Hershey also wanted to know how well a hospital organized its delivery of care. For example, How long was the average hospital stay? What was the rate of cesarean sections? How often did the hospital perform back surgery? This was a review that was not simply second-guessing but instead trying to put together a true cost-benefit analysis of care.

After tabulating the results, Hershey ranked the hospitals from one to twenty-three and picked the top ten to invite into its network. (One hospital, unhappy with Hershey's reimbursement, declined to participate and was not replaced.) Hershey Medical Center was approved as a referral center for certain complicated cases, but the hospital and its affiliated physicians did not make it onto the primary care network.

Still using its economic power, Hershey persuaded the local Blue

Cross and Blue Shield to provide performance data on physicians from claims records. That data helped Hershey picked 180 primary care doctors and 800 specialists to participate with the hospitals. That many doctors was deemed a large enough pool to make sure workers felt they had adequate choice of physicians.

Last, the company decided that high-quality care involved preventing illness as well as treating it appropriately and effectively. Beginning with management employees, Hershey initiated a wellness incentive program focusing on health risks workers could control. Cigarette smokers, those with high cholesterol or high blood pressure, and the morbidly obese paid extra health insurance premiums; those with good risk factors paid less. Workers who brought a letter from a doctor saying that their problem was uncontrollable, or that efforts to control it had failed, were exempted from penalty.

To persuade workers to join the new "HealthStyle" network rather than a conventional HMO or traditional fee for service plan, Hershey lowered the premiums to reflect the expected savings to the company. A little under a third of employees signed up in the first year alone, including such tough customers as Hershey chairman Zimmerman, vice president of human resources Lambly, and Richard Dreyfuss, then director of executive compensation and employee benefits.

The path Hershey chose was not easy. Before the first worker signed up, Hershey had spent two years in planning, committed its managers' time to hundreds of meetings, and written $1 million worth of checks. Even so, it took courage for the company to make purchasing decisions based on the information it found. Just as Sessa and Nash were warned that naming names was a surefire prescription for a lawsuit, so too did Hershey's lawyers caution the company that it might be sued by HealthStyle enrollees unhappy with their medical care. The company went ahead with the network anyway, and there have been no lawsuits.

Dreyfuss, Hershey Foods' benefits manager, says he and his family have been happy with their personal care. Company surveys show that general worker satisfaction has gone up even as company medical costs in the Hershey area have gone down. Although there has been nationwide pressure on health care costs during the same period, Hershey is convinced that its money and time have been well spent. "We made the business case that we looked at the million dollars [put into developing the network] as an investment, and we'll get a rate of return on it," Dreyfuss said. "We've probably saved seven million to ten million dollars" in the three years since the program began.

Despite Hershey Foods' satisfaction with its program, other companies have not jumped to copy it. Dreyfuss acknowledges he is disappointed. "Corporations are often their very worst enemies," he said. "Whereas they want to buy on quality, they get a little skittish because the data by some measures is not 100 percent conclusive, or, 'We haven't had it for 10 years.' I think . . . it's a combination of public relations and liability issues. They want an easy solution and an immediate solution. That's why they tend to buy whatever's on the shelf."

Dreyfuss, though, is convinced that the savings from Hershey Foods' aggressive use of information on the quality of medical care have been more than only monetary. "Have we saved lives? I think so," he said.

HOLDING THE MEDICAL COMMUNITY ACCOUNTABLE

In the world of the medical guild, success has long been linked to the "three *As*": availability (for helping out colleagues whose patients need to be seen quickly); affability (being easy to work with); and ability. The new paradigm of medicine adds a fourth *A* word: accountability. "Accountability is about individuals who are responsible for a set of activities and for explaining or answering [to others] for their actions," wrote Harvard Medical School ethicists Ezekiel J. Emanuel and Linda L. Emanuel in a January 1996 article given prominent play in the *Annals of Internal Medicine.*[29] Interestingly, Linda Emanuel was hired shortly afterward by the AMA to be vice president for ethics standards.

"The public trusts that hospitals will act in patients' best interests," wrote Haya Rubin, director of quality of care research at the Johns Hopkins Schools of Medicine and Public Health. "Therefore, hospitals must be accountable to demonstrate that they deliver high-quality care." Much the same reasoning applies to nursing homes, health plans, physician groups, and others. A growing number of state governments recognize this. By the end of 1996, thirty-seven states had medical data commissions, many of which were collecting and publishing some sort of quality of care information, according to the National Association of Health Data Organizations.

This public accountability on the part of physicians represents an extraordinary change, one inconceivable even a couple of decades ago. Medical sociologist Eliot Freidson noted then that physicians had their own set of rules. When doctors were asked what they would do about a colleague whose behavior violated technical norms of conduct, the most common response was "nothing." Asked what they would do if the offense was repeated, doctors answered: "I'd talk to him." Freidson described this informal disciplinary technique:

> Talking-to seemed to involve various blends of instruction, friendly persuasion, shaming and threats.
>
> The incidence of talking-to varied with social distance. . . . Talkings-to were also graded according to severity. The mildest (and by far the most common) talking-to was a simple man-to-man affair—one person informally raising the issue with another. If the offender did not mend his ways, the offended man might enlist the aid of other talkers. . . .
>
> In sum, the characteristic sanctions were never so strong as to reduce income and minimize or prevent work on the part of offenders, and they were rarely organized.[30]

Later on, Freidson noted:

> The benefit of the doubt is given to colleague performance. . . . "After all," the argument goes, "nobody *wants* to kill a patient." But if one does kill a patient, perhaps good intentions are not enough. . . . So long as [the profession] emphasizes good intentions rather than good performance . . . the profession cannot really regulate itself.[31]

And in fact the profession has proved incapable of effectively regulating itself. In that regard, of course, medicine is hardly unique. It is easy to understand the anger and outrage of cardiac surgeons in New York and Pennsylvania. Performance reports do not talk quietly in a hallway and respect a person's need to earn an income. Performance reports do not respect the "three *A*s." Worse, they represent interference in a "learned profession" by (nonlearned) outsiders.

Publicly, doctors snub these "report cards." An article in the 25 July 1996 *New England Journal of Medicine* looked at the impact of Pennsylvania's *Consumer Guide to Coronary Artery Bypass Graft Surgery* on referrals by cardiologists and on access to surgery by severely ill patients. The authors concluded that cardiologists were not using the guide to make referrals. The surgeons, however, were paying attention.

About 60 percent of the cardiologists said it was more difficult for them to find a surgeon for severely ill patients. About the same percentage of surgeons said they were less likely to perform surgery on severely ill patients.

Was that good or bad for patients? The authors did not address the question.[32] However, researchers at the University of Pittsburgh and Carnegie Mellon University found that hospitals that performed poorly in the 1990 Pennsylvania report improved their results by the time of the 1992 report. The authors saw this as quality improvement and noted that the hospitals that got better also gained market share.[33] Whether quality actually improved would require a clinical analysis—the mortality rates might have gotten better for other reasons. Still, other anecdotal evidence supports the theory that hospitals did respond to the public performance data.[34] So does the state's contention that the risk-adjusted mortality rate for bypasses declined by about 25 percent from 1990 to 1993.[35]

Apart from the effect its reports have had on patients, Pennsylvania's most important accomplishment may be the breadth of its activities. Accountability need not have a narrow clinical focus. From 1989 to 1996, the council published nine regional *Small Area Analysis Reports* looking at practice variation. It put out thirty-six regional *Hospital Effectiveness Reports* that reported comparative data on fifty to sixty diagnoses. There have also been focused reports examining cesarean sections, organ transplants, and other issues. Outside public view, the council has produced hundreds of customized reports for business, researchers, hospitals, and government organizations. In other words, the council is doing everything possible to make the use of its information accepted and routine. It is also changing with the times.

The council's June 1996 "Focus on Heart Attack in Pennsylvania" report attributed deaths to individual physicians, hospitals, and health plans. By doing so, it addressed issues of health care quality related to cost and access as well as to the technical quality of care. For instance, the council's data showed that a heart attack patient's chances of surviving could depend on his or her health insurance. In the western region of the state, patients with a managed care plan fared better than expected, but in the Philadelphia region they had a higher than expected death rate. Medicaid recipients in the region received even fewer procedures than did patients belonging to managed care plans. The report also found enormous differences within regions. In one poor section of Philadelphia, for example, a heart attack patient was eighteen times more likely to die in the hospital than someone living in a more affluent part of town. Whether that was due to a delay in seeking treatment or some other factor was unclear.

There is no doubt that the influence of performance information on the decisions made by large corporations and individual consumers has grown more slowly than anticipated. Just as many physicians and hospitals took time to acclimate to the new data, so too is the public just starting to focus on the availability of this kind of information. "We built up credibility, [but] it's a longer learning curve [to use the information] than we thought it would be," acknowledges Sessa. "[Quality measurement] is still new. If you want to use it, it's going to take a little work on your part. You've got to involve yourself, you've got to understand it. It's not just point and click."

But when financially powerful groups of purchasers take the time to delve into information on quality of care with the same intensity they have brought to cutting costs, the changes that result can begin to transform an entire metropolitan area's system of health care.

CHAPTER ELEVEN

Show Time

Come, give us a taste of your quality.
—William Shakespeare, *Hamlet*

In the kind of Hollywood movies that used to star Mickey Rooney and Ann Miller, a group of friends come together to gripe and groan about the indignities of everyday life. Suddenly one of them brightens with an inspiration. "I know," he shouts. "Let's put on a show!"

At its most basic, the appeal of the theater lies in the way the world created within a show takes the place of the world outside. The actors can say and do things they would never say or do in real life. In business or in government, one way to achieve much the same effect is to stage a demonstration or "pilot" project. By design this is an experiment. It demands a new script.

Six middle-aged, midcareer middle managers who gathered in a Minneapolis office tower in the fall of 1991 were ready to write that kind of script. They did not shout to each other, "Let's put on a show!" Benefits managers, as a rule, do not sing or tap-dance. But this group was definitely in a mood to step out and strut its stuff. The members had just been "dissed" by the state legislature. Even though the managers represented some of the Twin Cities' largest and oldest employers, the legislators had turned up their noses at the group's suggestions for health care reform. "If you know so much about controlling costs and improving care, how come you're not already doing it?" the legislators asked. The rebuff stung, not least because it contained a kernel of truth. The members of this loose-knit coalition called themselves the Business Health Care Action Group (BHCAG), but there had been a certain paucity of action.

How, the benefits managers wondered, could they turn the situation around? As they ate their doughnuts and drank their coffee, indignation slowly became determination. They'd put on a show, a demonstration project so exciting the politicians couldn't ignore it. It would reward good medicine, not just cheap medicine, yet it would save money too. "Not only that, all the main actors is this play could be "good guys." After all, this *was* Minneapolis–St. Paul, the headquarters of "Minnesota nice."

In this project, benefits managers who normally grasped at dollars and pinched every outgoing penny would get the chance to practice enlightened capitalism. Health plans that mostly tended to their own financial health had an opportunity to don the mantle of noble self-improvement. And physicians could star as the principled advocates of better medicine.

Before the production could take to the stage, there were more businesses to recruit, money to raise, and a detailed script to write. But in early 1992 the six-person cadre of benefits managers from BHCAG (pronounced BEE-kag) was ready. Was this kind of effort really believable other than in an old movie? Soon enough, newspapers and magazines across the country were sending reviewers to the Twin Cities to find out.

THE WRITER

"Write what you know" is the first advice given fledgling authors. John Burns, chief "scriptwriter" for BHCAG, certainly knew medicine. Burns trained as a general internist with a subspecialty in kidney disease, but he had learned flexibility at an early age. His father taught math and physics in the emptiness of depression-era South Dakota before moving the family to Virginia and then to Tennessee for a research job at the Oak Ridge national weapons laboratory. The senior Burns never settled into a predictable rut. At age fifty, he earned his Ph.D. in nuclear physics.

John Burns was forty-nine when he decided to take his own career into uncharted territory. Outwardly, everything was going well. He was senior physician of a five-man internal medicine practice in St. Paul and was also an officer of the Ramsey County Medical Society. Still, Burns could see that the days of the medical guild's ascendancy were numbered. Physicians' autonomy and earnings were under increasing attack, and Burns did not like the choices he had to make to maintain his standard of living. "Target income," the economists called it. If you froze physicians' fees, the volume of services would rise so that doctors' incomes stayed constant.[1] Doctors, like everyone else, had bills to pay and a lifestyle to maintain.

"I realized for me to make a living in the practice of medicine, I could have two routes," Burns said. "I could work harder and harder, get up earlier and stay up later, or I could start 'working the system,' putting patients in the hospital for borderline indications, doing more procedures, telling the patient to see me every two months instead of every three months. I'd ask colleagues how much of what they did was medically unnecessary. They'd say, 'I don't know, 40 percent.' Then they'd talk about the patients' demanding it or the standard of the community, another way of saying there was no standard. I participated in conversations where people said, 'John, until we change the rules of the game, this is what I need to [do to] support my family.' "

To supplement his income, Burns was consulting on occupational medicine for the local phone company. When a headhunter called to sound him out about a full-time job elsewhere, Burns decided to take the plunge. In 1981 he joined controls and electronics maker Honeywell Incorporated as director of occupational and environmental health. As medical costs soared, the outspoken Burns moved up to corporate vice president of health management.

As a newcomer to corporate America, Burns was not bound by the old ways of thinking; he was primed to be a paradigm "revolutionary." His determination to break out of the mold, however, had emerged even earlier. When it was Burns's turn to be president of the medical society, he brought unusual speakers to the meetings: a labor leader; the head of a Baptist seminary; a corporate chief executive; and Walter McClure, the tireless advocate of the "Buy Right" approach. McClure told the doctors they could either measure the quality of their work in a manner understandable to purchasers or could end up being treated as a commodity. Some physicians in the audience exploded in rage, while others stayed after the meeting to berate Burns personally for bringing in McClure.

Thanks to his experience as a practicing physician, Burns possessed an insider's knowledge of medical waste and featherbedding. Honeywell soon joined with Cummins Engine Company, John Deere and Company, and the Mayo Clinic in a project to examine just how much inefficiency permeated everyday care. The corporations compared the treatment of their employees seeing local fee for service doctors with the care of similar patients treated by Mayo physicians. Fee for service from august Mayo, with its salaried physicians working collaboratively in a group, turned out to be considerably cheaper than community care.

Burns used that lesson to his advantage. Health maintenance organizations (HMOs) were infamous among corporate customers for "shadow pricing": the HMO figured out what the average worker's medical bills would cost a company under fee for service, then it set its own flat rate slightly below the "shadow" cast by that larger figure. To foil that tactic, Burns signed an unusual contract with two multispecialty groups in the Twin Cities: the Group Health HMO, whose doctors were employees working for a straight salary, and the Park Nicollet Medical Center, whose fee for service physicians also treated HMO patients. Burns knew that both groups practiced a conservative style of medicine similar to Mayo's. So Honeywell told the organizations it wanted not their all-inclusive HMO rate, but their fee for service rate. Just as Burns suspected, paying the actual costs of care was 25 to 30 percent less expensive than the "shadow" rate from an HMO.

Burns also took a daring approach to the emotionally charged issue of organ transplants. Transplants can cost tens or even hundreds of thousands of dollars. They are also risky, with serious infection or complete tissue rejection a constant threat. As is true with more common surgeries, the transplant centers that perform a large number of procedures tend to get the best results. Since transplant services are prestigious and potentially lucrative, however, the number of hospitals offering them outstrips the number that have the experience to provide the best care.

Sick people desperate for a new heart, lung, or kidney are hardly in a position to comparison shop between institutions. Honeywell was. By doing so, Burns entered uncharted waters. This was vastly different from just paying bills. Without a government data commission to provide political cover (as in Pennsylvania and New York), Honeywell decided to select a few hospitals as its "centers of excellence" in transplants. The corporation examined the processes of care and patient outcomes at transplant centers around the country. For example, Honeywell looked at what percentage of patients survived for a year. At one point, a large medical center passed the word to its Honeywell sales representatives that it would switch its purchases of environmental control equipment unless it was accepted as a transplant site. The threat was ignored.

After Honeywell made its choices, the company took another bold step. It told its workers that it would pay for organ transplants only at the designated institutions. Given the high costs, the implications were clear. A large corporation had literally made a life and death medical decision on behalf of its employees.

Burns next tried to move from the esoteric realm of transplants to the more mundane territory of everyday care. As Honeywell's medical director, Burns had hired a veteran of the health care field to oversee health benefits administration. Laird Miller was a former operating room technician and had been an administrator of both a hospital and a physician group practice. Like Burns, Miller was unintimidated by medical mystique. Together the two worked out a plan to apply basic corporate purchasing tools to health care.

When a large organization makes an expensive purchase, it is common for it to write up a formal description of what it wants to buy and then invite vendors to submit bids. This detailing the specifications of a product or service is called a "request for proposal," or RFP. An RFP asks vendors to compete based on price and quality, whether what is being bought is a jet fighter or ballpoint pens. Burns and Miller reasoned that the same principle of adherence to specifications should apply to the purchase of health care. If state or federal "performance reports" represented one kind of accountability—here's how you're doing, you could be better—then contract specifications represented an even more concrete step in the same direction: here's what you *must* be doing to get our business.

As with any decision involving medical service, designing an RFP was not simple. For one thing, health care services can be hard to describe in detail. For another, an RFP reverses the usual balance of power between those providing care and those buying it. Traditionally the price, quantity, and quality of health care services have been defined by doctors, hospitals, and health plans. The professionals used their best judgment, and the laymen accepted it. An RFP meant that the purchasers set the ground rules. If it wasn't exactly "commoditization" of medicine, it was certainly "corporatization," even if the corporate bureaucrat signing the contract was a physician such as Burns.

At Chrysler, Joseph Califano used a crude kind of RFP for hospitals in 1982. But Chrysler's corporate survival was at stake, and Califano was no midlevel manager: he was a board member with the personal backing of the company chairman. In 1986, by contrast, Honeywell was prosperous. Taking on a few transplant centers was one thing. Angering hundreds of local doctors and a score of local hospitals was something else again. Honeywell's top brass said no to the RFP idea.

Although Burns couldn't get an RFP through the Honeywell front door, the project with the Business Health Care Action Group offered an opportunity to sneak the same thing in through the stage door. Putting on a demonstration project, a "show," gave Burns the freedom to write a script that imagined the world the way he wanted it to look. Burns worked hard to make sure his BHCAG colleagues would share his vision. At meetings, he regaled the assembly with tales of inappropriate treatments and wrongheaded economic incentives. He brought in articles from medical journals that documented variation in treatment divorced from scientific evidence. And he persuaded the group to look at some real numbers that directly involved their own friends, neighbors, and families.

At the request of the business group, Blue Cross and Blue Shield of Minnesota assembled a study that showed stunning variations in care. The study was the familiar one we have seen so many times in this book. The rate of cesarean sections done on Minnesota women in different parts of the state ranged from 9 to 48 percent. There was a fourfold difference in the frequency of hysterectomies. For a couple of diagnoses, the likelihood of being admitted to the hospital varied by as much as a factor of thirteen. It was all a damning commentary on the inconsistency of individual physicians' judgment.

BHCAG members agreed that something had to change. In early 1992, with the help of several consultants, the Business Health Care Action Group was ready to issue a sweeping "request for proposal" to the medical community. The participating BHCAG members now included fourteen companies whose workers and their families added up to 150,000 lives. This was a big-time production. BHCAG had taken center stage.

THE ORGANIZER

Fred Hamacher, vice president of compensation and benefits at Dayton Hudson Corporation, gave a stock reply to anyone who asked how he became BHCAG's chairman. Referring back to the nascent group's 1991 meeting, which was held in a Dayton Hudson corporate conference room, Hamacher explained: "I bought the doughnuts."

Every theatrical production needs financial "angels," so perhaps Hamacher's doughnuts provided as good a reason as any for his prominence. A more likely explanation was Hamacher's "can-do" attitude and bulldog persistence. Though his 1950s haircut and straight-arrow free-market beliefs seemed to signal ideological rigidity, Hamacher was a conservative pragmatist. He was in favor of whatever it took to get a job done. His boyish enthusiasm helped take the edge off the occasional shoot from the lip remark, which was an operating style several in the BHCAG group shared.

Hamacher, a native of a small Indiana farming town, joined Dayton Hudson as a benefits analyst in 1970. It was a time when the retailer was grappling with a momentous cultural change. In 1969, Minneapolis-based Dayton's (a department store formed in 1902 by a banker turned dry goods dealer) had bought out Detroit-based Hudson's (which traced its origins to a men's clothing store begun in 1881).[2] The new Dayton Hudson Corporation grew rapidly, fueled by its department stores (including Mervyn's and Marshall Field's), discount stores (Target), and bookstores (B. Dalton). Hamacher learned to act quickly and decisively as he oversaw benefits administration for an ever-expanding workforce.

In the early 1970s, many corporate managers shared the feeling of organized medicine that prepaid health care was a stalking-horse for socialized medicine. Hamacher, though, was willing to give this new system a chance. In 1972 Dayton Hudson and fourteen other employers joined with community leaders to create the Twin Cities Health Care Development Project. The coalition helped defeat a plan by traditional insurers to limit the number of prepaid plans in the metropolitan area to one large community group. (Nonprofit Group Health had been operating in the Twin Cities since 1957.) The employer-community alliance endorsed competition among many smaller plans and then helped some newer ones get off the ground. Members also lobbied successfully for state legislation that encouraged the formation of what came to be called health maintenance organizations.[3] Within three years, the number of HMOs in the Twin Cities area grew from one to six.

Minneapolis–St. Paul presented an ideal environment for HMOs. Prepaid care historically drew strong union support, which blended nicely with the ideology of Minnesota's unique Democrat–Farm Labor Party. At the same time, the concept remained acceptable to Republican progressives as a free-market alternative to state control. Indeed, HMO advocate Paul Ellwood deliberately shifted from the vocabulary of medicine to the vocabulary of business. Said Ellwood:

> We were reasonably calculating in our approach. We consciously developed a new rhetoric, for one thing. We began using the language of the marketplace, rather than the language of medicine. We began talking in terms of "providers and consumers" instead of "doctors

> and patients," for example. This, of course, was and still is highly offensive to many people in medicine, but we felt the old language was almost like the language of religion, and, thus, harder to use when trying to effect widespread change.[4]

Ellwood set up a think tank called InterStudy (where "Buy Right" advocate Walter McClure eventually worked) in the western Minneapolis suburb of Excelsior. *Fortune* ran a color photo showing Ellwood happily paddling a canoe from his home on one side of Christmas Lake to his InterStudy office on the other. The magazine called Ellwood a man "making waves" in American medicine.

Ellwood's proselytizing and the passage of federal and Minnesota laws encouraging the formation of HMOs made an impact. Plans with names such as Share, HMO Minnesota, and MedCenter began knocking on the doors of Twin Cities businesses, asking for a chance to enroll workers. The medical society, figuring if you can't fight 'em, join 'em, bankrolled its own Physicians Health Plan. Dayton Hudson showed the way for the corporate community; at a time when many workers were still trying to figure out just what an HMO was, it offered its workers a choice among regular indemnity health insurance and two different HMOs.

The outburst of HMO competition in Minneapolis–St. Paul pushed overall HMO enrollment upward at a dizzying 27 percent annually from 1971 to 1978.[5] By the early 1980s, the percentage of Twin Cities residents belonging to HMOs was six times that of the rest of the country—roughly 25 percent to 4 percent. The Reagan administration's support of "competitive health plans" helped HMOs spread nationally, but HMO membership remained three times higher in the Twin Cities at the end of the decade—about 50 percent of the population versus 16 percent.[6]

Twin Cities hospitals were the first to feel the effects of this HMO boom. HMOs had always been more frugal with hospital care than fee for service doctors. The rate at which local residents were admitted to the hospital slid by nearly a quarter from 1980 to 1986, while the average time a patient remained in the hospital dropped by nearly 40 percent.[7] As beds emptied, Twin Cities hospitals began to consolidate into companies such as Health One, LifeSpan, and (when those two combined) HealthSpan. HMOs, too, began to consolidate and change. Unrestricted fee for service medicine was slowly beginning to die.

Still, large employers based in the Twin Cities remained unhappy.

Costs were below national norms, but they were beginning to rise at the same double-digit pace. Hamacher came up with a statistic everyone could understand. Dayton Hudson, he said, had to sell 39,000 Teenage Mutant Ninja Turtles action figures to pay for an appendectomy. Meanwhile, the state of Minnesota was threatening to finance its own reform plan with a tax on business.

"We [benefits managers] would see each other at meetings for years," said Hamacher. "We'd say we ought to do something, but the pain wasn't bad enough." Once the pain reached a critical level, however, Hamacher and BHCAG were ready to act.

THE CURTAIN RISES

> It is a familiar failing of visionaries and people who live in the realm of ideas and issues that they are not inclined to soil their hands with the nuts and bolts of organization or social functioning. . . . Every leader needs some grasp of how to "work the system."
>
> —John Gardner, 1986

In a play, actors must recite the lines written for them. In a musical, the singers cannot choose their own tunes. Using similar logic, BHCAG laid down a set of rules that all the companies in the demonstration project had to follow. First, all BHCAG participants had to offer the new plan that the group designed without any changes, although members could offer additional plans as well. Before joining BHCAG, its founding members (Dayton Hudson, Honeywell, First Bank, Norwest Bank, Pillsbury, and General Mills) each provided employees with a slightly different benefits package, and each required somewhat different forms and procedures. The result was massive unneeded paperwork. "I hate like hell to spend money on administrative overhead," growled an unhappy Hamacher. "A dollar for health care is OK, but ten cents for administration drives me nuts."

Second, the group made clear that it wasn't just looking for discounts. BHCAG was going to purchase health care on "value"—the combination of cost and quality—not just price. Potential BHCAG members were interviewed before being allowed to join; companies looking for "cheap, cheap, cheap" were given the hook. Finally, the group adopted a rule that required a great deal of self-control. It said there were to be no confrontations. There would be no confrontations with each other—decisions would be made by consensus—and no deliberate confrontations with doctors or hospitals either. There would be no grandstanding, no looking for a fight—just a practical midwestern focus on finding answers to some tough questions.

Doctors, hospitals, and health plans "were frustrated as heck, too," recalled Hamacher. "So we told them, 'Here's what we're thinking of doing. We don't have the keys to wisdom. Give us some input.'" Hamacher reflected, then added dryly, "That caught them off guard."

The first "request for proposal" issued by the Business Health Care Action Group bore the upbeat title "the Quality of Care Partnership." A partnership it may have been, but it was one whose basic terms were unmistakably dictated by business. The proposal began by putting the profit maximizers (business) and the professionals (the medical community) on equal ground, pointedly noting the large number of studies on unexplained practice variation and the glaring absence of outcomes information to justify many common medical practices. This state of affairs "confuse[s] employers," the proposal continued, although BHCAG didn't sound very confused. The tone was set by an approach that Honeywell's Burns called "specify, but verify." An excerpt from the RFP, with emphasis added, illustrates the point.

> Most employers recognize that documentation of the clinical quality of medical care is an extremely complex and difficult process. Yet we are convinced that is both possible and necessary for employers and employees to better understand the *product being purchased* when they contract for such services. Additionally, just as *the products and services offered by employers are subject to continuous quality improvement,* it is urgent that employers be assured that *the services of their affiliated health care delivery systems undergo the same continual scrutiny.* To that end, we propose the employer enter a long-term partnership with one or more health care delivery systems to provide *objectively documented* high-quality medical services to employees. *Quantification of quality in this arena will require increasingly sophisticated monitoring processes and instruments* over time and will involve a high degree of cooperation between providers, employers and employees.[8]

The BHCAG proposal was designed to ensure that health plan doctors would pause and consider whether an intervention was necessary (the patient would worsen without the treatment) and appropriate (the intervention was the best one justified by the medical evidence). The next step was examining how well the intervention was performed and whether it achieved the expected improvement in the patient's health.

BHCAG's demands for information were formidable by any measure. In the context of the historical reluctance of American business to truly manage health care, they were extraordinary. This was a full-blown bureaucratic inquisition, designed to systematically expose how hospitals, physicians, and health plans really operated. A taste of just "phase 1" of the proposal, which listed the functions the winning bidder for the BHCAG business should be able to perform immediately, shows the depth and breadth of information being demanded.

- Is there a written Quality Improvement (QI) plan? If yes, when was the last time it was updated?
- Who is the individual responsible for program implementation, and to whom does he or she report? Please provide a resume of this person.
- To whom does the [QI] committee report? What is the Board of Directors' role in the QI plan?
- Are practice guidelines used? Describe the method of establishing guidelines and communicating them to plan providers.
- Is performance assessed against the guidelines?
- How do you examine the continuity of care received by participating [HMO plan] members? How do you detect underutilization?
- What improvements have been implemented during the past two years as a result of the [QI] program? How have these changes improved the quality of care?
- Do you perform an initial on-site visit at a prospective primary-care physician's office? Please provide a copy of your office survey form.
- Is there a process for periodic verification of clinical credentialing . . . ? Does the re-credentialing process include review of data from:
    - Member complaints; utilization management; member satisfaction surveys; individual quality performance; individual utilization performance.
- For the following procedures, do you maintain formal, written, procedure-specific standards?
- Heart transplant; lung transplant; liver transplant; kidney trans-

plant; pancreas transplant, autologous bone marrow transplant; coronary artery bypass graft; angioplasty; cardiac valve replacement; brain and spinal cord rehabilitation; selected neurosurgery; air ambulance transport.

- What are the specific standards for each of the above procedures for [the following indicators of quality]:
  - Annual institutional volume [of the hospital]; annual surgeon volume; average length of stay; in-hospital mortality; surgical complication rate; annual patient survival; annual graft survival (as appropriate); ten-year reoperation rate (for CABG); graft vessel type (for CABG).
- Are the standards reviewed and changed each year? Please provide a copy of last year's standards on a few of the procedures demonstrating this change.

BHCAG's "phase 2" requirements advanced a step further. The winning bidder was required to collect medical practice variation data on the rate of selected medical and surgical procedures among the health plan's total membership; data on outpatient services for acute and chronic diseases; and data on the preventive care provided to adults (such as breast cancer screening) and children (such as immunizations).

Separately, the coalition turned a rare spotlight on the sensitive topic of medical mistakes. The RFP told health plans to document the frequency of certain worrisome events that could indicate trouble at a hospital; for example, a patient's unscheduled return to the operating room, unanticipated transfers to the intensive care unit, or significant medication errors.

Finally, there was the phase 3 "wish list." These items were not on the near-term horizon. They were mentioned mostly to send a signal about the direction in which the coalition expected health care to evolve. BHCAG wanted to contract with someone who looked ahead to providing clinical outcomes of care (death, complications, and the like) and patient-perceived outcomes; for example, how well patients functioned in their daily lives after medical treatment.

Hamacher rightly called the sweeping BHCAG proposal "a whole new way of thinking." Even Honeywell had not gone this far. On its own BHCAG wasn't merely seeking to buy "good" care, as Honeywell, Chrysler, and others had done. The BHCAG corporations were trying to push the entire Twin Cities health care system, from the office examining room to the hospital's operating room to the health plan's boardroom, in the direction of "best" medical care. In that sense this effort truly demanded a partnership; to succeed, the business community had to persuade those who provided care to go along.

BHCAG also decided that an agenda this ambitious required a full-time executive director to guide its implementation. Steve Wetzell was vice president for benefits and payroll at First Bank System, a founding BHCAG member. Wetzell, then just thirty-seven, brought academic training in business administration and human resources, tactical savvy, and the ability to turn a phrase. These were not inconsequential talents in a high-visibility project where the public image of being "good guys" brought measurable political benefits. "We don't want health plans to manage care," Wetzell said, "we want providers to improve care." Another time, he summarized the coalition's attitude toward doctors and hospitals this way: "In God we trust. All others bring data."

For all of BHCAG's swagger, the group realized there was no guarantee that anyone would or could meet all the coalition's requirements. BHCAG might write a script, but it could not be certain that all the other actors would read their parts as written. Although BHCAG members collectively spent some $200 million a year for health care, their employees constituted less than 10 percent of the area's insured population. Privately, coalition members acknowledged that their influence came as much from the name recognition of the group's blue-chip partners as from economic clout.

Similar efforts elsewhere to force accountability in medicine had started out with more of an edge. In New York State, hospitals with open-heart surgery programs joined with the state health department as partners in data collection because they had little practical alternative. In Pennsylvania, requests to hospitals and doctors by the Health Care Cost Containment Council had the force of law. Meanwhile business coalitions in some other cities, such as Cleveland and Cincinnati, held such economic power that the medical community made at least a minimal attempt at cooperation to avoid a showdown.

To compensate for BHCAG's weakness, Burns practiced psychological warfare. For example, he dropped a few ostentatious public hints that the coalition might build its own hospitals and bring in new doctors if its proposal found no takers. The suggestion was mostly useful as a bluff. The benefits managers had neither the money nor the authorization from their corporate bosses to do any such thing.

In the end, though, the changing economic and social environment of medicine in the 1990s allowed the show to go on. With managed care on the rise, doctors and hospitals were eager to try out a new script that would preserve their independence. Health plans, meanwhile, lusted after BHCAG's business. Rather than facing an empty stage, BHCAG found itself auditioning the local medical community in a careful search for the right actors for its play.

TIMING IS EVERYTHING

Suppose for a moment that you are the manager of travel services for a Chicago corporation with hundreds of employees on the road at any one time. Some days it seems that half your workers live at O'Hare International Airport. Since three major airlines have hubs there, you decide to see which of them will offer you the best combination of service and price. When you call them, however, you find you have entered the Twilight Zone. It turns out that the airlines believe their main job is keeping the pilots happy.

Schedules? "Each of our captains uses his professional judgment as to when the plane should leave, where it should go, how fast it should fly, and when it should arrive." The type of aircraft? "That's really the kind of technical decision we feel is best left to the pilot. After all, he's the one who has to fly it." Fares? "The pilot, copilot, and navigator charge each individual passenger what they feel their professional services are worth." Safety oversight by the airline? "Our pilots and planes are certified by the Federal Aviation Administration. If there are any questions about safety, the pilots are ethically obligated to discuss the matter confidentially among their peers and then take any necessary corrective action."

On second thought, you decide to call Amtrak.

The success of any innovation depends on the environment in which it is introduced. Corporate contracts with airlines would make no sense in an aviation industry populated by thousands of tiny airlines that make a few flights a day at irregular intervals. Once a large airline offers a standardized schedule to a preset list of destinations on a certain type of aircraft, then a contract is possible.

Even then, however, other elements need to be present. When government regulation meant that the airlines charged much the same fare on the same routes, a large buyer got no discount. Even with a permissive government attitude, however, there has to be marketplace demand for contracting. The airplane was a luxury form of travel for many years. When it became a common business tool, with hundreds of thousands of business travelers each flying tens of thousands of miles annually, the economic and social equation changed.

The request for proposal from the Business Health Care Action Group was important because it signaled the entry into the health care marketplace of a powerful and sophisticated buyer. The coalition specified in detail exactly what *it* wanted to purchase rather than leaving it to the medical professionals to define the health care services they would sell. And like a company that might contract with a big airline over a less expensive but smaller start-up, the coalition members were free to evaluate both the cost and the quality of the services they were offered.

What made BHCAG's strategy possible in the first place, however, was a sea change in the economic and social environment of medicine. A big buyer needs a big seller. A corporate travel buyer needs to deal with an airline company, not thousands of individual pilots each flying their own planes. Although Minnesota had a long tradition of group practices, the ascendancy of HMOs accelerated the consolidation of the health care marketplace. Health plans collected doctors and hospitals into organized groups to "produce" medical services, and the "scientific management" envisioned for the hospital industry in the early part of the century emerged as something that applied to health systems instead. The corporate benefits manager, by manipulating the health insurance premium the worker paid, could "steer" workers to one or another plan. Or at least benefits managers could do that if they were willing to take the trouble to evaluate the differences between the plans. The name for that evaluation is "cost-benefit analysis."

Today, physicians and hospitals increasingly see cost-benefit analysis as a friend and protector against thoughtless pressures to blindly cut costs. That attitude represents a complete turnabout from the way the concept was initially viewed. Stanford University economist Alain Enthoven first laid out the details of what he called "managed competition"—bringing marketplace analysis to health care—in a 1978 article in the *New England Journal of Medicine.*[9] The reception was decidedly low key. Neither policymakers nor the medical community took the idea very seriously.

Enthoven was not surprised. Health care is not unique either in its suspicion of new ideas or in its insistence that its practices cannot be adequately assessed by objective criteria. Enthoven had already experienced much the same objections when he tried to control a segment of the American economy as resistant to change as medicine: the defense industry.

The reserved and intellectual Enthoven is the Dr. Strangelove of health care. Before turning a gimlet eye on the economics of health, he analyzed the costs and benefits of war as one of Robert McNamara's "whiz kids," recruited by McNamara when he left the presidency of Ford Motor Company in 1961 to become President John F. Kennedy's secretary of defense. McNamara was determined to show that modern management techniques could be applied to the Pentagon. At McNamara's behest, Enthoven created the Office of Systems Analysis to provide an objective economic appraisal of weapons and strategies. It was not a task for the faint of heart. The Cold War confrontation with the Soviets constantly threatened to ignite into a hot one, while the "hot" conflict in Vietnam steadily escalated. Discussions of defense spending, like debates over medical spending, came cloaked in emotionalism. If medical "captains" do not like having their judgment second-guessed, real captains (and generals and admirals) are even more vehement. That didn't bother Enthoven. His mandate came from the top.

Kennedy and his successor Lyndon B. Johnson "were trying to protect money for domestic programs," Enthoven recalled. "They knew that money spent for national defense would not be spent on domestic programs." The government could not afford to let the military and the defense contractors write their own specifications for weapons the government would buy. That was Enthoven's job, and he set to it with a vengeance. Success, however, turned out be transitory.

Just as the national preoccupation with high medical costs waxed and waned, worries about Defense Department waste proved similarly cyclical. The Nixon administration, which took over in 1969, cared more about appeasing southern conservatives than clamping down on inefficient military contractors. Besides, the Vietnam War was winding down. "Value purchasing" in defense would not capture public attention again until another Republican president, Ronald Reagan, began pumping unsupervised dollars into defense and promptly got $500 hammers and $1,000 toilet seats in return. Enthoven learned a valuable lesson. When the financial pressure was on, the politicians were interested in cost effectiveness. When it wasn't, other factors took over.

Being a logical sort, Enthoven sought out another field plagued by out-of-control costs. Ignoring Stanford colleague Kenneth Arrow's opinion that the term medical marketplace was an oxymoron (as discussed in chapter 10), Enthoven developed managed competition. By this time Democrat Jimmy Carter was in the White House; his administration was interested in regulatory controls, not cost-benefit analysis. Only in the late 1980s, as worries about double-digit medical inflation again brought health care costs to the top of the national agenda, did Enthoven start to find an audience.[10] Savvy in the ways of Washington, Enthoven hooked up with two politically experienced partners, HMO advocate Ellwood and Washington political consultant Lynn Etheredge. Their timing was excellent.

The original idea behind HMOs was that they were supposed to compete on price and quality. The Nixon administration had embraced them as an alternative to a government-run health care system. Managed competition amounted to a more sophisticated tinkering with the HMO concept, but the audience appeal remained the same. Rising health care costs had brought the idea of a government-financed health system to the forefront of public policy once again. Managed competition was a way to head it off at the pass. In 1991 a group of congressional "new Democrats" introduced managed competition legislation as an alternative to either a Canadian-style "single payer" system or a convoluted government mandate for universal coverage known as "pay or play." (Businesses had to provide coverage to all workers or pay the government to do it.) In 1992 a bipartisan coalition of legislators seized on the approach, and an ambitious "new Democrat" candidate for president took notice.

Bill Clinton was looking for a way to separate his approach to health care reform from the tepid market tweaking of the conservative Bush administration (health reform was an issue that George Bush personally cared little about) and the aggressive market abandonment of the Democratic left. Clinton decided to endorse a modified version of managed competition (critics preferred "bastardized") and make health care reform a centerpiece of his campaign. What all versions of managed competition shared was a vision of the end of the cottage industry, medieval guild structure of American medicine. In its place would arise large-scale "accountable health plans" that would compete for patients' business.

The long and intense national debate on health reform that ensued did almost as much to change the perceptions of what was possible as actually passing legislation would have done. Only six years before, Honeywell's senior management hesitated to use an RFP to buy health care. Now, "accountability" was tossed around in common conversation by political pundits and other members of the in-the-know, inside-the-Beltway crowd. Competition was "hot," and the Business Health Care Action Group found itself riding the crest of a national wave. What had been a local demonstration project, the equivalent of an off-off-Broadway revue, became a "must have" ticket. Managed competition was coming to Main Street USA, and a preview could be seen, heard, and touched in the Twin Cities.

The news media flocked northward. "Employers' Attack on Health Costs Spurs Change in Minnesota," wrote the *Wall Street Journal.* "While Congress Remains Silent, Health Care Transforms Itself," advised the *New York Times.* "Results-Based Competition Injected into Health Care," said the *Chicago Tribune.* But it was left to *Medical Economics* magazine, with a bow to a famous *New York Daily News* headline (Ford to City: Drop Dead), to accurately summarize why BHCAG's purchasing program was such an important model for the rest of the nation. *Medical Economics* warned its physician audience: "Business to Doctors: Show Us You're Doing It Right."

But how could doctors demonstrate with data something they had so long believed was too elusive to quantify? That was the challenge facing the coalition of health plans and physician groups that captured the BHCAG business in June 1992. The coalition included the Group Health Incorporated HMO, Park Nicollet Medical Center, MedCenters Health Plan (an HMO affiliated with Park Nicollet), and the Mayo Clinic.[11] What attracted BHCAG to the group was not only its price, but its leadership's commitment to a key business technique for turning scientific management into solid results. The technique is called CQI, or continuous quality improvement.

CHAPTER TWELVE

Changing the System from Within

Ideas . . . both when they are right and when they are wrong, are more powerful than is commonly understood. . . . I am sure that the power of vested interests is vastly exaggerated compared with the gradual encroachment of ideas.
—John Maynard Keynes

It takes a certain self-confidence to travel to the Mayo Clinic, stand up in front of its clinicians and administrators, and calmly lecture on the urgent need for them to improve the quality of their professional work. Donald Berwick, however, is a man whose courage is based on an unshakable sense of mission. The son of a small-town Connecticut general practitioner, Berwick holds a bachelor's degree in social systems (summa cum laude), a master's degree in public policy, and a doctorate in medicine (he's a pediatrician)—all from Harvard. He is also founder and president of the Boston-based Institute for Healthcare Improvement. As IHI's president, Berwick determinedly crisscrosses the country spreading the word about a new paradigm of medical practice, one whose central tenet is "continuous quality improvement" (CQI).

The quality improvement movement says that the delivery of health care services to patients must be viewed as a system. Physicians play a central role, but their ultimate success depends on nurses, technicians, and others within the system. The heart attack improvement project at Anderson, the pneumonia improvement at Forbes, the guideline use at Cedars-Sinai, and the bypass surgery improvements at Winthrop-University are all examples of CQI efforts. In articles and speeches, Berwick returns repeatedly to this theme of interdependence, in a conscious attempt to change the physician's worldview.

"The solo doctor who embodies [by himself] every process needed to ensure highest-quality care is now nearly a myth," Berwick writes. "All physicians depend on systems, from the local ones in their private offices to the gargantuan ones of national health care. . . . Those who speak for the profession, for health-care institutions, and for large-scale purchasers must establish and hold to a shared vision of a health-care system undergoing continuous improvement."[1]

As an unabashed member of the medical establishment, Berwick has won respect for views that could be very threatening coming from someone else. When the *New England Journal of Medicine* changed its longtime typeface in mid-1996, an explanatory editorial even justified this jolt to readers' sensibilities by citing a Berwick exposition on the need to constantly improve one's work. Despite CQI's inroads among the medical intelligentsia, however, it is still regarded suspiciously by many practicing physicians.

"The idea of measuring quality [in health care] in a systematic way is still a matter of enormous contention," Berwick acknowledges. "There is a continuing lack of conviction [by doctors] that improvement is needed . . . The conviction is, 'We're darn good, why don't people pay us what we want?' [But] how good you are doesn't say how good you could be."[2]

It is the fervent belief in this ideal of "how good you could be" that drives Berwick and that has brought him to Mayo to keynote a special meeting titled "Moving Forward: The Mayo Conference on Quality." In addition to the several hundred people who sit in the auditorium, hundreds more watch this meeting on closed-circuit television at other Mayo locations. Economic concerns—including pressure from the Business Health Care Action Group—is what prompted Mayo to first consider continuous quality improvement. But economics is not why the clinic leadership has finally embraced the "clinical evaluative sciences" (the science of examining the impact of everyday care) as a proper intellectual companion to the "biomedical sciences" (traditional research). This is why Robert Waller, Mayo Foundation president and chief executive officer, who came to the clinic from the National Institutes of Health, has invited Berwick to speak first.

"Those who provide medical care must lead in [changing] medical care," Waller says in his introduction. He then adds what, within the low-key Mayo culture, amounts to an effusive endorsement. Berwick, he says, "is an individual of compassion and honesty and integrity." "My awe in coming here each time is real," Berwick responds. "Mayo, among a very few, can lead the country by force of sheer example. . . . If you succeed [in implementing continuous quality improvement], you'll show the way to getting out of this [health care] mess." But almost immediately a hint of heresy sneaks into the deferential tone. "The challenge is to honor your heritage, but to move on from it."

But move where? Ever so gently, Mayo CEO Waller suggests that the end of reputation-based medicine is at hand—even for the Mayo Clinic. "[The issue is], can we manage quality, and if so, how?" Waller asks the group. "[And] can we develop systems that provide solid data?" To some clinicians, Waller's words have a foreign sound. Yet "data systems" and "managing quality" are really what the Mayo Clinic has always been about.

THE ASSEMBLY LINE

The most important factors affecting a physician's performance are "determined mainly by [the doctor's] work environment."[3] That's hardly a surprise to Mayo. As carefully as the clinic screens the physicians it invites to join its staff, what is called the "Mayo way" is still seen as the ultimate guarantee of consistent, high-quality care. In one sense the Mayo way is a statement of values and principles summarized in a glossy wallet-sized card given to all employees. Under the heading "Our Primary Value" there is just one statement: "The needs of the patient come first."

In a broader sense, though, the "Mayo way" refers to the accumulated weight of the Mayo tradition. Doctors, nurses, and administrators constantly ask themselves whether a course of action is consonant with the way the clinic's founders would want things done. The Mayo Clinic system of care is viewed as a kind of collective continuation of the medical practice of the Mayos themselves.

"From the patient's perspective, you turn yourself over to the system, and it analyzes you and tells you in its collective wisdom what is the best thing to do," explained one clinic official. "We view Mayo as a method of providing care."[4]

Mayo is unique even among group practices in its reliance on a kind of enlightened assembly line. The approach is adapted from the "scientific management" of Frederick Taylor's turn of the century time-and-motion studies. Patients are sent from laboratory to examining room to hospital in a carefully choreographed routine. To allow doctors to move quickly from patient to patient, the examining rooms themselves are arranged along a corridor. Colored lights outside each room signal whether the room is empty, contains a patient waiting to be seen, or is occupied by a physician and patient together.

This Model T–like production system was introduced in 1907 by a Mayo physician named Henry Plummer, about the same time the real Model T was rolling off its assembly line. Plummer conceived the idea of standardizing not the decisions made by doctors—that always depended on the patient's individual needs—but the raw material doctors used to make their decisions; that is, the information contained in the patient chart. It is a crucial distinction. Plummer set in motion a series of events that conspired to keep unwanted variation low and the quality of care high. His most important innovation was called the "unified medical record."

The Mayo medical record, conceived in a world of inkwells and blotting paper, remains unique even as today's multibillion-dollar health systems rush to put the same concept into electronic form. In the rest of the medical world, every doctor's office and hospital generally keeps its own records of an encounter with a patient. Sharing of information is hit or miss. At Mayo, by contrast, every doctor works off the same paper chart. Each doctor, whether in or out of the hospital, views the complete spectrum of patient information, including everything from outpatient diagnostic tests to in-hospital nursing notes. And each doctor adds new information to the chart in a standardized format that colleagues can understand and use.

This elaborately cross-referenced record of every patient encounter with any Mayo doctor was conceived as something permanently available for both patient care and research. Plummer ordered paper for the medical charts that was guaranteed to last a century, and he personally tested the pens and ink to be used in making notes. Thanks to Plummer's prescience, Mayo has more than 4.5 million patient files.

Not surprisingly, clinic founders William and Charles Mayo were early and enthusiastic boosters of hospital standardization. William Mayo served on the American College of Surgeons' Committee on Standardization of Hospitals—the committee chaired by Ernest Amory Codman. At a 1915 meeting of the fellows of the College, Charles Mayo singled out Codman's "end result idea" for special praise. "The greatest stimulus [for standardization] has come from accomplishments in Boston," declared Mayo, "and I give great credit to Dr. Ernest Amory Codman for his pioneer work."[5]

Just as the Mayo system was inspired by industry, at least one famous industrialist was inspired by Mayo. Henry Ford is said to have recruited Mayo physicians to come to Detroit from the clinic's Rochester, Minnesota, home to help establish the Henry Ford Hospital.[6]

The unified medical record does more than ensure "efficiency, thoroughness, and replication in examinations and reporting [of results]."[7] It also provides a subtle but powerful form of quality control. In a typical community setting, independent fee for service physicians have only a general idea about the practice patterns of their colleagues—as we saw in Maine in chapter 1. Mayo doctors, on the other hand, metaphorically peer into each other's examining rooms all the time. The medical record shows every Mayo doctor how every other doctor makes diagnoses and prescribes treatment. By tradition, Mayo doctors do not wear the white coats of "scientific" medicine. But the unrelenting peer pressure of the common medical record pushes them to keep up with the latest scientific studies much more than is true in many places where the white lab coat is common. Understandably, no one wants to be known to peers as the person who can't keep up.

The clinic's commitment to "evidence-based medicine" similarly traces its roots to the clinic's early days. "Dr. Will" and "Dr. Charlie" stressed a constant search for "best practices" even after the clinic's reputation was comfortably established.[8] The present Mayo leadership invokes the founders' blessing on continuous improvement projects with a quotation from Dr. Will: "The glory of medicine is that it is constantly moving forward, that there is always more to learn."

One thing the original Doctors Mayo did not learn was that there was an alternative to Taylorism for managing industrial processes. It wasn't their fault; this alternative method of quality control was not well publicized or accepted at first. The reasoning behind it was unconventional. But over time it would have an extraordinary impact on both industry and medicine by becoming the foundation of continuous quality improvement.

A PHYSICIST MAKES A TELEPHONE

For a man whose ideas would eventually reshape American industry, Walter Shewhart was a reticent revolutionary. Contemporaries described him as gentle, benign—even "radiant."[9] A native of the small town of New Canton, Illinois, Shewhart earned a Ph.D. in physics in 1917 at the University of California, Berkeley, then spent a year teaching at a secondary school in Wisconsin. He moved back to Illinois to join the Western Electric Company, forerunner of the famous Bell Telephone Laboratories. It was the start of an "information revolution." New automated dialing systems were giving more and more Americans access to Alexander Graham Bell's revolutionary communications device. Shewhart's tasks included ensuring the reliability of the fast-growing national system of phone exchanges (the nerve center for switching all calls coming into and out of an area) and the production of the phones themselves.[10]

Shewhart decided to apply what he had learned about statistical techniques in graduate school to the mundane but important task of producing a consistently high-quality telephone. The solution he came up with was nothing less than an intellectual tour de force. Shewhart's insights were astounding for both the way he arrived at them and the influence they continue to exert many decades later. For example, Shewhart was inspired by an early scientific paper by Albert Einstein on the movement of atomic particles. Future generations then applied Shewhart's work to everything from the manufacture of automobiles to improving service at luxury hotels to, as we shall see, treating stroke patients at the Mayo Clinic.

Unlike the phone company's industrial engineers, Shewhart did not expect a factory to turn out "perfect" phones all the time. He believed the specifications of any manufactured product would always vary to a certain irreducible extent. He called this normal difference "common cause" variation. Attempts to eliminate common cause variation and make every production run identical not only were a waste of time and money, they also risked making things worse rather than better. In contrast to common cause variation, "special cause" variation, traceable to something other than the normal vagaries of manufacturing, needed to be addressed immediately. By eliminating "special cause" variation, a company increased its productivity, the quality of its product, and as an inevitable result, profits. When production consistently met specifications, a company did not have to spend so much time and money repairing or replacing defective items.

The key question, of course, was how to differentiate the two categories of variation. This was where Shewhart's training in physics came into play. In breaking with the accepted mind-set about industrial production, Shewhart found support in, of all places, the writings of another master of unconventional thinking—Einstein.[11] The common thread linking the two men was their interest in the seemingly paradoxical concept of the predictability of randomness.

In the early nineteenth century a Scottish botanist named Robert Brown demonstrated that pollen randomly dispersed in water moved constantly in an unvarying pattern unless disrupted by an outside force—for example, a rock thrown into a pond. This movement, at once constant and random, was dubbed "Brownian motion." In 1905 Einstein used statistical techniques to reveal the cause of this puzzling phenomenon. In demonstrating that the pollen pattern resulted from the collision of individual atomic particles, Einstein helped prove the existence of molecules and atoms to a still skeptical scientific community. Einstein was able to show that although the specifics of which atom knocked into which other atom constituted a series of chance events, the overall pattern of movement stayed within certain calculable boundaries.

This strange notion of controlled randomness is what inspired Shewhart with a solution to the telephone manufacturing problem. On 16 May 1924, the thirty-three-year-old physicist presented his boss at Western Electric with a one-page memorandum that included a diagram Shewhart called a control chart.[12] This diagram, in an easy-to-understand format, graphically represented the principles of Brownian movement ("common cause" variation) and movement that was not within Brownian limits ("special cause" variation). However, the control chart applied these principles to a practical business problem—it married the insights of Browning and Einstein and turned them into something that could be used by a high-school graduate overseeing the production of telephones.

Here is how it worked. Shewhart calculated mathematically valid upper and lower limits of "normal" variability of a process. In the case of making telephones, Shewhart gave his theoretical calculations a reality check by studying the actual Western Electric production process. On the control chart, Shewhart drew the upper and lower bounds of normal variability as horizontal lines. These were the borders of common cause variation. Precisely halfway between those limits, Shewhart drew another horizontal line. That line represented zero defects—precise conformity with specifications, or "quality."

To tell whether the production process was "in control," a plant foreman had only to glance at this chart. If the number of defects remained between the borders set by the upper and lower lines, then the variation was normal and the product could be sent out to customers. (Of course the specifications themselves could be altered by changing the values represented by each line.) If the defect level crossed the boundary lines—by either going up too high or dropping unexpectedly low—it signaled special cause variation. Then it was management's job to find the source of the problem.

As a physicist, Shewhart viewed his approach as comparable to the classic teachings of the scientific method. A company first specified what its product should look like (the hypothesis), then produced the product (the experiment); finally, it used a control chart to see whether the specifications had been met (the test of hypothesis).[13]

Not only did the control chart turn factory managers into scientists, it also changed their jobs from spotting "bad" products to improving the entire system. Once a process was "in control," managers could use the chart to systematically examine ways to make production even better; in essence, taking on "normal" variation in a holistic way. The control chart turned out to be a tool for both continuous measurement *and* continuous improvement.

A 1939 book of Shewhart's lectures edited by W. Edwards Deming, an avid Shewhart follower, highlighted the importance of this new method. "Most of us have thought of the statistician's work as that of measuring and predicting and planning, but few of us have thought it the statistician's duty *to try to bring about changes in the things that he measures,*" wrote Deming, a Ph.D. physicist working as a senior mathematician at the U.S. Department of Agriculture (emphasis added). Added Deming: "It is evident, however, from the first chapter [of this book] that this viewpoint [of Shewhart's] is absolutely essential.[14]

Although Shewhart's writings dazzled mathematicians and statisticians, contemporary industrialists were not so smitten. Even Bell Labs preferred to stick with the tried-and-true sampling and inspection techniques it knew so well. The full implications of Shewhart's insights into the opportunity presented by systematic improvement, written during the first third of the twentieth century, began to be realized only in the century's final third. In midcentury, Shewhart follower Deming also encountered problems in getting American industry to understand the potential of the process control idea. But unlike Shewhart, Deming was finally able to find a receptive audience. Unfortunately for American business, that audience was Japanese.

FROM JAPANESE CARS TO AMERICAN MEDICINE

The turmoil of the 1960s and early 1970s shattered many of the old ways of thinking in American politics and popular culture. In the late 1970s and the early 1980s, it was the turn of American business to face upheaval. From steel to machine tools to consumer electronics, Japanese companies were everywhere ascendant. It wasn't just that Japanese products often cost less. In a sharp rebuke to American management and workers, consumers also bought Japanese because the products were better made. In automobiles, for instance, Toyota and Nissan (maker of the Datsun) had learned well the painful lesson that low cost, low quality wouldn't sell. By the mid-1970s, both Japanese automakers were selling more cars in the United States than onetime import leader Volkswagen. By the end of the decade, amid rave reviews from consumer magazines for their quality, nearly one in four cars sold in America were Japanese.

Even American businesses began altering their purchasing patterns. Electronics manufacturer Hewlett-Packard found that fifty to one hundred of every fifty thousand semiconductor chips it bought from American companies failed inspection on arrival at the Hewlett-Packard factory; none of the Japanese chips did. In the field, American chips were twenty-seven times as likely to fail as Japanese ones.[15]

In late 1979 NBC News decided to make a documentary exploring the reasons behind this humbling of American industry. The documentary's producer, Clare Crawford-Mason, was an experienced print and television reporter, but she soon found herself despairing at the tedious explanations of trade and manufacturing minutiae she encountered. Then a faculty member at American University in Washington, D.C., suggested she speak with an elderly consultant who lived nearby. Deming was then seventy-nine years old. As he pulled out yellowed newspaper clippings, the stunned Crawford-Mason could hardly believe the story unfolding before her.[16]

This obscure elderly consultant had worked with the United States military during World War II, enthusiastically teaching American factory workers and managers to use statistical process control methods to boost production while keeping quality high. But when the war ended, his lessons were forgotten during the ensuing years of plenty. American business could sell everything it could make. In Japan, however, the war's legacy lingered. The nation's industrial base was in ruins, and the label "Made in Japan" was a badge of shame signifying that a product was poorly made. In 1950, Deming was invited by the Union of Japanese Scientists and Engineers to share his insights on how their local industry could improve. As a gesture of friendship to a country that was now a United States ally in the Cold War against communism, Deming's visit was sponsored by the Supreme Commander of the Allied Powers—the occupation force that was still overseeing postwar reconstruction.[17]

Deming's seminars were so popular that just one year later Japanese industry established an annual Deming Prize to recognize companies that implemented his methods. In 1960 Japan's prime minister personally pinned a jeweled solid gold medal on Deming's lapel and presented him with the Second Order of the Sacred Treasure, given under the authority of the emperor. Although Deming was the first American ever to receive this honor, the Sioux City, Iowa, native remained virtually unknown back home. A typical consulting project called on him to make a statistical analysis of accounts receivable in the trucking industry. As NBC's Crawford-Mason probed for details of Deming's life story, his frustration spilled over. "He kept going on and on and on that nobody would listen to him," she recalled to fellow journalist Mary Walton, author of *The Deming Management Method.*

The ninety-minute NBC documentary "If Japan Can . . . Why Can't We?" aired on the evening of 24 June 1980. The show's final fifteen minutes—an eternity in television time—showcased Deming's work in postwar Japan and his more recent success at a major United States company that had heard about him through a Japanese business partner. Narrator Lloyd Dobyns asked the blunt-spoken Deming whether the methods that worked there could succeed here. "Everybody knows that we can do it . . . [but] there's no determination to do it," Deming replied. "We have . . . no goal."[18]

The next day the phone in Deming's office, in the basement of his home, rang relentlessly. The year before the NBC documentary, about fifteen people had showed up at Deming's one annual seminar. Afterward he invited the group to his home for drinks. A year after the documentary, Deming's roster of clients included the likes of Ford and General Motors. By 1985 nearly four thousand people were attending one of Deming's four-day presentations.[19]

One of the many calls Deming received came from an unlikely source. Paul Batalden was a midlevel administrator at a large multispecialty physician group in suburban Minneapolis. The thirty-nine-year-old pediatrician had not seen the television documentary on Deming, but he had read about it later in the *New York Times*.[20] Batalden immediately sensed a kindred spirit.

Batalden was an unusual mixture of successful medical insider and antiestablishment outsider. While still in his twenties, he had practiced at the National Cancer Institute, served as medical director of the federal Job Corps, and become assistant surgeon general responsible for the federal Community Health Service. At the time, the Community Health Service oversaw everything from neighborhood health centers to quality standards for Medicare. It was also given the task of promoting the development of health maintenance organizations, the chosen private sector path to national health reform.

In 1975 Batalden left government for two jobs in the Twin Cities. Part of his time was spent as an outsider, working for Paul Ellwood's InterStudy think tank. Simultaneously, Batalden headed the pediatrics and quality assurance departments at the St. Louis Park Clinic, a group practice of medicine. On his own, Batalden began mapping some of the clinic's processes of care. He introduced doctors to the odd idea that the patient was a "customer." Patients were even polled about their experiences with their doctors. One physician was so unnerved by complaints about his persistent hostility that he voluntarily enrolled in psychotherapy. Eventually Batalden dropped out of InterStudy and devoted himself full time to quality improvement, even obtaining a grant from the Kellogg Foundation—the same group that had funded Vergil Slee's pioneering professional activity studies back in the 1950s.

Like Deming, Batalden believed that people were often prevented from doing their best by poorly designed workplace systems. Batalden's belief in "patient power" also resembled Deming's belief that the customers who used a product should have a say in its design. Deming, intrigued by a phone conversation with this unusual physician, invited him to attend an upcoming seminar in Atlanta. Batalden accepted and brought along another clinic doctor, Loren Vorlicky. The result was culture shock.

Reading about quality improvement in the *New York Times* was not the same as sitting in a ballroom filled with six hundred industrial engineers learning the nuts and bolts of the subject. "These engineers were smoking, and Deming was reading from his book, and he was talking about ball bearings," Batalden recalled, "and I was wondering what in the world we were doing there."

At the end of the first day, Batalden and Vorlicky joined Deming for dinner and encountered his famous work ethic firsthand. "What was very unusual about this thing was this guy who was eighty years old and had been lecturing for nine hours," said Batalden. "He gave himself an hour and a half for dinner because he had work to do when he got done with the meal."

As the seminar continued, Batalden began to look beyond ball bearings to the underlying principles Deming was trying to teach: "It dawned on me that what Deming was talking about was a theory of work and a theory of the workplace and a theory of the worker. If people in health care were ever going to understand what he was talking about, we had to move out of the language of manufacturing, back into the theory, and then back out again in health care talk."

A cornerstone of the "Deming method" was his fourteen points to guide managers in a "transformation" of American industry. The list began, "Create constancy of purpose toward improvement of product and service, with the aim to become competitive and to stay in business, and to provide jobs." It ended, "Put everybody in the company to work to accomplish the transformation. The transformation is everybody's job."[21] Batalden went home and adapted the list to apply to the kind of work performed by clinicians and health care administrators. Deming was pleased, but back at the St. Louis Park Clinic, Batalden's colleagues were mostly puzzled.

A new way of looking at the world succeeds only when the old way painfully and obviously fails, wrote science historian Thomas Kuhn. The much-touted health care "crisis" was mild compared with the crisis affecting American industry. Ford's Japanese competitors threatened the company's very existence. Aware of the yawning quality gap between its products and those made by the Japanese, Ford applied Deming's advice to the design and production of a new family sedan it called the Taurus. With a few exceptions, a similar sense of urgency was lacking in American medicine. When Medicare changed to a fixed-price reimbursement system, hospitals and doctors initially panicked. Then they realized there was so much waste in the system that they could easily reduce their costs enough to profit from the government's "average" payment. At academic medical centers, Medicare profits soared to record levels.

Batalden persisted. In the mid-1980s, the St. Louis Park Clinic merged with another large physician group to become the Park Nicollet Medical Center. Batalden was promoted to chief operating officer, then quit. He wanted to work full time as a missionary for the systematic improvement of medical care.

Unfortunately, although a few businesses might rant and rave about waste and a congressional committee would hold an occasional hearing, most of the medical establishment believed as always that everyday care "was the best in the world." Batalden's requests for financial support to improve quality were rebuffed by academic medical centers and by government agencies. A prominent health care foundation told him the whole thing sounded "far out." What saved his dream was a for-profit business begun by a father-son doctor team and an entrepreneur who had earned his wealth by franchising Kentucky Fried Chicken outlets. Together this team had built a hospital chain called the Hospital Corporation of America (HCA), headquartered in Nashville, Tennessee, far from the medical establishment.

HCA had a special interest in advocating the development of objective measures of health care quality. Investor-owned hospital companies were under relentless attack from critics who accused them of profiteering at the expense of good medicine. The careful tracking of care proposed by Batalden could give HCA the ammunition it needed to respond. Besides, the techniques promised to cut costs and increase profits.

HCA's chief executive, Thomas Frist Jr., the younger of the two doctors who helped start the corporation, was intrigued. In the early 1980s intimate gatherings of top corporate executives invariably included talk about the work of Deming or of other Shewhart followers such as Joseph Juran and Philip Crosby. At one such meeting, Frist buttonholed Robert Stempel, then chief operating officer of General Motors, to ask his honest opinion about "total quality management" (TQM) and "continuous quality improvement" (CQI). Stempel strongly endorsed them, and the top executives at companies like Ford and IBM gave similar replies.

Frist was a realist. If HCA spent a lot of money on some quixotic quest for statistical perfection, it might raise its costs and get nothing in return. After all, Frist recalled, "U.S. hospitals were in the service sector. We were not competing in a global marketplace, and I did not believe that either states or the federal government would place quality before cost. . . . I was worried about whether we could afford to undertake a major new program when our competition was not. Furthermore, no one had a model for hospitals. If we wanted to do it, we would have to look outside the industry for guidance."[22]

In 1986 Frist hired Batalden but gave him a limited mandate. "Pick seven or eight hospitals," Frist told him. "Let [quality improvement] prove itself" before rolling it out to the whole HCA system. What Frist meant was "prove it to me."[23] Batalden did.

In 1966 Avedis Donabedian, a Lebanese-born physician-researcher at the University of Michigan, had developed the first true conceptual model for evaluating everyday care. In Donabedian's formulation, medical quality rested on a tripod formed by the interaction of three elements: structure (having the right equipment in place), process (doing the right thing), and outcome (the results).[24] This model can be seen in complicated hospital therapies or in something as prosaic as the bandage (structure) a mother puts on a child's hand (process) to stop a cut from bleeding (outcome). Continuous quality improvement took the structure more or less for granted, honed in on every step of process, then measured the resulting alteration in outcome.

Within a few years Frist was publicly boasting about the ways HCA had improved its clinical processes. An HCA hospital in Portsmouth, New Hampshire, altered its management of pain control for patients undergoing hip replacements and similar surgery. The new approach let patients walk unassisted sooner and leave the hospital two days earlier. This was better for the patients and, under Medicare's fixed payment system, more profitable for HCA. (In the old cost-plus environment, by contrast, that process improvement would have emptied more HCA beds and cost the chain money.) In Wichita, Kansas, an HCA hospital studied its care of diabetics and learned to stabilize blood sugar more quickly, again getting patients home sooner. And in Pensacola, Florida, an HCA hospital found it could use less sophisticated, and less expensive, antibiotics for many patients without any difference in the results of care. The switch saved money and reduced the chances of resistance to antibiotics.[25]

A pleased Frist opened his wallet. From 1987 to 1992, HCA cut its corporate overhead by almost 80 percent, but the budget of Batalden's Quality Resource Group was increased. Batalden trained HCA managers as well as interested outsiders from all over the country in applying statistical process control techniques to health care. One of Batalden's most attentive students was a slightly younger pediatrician who was on the staff of the Harvard School of Public Health in Boston. The student's name was Donald Berwick.

Berwick had followed Batalden's example and attended one of Deming's industrial seminars. As had happened with Batalden, Berwick found the exposure to Deming initially frustrating. He recalled, "Something fundamental was at stake, some set of assumptions so wide and so pervasive that, psychologically, defense seemed more convenient than learning."[26] Like Batalden, however, Berwick stuck with it. Slowly, understanding dawned. A Berwick colleague, David Blumenthal, described running into him a short time after his return to Harvard. "Normally calm and contained, Berwick radiated an excitement bordering on elation as he described his experience. Anything that could do that to Don Berwick, I decided, was worth checking out myself."[27]

Berwick and Batalden would talk for hours about ways this new tool could be applied to improving patient care, and it was clear that the missionary spirit burned at least as strongly in the younger man. In 1991, as the health care establishment finally began to perceive the urgency of linking cost controls to quality measurement and management, the two men were able to obtain foundation funding for a new Institute for Quality Improvement (later the Institute for Healthcare Improvement). Berwick left his job at a health maintenance organization in Boston and became the institute's future president; Batalden was named chairman of the board.

Tom Frist's HCA hospitals did not have any foreign competitors, but the American companies coping with theirs gradually made it just as difficult to turn an easy profit. The shifting tides of economic fortune washed away Frist's dream of turning HCA into IBM (or perhaps fulfilled it in an unintended way). In October 1993 HCA was merged into an aggressively managed for-profit chain called Columbia Healthcare. The corporate culture at the new Columbia/HCA Healthcare Corporation changed, and Batalden decided to leave.

Fortunately, Batalden found a pleasant job at Dartmouth Medical School. The director of the Center for the Evaluative Clinical Sciences happened to have worked briefly at Harvard with Don Berwick and, from his own career, fully understood Batalden's obsession with reducing unnecessary variation and improving medical quality. Batalden's new boss was Jack Wennberg.

THERE'S NO "I" IN "TEAM"

> Everyone connected with the hospital must be in thorough accord with the new order of things. One balky horse in a team will stop the wagon.
>
> —A North Carolina surgeon, speaking of hospital standardization, at the 1923 meeting of the American College of Surgeons[28]

Despite the Mayo Clinic's connection to the industrial progenitors of "scientific management," the clinic did not take easily to continuous quality improvement. Success breeds conservatism, not paradigm breaking. Wennberg's variation studies were not welcomed by the doctors of New England, Batalden's improvement efforts encountered few enthusiasts at the St. Louis Park Clinic, and even Don Berwick was unable, in the mid-1980s, to transform the health maintenance organization where he was vice president of quality of care measurement. At Mayo, a group called the Academic Medical Center Consortium finally provided the needed wake-up call.

The twelve hospitals that made up the Academic Medical Center Consortium included members whose names—Mayo, Johns Hopkins, Duke, Massachusetts General—were synonymous with medical excellence. Consortium members agreed to jointly develop methods to measure the appropriateness and outcomes of four important surgical procedures and then benchmark their individual performance against that of the group. In 1993 the group reported its findings on carotid endarterectomy, a common treatment for patients who have suffered a stroke; Mayo's leaders were shocked by the results. Mayo stroke patients stayed hospitalized almost seven days, while patients at the other institutions averaged just four days. Moreover, the outcomes data provided no evidence that Mayo patients fared any better.[29] Since Medicare reimbursement was fixed, Mayo (which owned the two Rochester hospitals) was unnecessarily losing thousands of dollars every time it treated an elderly stroke victim. The clinic's leadership had been cautiously experimenting with quality improvement for administrative functions like answering telephones. Now Mayo's leaders made stroke care one of the clinic's top quality improvement priorities.

Gilbert Korb Jr. knew none of this when he arrived at Mayo in an air ambulance. He had come to the clinic for the first time back in 1951 as a scared twenty-three-year-old facing the grim diagnosis of testicular cancer. He made the trip to Rochester from Evansville,

Indiana, after his father confronted him with this question: Where do the doctors go when they have a problem? Korb's treatment was successful, and he returned to Mayo for regular checkups for five years, stayed away for many years after, then came again in the mid-1980s for treatment of atrial fibrillation, a condition in which the heart beats erratically. But the health problem Korb feared most was not cancer but stroke, with its often crippling aftermath. On Thursday, 13 April 1995, a few weeks shy of Korb's sixty-eighth birthday, his nightmare came true.

The interruption of the blood flow to the brain lasted only a moment or two, but the effect was striking. Korb's speech became garbled, his words slurring indistinguishably into each other. His right hand turned weak, and a handkerchief slipped from his grasp. Korb was preparing to go to work. Instead, he shakily telephoned his son. "I believe you ought to take me to the hospital," he said. "I think I'm having a stroke."

Korb did not stay there long. By Sunday night, at his request, he was on his way to Rochester. In choosing the Mayo Clinic, Korb was unknowingly participating in an ongoing experiment with continuous improvement techniques. The challenge Korb's doctors faced was to take the hallowed Mayo way, add just the right amount of industrial quality control techniques, and then seamlessly apply the resulting mixture to patient care. In Korb's case his neurosurgeon, David Piepgras, was the man with primary responsibility for accomplishing this tricky task.

Piepgras was a traditionalist—a black-and-white portrait of neurosurgery founder Harvey Cushing hung in his office—and a loyal Mayo soldier. After nearly a quarter century as a surgeon and medical school professor at the clinic, he had strong individual opinions that were matched by an equally strong dedication to clinic collegiality. Because he was chair of the department of neurosurgery, Piepgras was asked to serve on the nine-person quality improvement team assembled by the Juran Institute, Mayo's consultants. (Joseph Juran, like Deming, was a disciple of Walter Shewhart.) To manage a process, you must first "listen to [its] voice," Shewhart had said. Piepgras thought he knew a thing or two about the process of neurosurgery, but he reluctantly agreed to go along with the quality improvement team as its members set out to become good listeners.

A process—be it making telephones or performing surgery—cannot literally speak, of course. Its "voice" must be heard in other ways. Just as the notes on a sheet of music provide a pictorial representation of the sound of a song, the continuous improvement team used different types of charts to pictorially represent how stroke treatment at Mayo "sounded." The first kind of picture was a "flowchart" that divided stroke treatment into separate stages that "flowed" into each other. By breaking work into smaller parts, one can examine each increment more closely to see how it fits with what comes before and after. The flowchart for the hospital stay of carotid endarterectomy patients had three sections. The first ran from the patient's admission until the angiogram, a diagnostic procedure in which a contrast material is injected into the carotid artery so the artery shows up on X rays. The second went from the angiogram until surgery. And the third stretched from surgery to discharge.[30]

As the team analyzed each section of the hospital stay, it drew another picture, called a Pareto diagram. Vilfredo Pareto was a nineteenth-century economist and sociologist who calculated that 20 percent of a nation's people possess 80 percent of its wealth. He displayed this conclusion graphically. The connection between distributional economics and process control is this: some 80 percent of the difficulties with a process are typically caused by 20 percent of the possible factors. In a Pareto-style bar graph, it is easy to spot these "vital few" causes because the size of each bar corresponds to the frequency of a problem's occurrence. The taller the bar, the greater the barrier to efficiency it represents. At Mayo, the physicians' obliviousness to the economic consequences of their behavior accounted for the tallest bars of all.

There was, for example, the procedure for ordering an angiogram, which occurred during the first period of the hospital stay. First, a staff neurologist examined the patient. The neurologist then talked with a neurosurgeon, who also had to see the patient personally before ordering the test. Although this seemed reasonable, the patient wasted his first full day in the hospital being prodded and poked by a parade of medical students, interns, and residents. On day 2, the neurologist visited. The surgeon might not see the patient to discuss the angiogram until day 3, which delayed the performance of the test until day 4.

The obvious solution was to speed up the consultations and the ordering of tests. Less than twenty-four hours after Piepgras was asked to examine Korb, he did so and simultaneously ordered an angiogram. A cardiologist also made a quick appearance to order an echocardiogram, which provides an image of the beating of the heart.

During the second period of the hospital stay, thoughtless implementation of Plummer's principles of scientific management had degenerated into near-slapstick inefficiency. To make scheduling easier, Mayo assigns each surgeon a color, orange or blue, corresponding to alternate days of the calendar. "Orange" surgeons operate on orange days; "blue" surgeons on blue days. On blue days, the orange surgeons see patients at the clinic; on orange days, the blue surgeons see clinic patients.

Under the old Mayo procedures, a neurologist would refer the stroke patient to a neurosurgeon for a presurgery consultation after the angiogram. But if the neurosurgeon was an orange one and the next day was an orange day, the surgeon would be tied up in the operating room. After a whole day had been wasted, the neurosurgeon would see the patient and schedule the operation. It was enough to give an efficiency expert a bad case of the blues.

By the time Korb reached Mayo, the "color wars" problem had been conquered. His diagnostic tests were ordered on a Monday. Tuesday was "picture day." And then, Tuesday night, Korb's neurologist, neurosurgeon, and cardiologist—regardless of their "color"—met to compare notes.

"One of the messages that came out of this [continuous improvement] study was 'Let's not postpone things,' " acknowledged Piepgras. "The reason we show up there on Tuesday night at eight o'clock is not because we like to be in the hospital, but because we realize we've got all the information we need. . . . We're going to make the decision tonight, so if we're going to do anything, we're going to do it tomorrow." Indeed, although the specialists concluded their conference late Tuesday night, Korb was being prepared for the operating room by 6:00 A.M. Wednesday.

Piepgras and his colleagues concluded that Korb's "spell" was most likely caused by a carotid problem. The artery was less than three-quarters blocked, but it was highly irregular and clotted by ulcers. They decided it needed to be cleared out. And since Korb was going to be under general anesthesia for the carotid surgery, the cardiologist suggested it was a good time to "cardiovert" him—deliver a shock to his heart to stabilize its fibrillation. This meant Korb did not have to take anticoagulant drugs for his heart, drugs that thin the blood and need to be closely monitored. It also shortened his stay in the hospital after surgery, reducing the chance of a hospital-caused infection, and eliminated the risks of a second operation. In other words, Mayo was now getting better economic and clinical results.[31]

Even though Piepgras had already scheduled brain surgery on a different patient, he managed to juggle the timing of the two procedures. However, the pits and clots in Korb's carotid artery presented a special challenge. In an operating room in the basement of St. Marys Hospital, the same hospital where Will Mayo used to remove gallstones with a brass spoon, Piepgras and his surgical team spent more than four hours delicately clearing away obstacles to the flow of blood to Korb's brain. It was a display of skill and dedication that no "control chart" could ever accurately picture.

Half an hour past midnight, Piepgras walked in street clothes down the hospital's long and silent second floor hallway. A patient is not a collection of parts awaiting repair, and a surgeon is not a factory worker who punches a time clock and then goes home. "The needs of the patient come first." Even in the era of cost-conscious medicine, Mayo's leaders constantly repeated that slogan. After an eighteen-hour day, Piepgras remained faithful to that tradition. Arriving at his patient's room, he knocked on the door. Korb, his head bandaged, looked up to find the neurosurgeon inquiring how he was feeling. "I'm fine," Korb, replied, still groggy from anesthesia. Then he added a thought. "Go home," he told Piepgras, "and get some sleep."

The very next morning, the nurses began preparing Korb to go home.

Quality improvement techniques are easy to accept when they lead to doing the same old thing a little better. Doing things differently is more threatening. Discharging a patient who has just had surgery on the main artery bringing blood to the brain is serious business. Piepgras had no intention of risking a patient's life just to shave some time off the average hospital stay. Yet after combing through the data on the risk of postsurgical complications, Piepgras reached a conclusion that surprised him. Most complications happened in the first twenty-four to thirty-six hours. As a scientist, the neurosurgery chief found himself bending with the weight of the evidence. "I don't think patients need to stay in the hospital five, six, seven days after an operation any more," he acknowledged later. "Whereas, before [the continuous improvement team], I thought that they did. It's a mind-set." A "mind-set," of course, is another word for "paradigm," a way of viewing the world.

Although the neurosurgeon had to approve the discharge, the responsibility for getting the patient ready to go home more quickly, yet safely, fell to the nurses. On Thursday morning, the task of providing cost-effective caring for Gil Korb was taken on by neurology nurse Joye Nelson, a former elementary school teacher who had made a career change.

"We used to let patients laze around for a day or two, turn 'em over and baby 'em," said Nelson candidly. "It was nice, they loved it." Yet patient outcomes improved when the staff picked up the pace of rehabilitation. "Bed rest is what kills people," said Nelson. "They get better faster by getting up."

At the neurosurgery nursing station, veteran supervisor Kathleen Spoo remembered when her mother, a retired nurse, was hospitalized for more than two weeks after carotid surgery twenty years before. "After four days, she was off making patients' beds out of boredom," Spoo recalled. Even before the Mayo quality improvement team made its recommendations, added Spoo, the nurses "could see people didn't need to be here that long."

The average carotid endarterectomy patient at Mayo stayed in the hospital for 8.1 days in 1992, 6.8 days in 1993, and 4.6 days in April 1995, the month Gilbert Korb suffered his stroke—a decrease of 43 percent. Korb was discharged on Friday after a little over five days in the hospital.

The carotid endarterectomy experience at Mayo did not persuade every doctor. The leader of an improvement team examining surgery for brain tumors received several T-shirts with a cartoon showing a man car sticking his head out his car window into what looks like the drawer of a cash machine. The caption reads, "Drive-through Brain Surgery." Yet some physicians who began as skeptics became converts. One was Michael Ebersold, a mild-mannered neurologist who headed a team examining lumbar disk surgery, a common treatment for back pain.

Despite the "team" nature of Mayo practice, Ebersold nonetheless found wide differences among individual surgeons in the use of blood products and drugs. Because no one had ever tried to connect these differences to patient outcomes, the "peer review" encouraged by a unified medical record viewed the differences benignly. Ebersold, though, tried some "internal benchmarking," speaking to his surgeon counterparts at the Mayo locations in Jacksonville, Florida, and Scottsdale, Arizona. In his conversations, he discovered that the simplest of tactics, such as quickly getting back surgery patients up and walking, paid almost embarrassingly abundant dividends. Patients suffered fewer back spasms and needed fewer narcotics. The reduction in narcotics led to less urine retention, so they didn't need catheters. The early walking reduced phlebitis (blood clots in the leg) and the incidence of fever. That in turn meant that patients received fewer antibiotics, so there were fewer complications from antibiotic use. All these good things were happening to Mayo patients in Jacksonville and Scottsdale, but not in Rochester. Ebersold decided that had to change. Under his leadership, length of stay went down and care got better.

"The key word is humility of the physician," says Ebersold, who grew up on a farm a couple of hours' drive away. "Historically, we've been able to practice medicine with, 'Damn the costs, we're going to do everything possible.' But everything possible may not be good. It's not rational and it's expensive, and it often results in more problems [for patients]. We can no longer afford to do 'everything.' We can do what is appropriate, indicated and needed. And do that right."

THE MAYO WAY

Robert Waller, the Mayo Foundation's president and chief executive officer, knows that the world has changed since he was a young ophthalmologist. "Twenty years ago, people might say you're Cornell or Harvard or the University of Minnesota or Mayo, [and] therefore you must have good quality. That's in the past. Now it's, 'We think you're good quality, you've assured us you're good quality—now we ask you to prove it.' That's a quantum leap forward."

"Specify but verify" is the path John Burns told the Business Health Care Action Group to follow. Mayo, as a member of the HealthPartners team, wants to make sure its care can pass that kind of rigorous objective scrutiny. That seems to be why Waller brought in Berwick, a clinician who could help persuade other clinicians that the old-time religion of unlimited professional autonomy is dead.

"Improvement requires aim—or it doesn't happen," Berwick tells the group. "Improvement requires change." The change can be wrenching—"resetting" the system, the way an outside hand resets a thermostat. Except this thermostat is the trillion-dollar health care economy. "Improvement requires knowledge," Berwick continues—not just the kind of research knowledge the Mayo Clinic is famous for, but knowledge specifically designed to improve systems of care. The kind of knowledge that involves flowcharts and Pareto diagrams and control charts.

"Improvement requires a system to nurture [it]," Berwick concludes. "In a classic Deming model, an organization would Plan improvement, Do it, Check the impact of the change, and then Act on that knowledge to continue the cycle." In Deming-speak, PDCA.

A Mayo nurse tells Berwick that she tried to use continuous improvement techniques on her job, only to be told by a surgeon that what she was doing was not the "Mayo way." "The past is to be honored, but it is an obstacle," Berwick directly replies. "Your excellence is in your way. You're not alone in this. I come from Harvard." The Mayo way? "I would drop that," Berwick adds offhandedly, to nervous titters from the crowd. "The Mayo way is to help people."

Later, in the hallway, neurologist J. D. Bartleson, who chairs the clinic's continuous improvement council, admits that he sometimes tires of trying to explain to colleagues why this new way of examining their medical practice is important. "It's all a paradigm shift," says the earnest Bartleson, an eighteen-year clinic veteran. "We could have been scrutinizing this information earlier, but we didn't feel we had to, so we didn't."

You can't ask "unthinkable" questions, in other words, until something happens to make you think these questions need answers. In the 1990s, American businesses are doing to the American health care system what foreign businesses did to them in the previous decade—leaving them no choice but to improve or go out of business. In a 1993 poll, seven out of ten hospitals said they were involved with some sort of formal continuous quality improvement/total quality management activity. Attendance at an annual conference sponsored by Berwick's institute has soared to over one thousand, and exhibitors eagerly pay for the right to reach participants. Among the speakers invited to give a presentation was the Business (now Buyers) Health Care Action Group's Steve Wetzell.

The Mayo Clinic has adopted the ideas behind quality improvement into its formal vision statement, an action as serious to the traditionalists at Mayo as an amendment to the Constitution. One of the clinic's eight core principles is now a call to "continuously improve all processes and services that support the care of our patients." Meanwhile, the Mayo Conference on Quality has become an annual affair that grants continuing education credits to the physicians and nurses who attend.

For Mayo and other members of the HealthPartners group, however, working on a few projects was not sufficient. The next big step was to take their belief in a new paradigm of medical practice and devise a way to transform an entire system of care.

CHAPTER 13

The Early Worm Gets the Bird

We shall have to learn to refrain from doing things merely because we know how to do them.
—Sir Theodore Fox in the *Lancet,* 1965

The nineteenth-century Chicago architect Daniel Burnham proclaimed, "Make no little plans!" The consortium of medical practices, hospitals, and health maintenance organizations that captured the Business Health Care Action Group contract had little choice but to take a similar approach. The group's challenge was to bring clinical consistency to the practices of nearly 2,500 affiliated physicians. Its response was to set up an ambitious spin-off organization called the Institute for Clinical Systems Integration (ICSI).

ICSI's plans were certainly big enough. Its organizers pledged to help create "a living laboratory for continuous improvement in the quality and value of health care." The official vision statement was even grander: "ICSI will have succeeded if variation in physician practice is reduced, care outcomes are improved, providers enjoy working in the system, member satisfaction is high, costs increase at or below the rate of increase in the Consumer Price Index, use of information systems is embedded in daily physician practice and the Institute becomes an example of what is right in American medicine."[1]

More prosaically, ICSI's success in meeting the strict requirements of the BHCAG contract depended on a massive education campaign to promote the use of clinical practice guidelines. As a first step, local doctors were invited to help codify the scientific knowledge on which each guideline would be based. This was a relatively straightforward task, but it was complicated by the volume of guidelines demanded by BHCAG. The contract required the development of sixteen guidelines the first year, fifteen the second year, and another ten the year after. BHCAG also required the health plans to monitor how the guidelines affected patients.

"Continuous quality improvement (CQI) shouldn't be done for CQI's sake," said Steve Wetzell, BHCAG's executive director. "It should be done if it makes the product superior. Data don't solve the problem [of medical practice variation]; it's only if the data drive the way medicine is practiced in the community."

That was the tricky part, of course. Most health care organizations struggle to persuade physicians to adopt a few guidelines in a year. ICSI planned within five years to implement protocols affecting 80 percent of all conditions that doctors treat.

Overseeing this ambitious venture was Gordon Mosser, ICSI's executive director. A native Minnesotan, Mosser was an epidemiologist who had studied in England under Archie Cochrane, the founding father of evidence-based medicine. Back in the 1930s, Cochrane was struck by the waste in much of medical care. He eventually wrote a seminal book titled *Effectiveness and Efficiency* and came up with a slogan meant to illustrate what would be gained by providing only necessary care. Said Cochrane: "All effective treatment might be free." A framed letter from Cochrane hung on one of Mosser's office walls.

At Park Nicollet, medical director Rodney Dueck described his job as "trying to create the flicker of insight in the mind of our colleagues so that they draw their own conclusion that [the need for change] is true." On a larger scale, the same held true for Mosser. Mosser, who had studied philosophy before prudently settling on a career in medicine, visualized ICSI as helping physicians adjust to three fundamental changes in their professional lives.

The first was the shift from practice based on the experience of the individual doctor to practice based on scientific evidence. Just as Scott Weingarten had done at Cedars-Sinai, ICSI built support for this change by appealing to its doctors' sense of professionalism. The second change, linked to the first, was more difficult. The individual physician's near-unlimited authority to interpret the medical literature was being replaced with a group interpretation. Doctors had to trust their colleagues who drafted the guidelines, even if they did not know those colleagues personally. This leap of faith was tough enough when treatment of one clinical condition (pneumonia, heart attacks, tetralogy of Fallot) was at issue. It was even more difficult during a disruptive period when doctors were being told to standardize virtually their entire practice. To reassure doctors that standardization was not a weapon for forcing them into "cookbook medicine," ICSI adopted the rule used by Salt Lake City's LDS Hospital: if a doctor disregarded a guideline, the doctor was presumed right and the guideline wrong until it was shown otherwise.

The final change in medical practice was perhaps the most difficult of the three. W. Edwards Deming, the pioneer of continuous quality improvement (CQI), asserted that "knowledge comes from theory. Without theory, there is no way to use the information that comes to us."[2] ICSI's biggest challenge was to inculcate widespread acceptance of CQI theory among its front-line physicians. Those physicians had to accept a new way of thinking: that medicine was changing from an activity where continual improvement was sporadic, triggered by technological advances or the individual doctor's personal experience, to one where improvement was the result of constant attention to the processes of care.

As difficult as that paradigm shift was on its own, the BHCAG contract also mandated an unprecedented level of accountability by physicians to outsiders. Individual doctors were no longer the sole collectors and interpreters of clinical information. Paul Lembcke's medical audit in the 1950s had urged hospitals to compare themselves with other institutions "of acknowledged merit." ICSI, through the use of database and performance measurement systems, was forcing its members to do precisely that. Only the jargon had changed, to "benchmarking."

First-rank quality consultants like Deming and Joseph Juran routinely required the backing of a company's chief executive officer before accepting an assignment. A study by the U.S. General Accounting Office confirmed the wisdom of that decision. Corporate quality improvement succeeded only when it was "integrated into strategic and operational planning," said the GAO. "Gaining employee commitment to continuous improvement required a profound shift in the philosophy of senior management."[3] Fortunately for ICSI, the top executives at the consortium members—the Mayo Clinic, Park Nicollet Medical Center, and Group Health—all started out with a strong personal belief in the value of quality improvement techniques.

Mayo CEO Robert Waller, as discussed in the previous chapter, actively promoted quality improvement as part of the clinic's "toolbox." Waller even visited the Walt Disney Company and Marriott Corporation to study their approach to keeping customers happy. At Group Health (which eventually changed its name to HealthPartners), CEO George Halvorson promoted CQI as the cornerstone of health care reform.[4] Energetic and ambitious, Halvorson began his career as a newspaper reporter in North Dakota but ended up in health insurance after assuming that a want ad seeking an "underwriter" had something to do with journalism. (Underwriters rate the financial risk of insurance transactions.) Halvorson retained a journalist's affinity for publicity. In an opinion piece in the local newspaper, he challenged employers to use "financial incentives to create efficient, high-quality care systems. . . . [I]t's time for buyers to start demanding results—to start paying for health outcomes, rather than simply paying for the health care process."[5]

Park Nicollet CEO James Reinertsen had perhaps the deepest personal ties to the quality improvement movement. When Reinertsen first joined what was then the St. Louis Park Clinic, he became fast friends with another young physician who belonged to the same church. That colleague was Paul Batalden, the pediatrician who first brought CQI from industry to medicine. Years later, when Park Nicollet merged with Methodist Hospital to form HealthSystem Minnesota, Reinertsen created the title "chief quality officer" to go with his more conventional duties as co-CEO. Reinertsen helped conceive ICSI, and as board chairman he constantly reminded members that quality management was a means to an end. "Focus on transformation, not on 'doing continuous improvement,'" Reinertsen urged. "The biggest risk . . . is that people get inappropriately focused on tools [and] methods."[6]

If ICSI's leaders were ever apt to forget that, BHCAG was waving the checkbook to remind them. Most of ICSI's budget came from the consortium of care systems, which paid out $1 million for ICSI's planning stages and agreed to allocate another $1.8 million annually. But 15 percent of ICSI's operating budget came from BHCAG. That contribution entitled the employers to seats on ICSI's board, subcommittees, and work teams. Although employer representatives called themselves the "voice of the patient," no one forgot they were also the voice of the paying customer. "When participants' zeal for collaboration faltered," acknowledged Reinertsen, "the presence of BHCAG kept us focused on the promise we had made to them."[7]

The need for a continued outside threat was not unique to medicine. Deming repeatedly asserted that the scope of change demanded by CQI was too sweeping and too painful for any organization to take on unless the alternative was palpably worse. A 1991 book on Deming encapsulated that view in its title: *Quality or Else.*[8] Deming's personal history had shaped that belief. His first big chance to demonstrate what his methods could accomplish for industry came when the United States was trying to win World War II; his second chance came when Japanese industry was recuperating from losing the world war; and his third opportunity arrived when United States industry found itself on the losing end of a trade war with the Japanese companies that had listened to Deming when American companies had not.

The same dynamic has played out in health care. In private, industry executives acknowledge that without outside pressure they would be unable to get their organizations to change.

"CQI is a survival strategy," says a physician-executive active in the quality field. "Cultural change is unpleasant. You don't engage in it unless you're in a competitive environment. It's tough to get people to change for altruism."[9]

"CQI is like therapy," adds a quality analyst for a hospital association. "Your therapist can't cure you. You've got to do it yourself. But business is telling the providers to do CQI or risk losing patients. In other words, 'Go to therapy or be fired.'"[10]

In a rural town thirty miles southwest of the Twin Cities, a small group of general practitioners accepted the challenge to effect wholesale change. The four-man practice, associated with an HMO in the BHCAG consortium, was able to demonstrate that medical excellence and accountability can be achieved by any group of physicians willing to pay careful attention to the many details of changing their patterns of care. But being the first to do something important does not necessarily translate into being the first to reap financial rewards. In folk wisdom, "the early bird gets the worm." The early worm, on the other hand, may just get eaten.

GOD IS IN THE DETAILS

> Tell me and I will forget.
> Show me and I will remember.
> Involve me and I will understand.
> —Chinese proverb

Northfield, Minnesota, a community of just a few thousand people, is home to two liberal arts colleges (St. Olaf's and Carleton), one of the country's largest manufacturing plants for breakfast cereal (Malt-O-Meal), and an old bank building where the Jesse James gang once botched a robbery. The resulting shoot-out has been chronicled with varying accuracy in several Hollywood movies and is reenacted in Northfield every September for the benefit of tourists.

To ICSI members, the old river milling town had another claim to fame. At least until the middle of 1995, Northfield was celebrated for being on the leading edge of medicine's industrial revolution.

Although no medical specialists practice full time in Northfield and Northfield Hospital has only forty-seven beds, the town was the home of the four doctors of Family Physicians of Northfield. In all of ICSI, the group consistently finished at the top in actually using guidelines to change the practice of medicine. Indeed, a good case could be made that Family Physicians of Northfield's achievements set a national benchmark.[11]

In many ways, medical practice outside the hospital is far more difficult to standardize and improve than practice inside it. The analogy of the hospital and the factory is not so far-fetched. The doctor's office, by contrast, is more like an open-air market. The interaction between patient and physician is less clear-cut than in the hospital. The patients who come to the doctor's office often have no well-defined disease, yet the physician must still respond and provide appropriate and effective treatment.[12] A string of studies shows that often doesn't happen. As long ago as 1957, researchers criticized a group of family practitioners for failing to properly examine women patients for breast cancer despite "the considerable publicity given to breast cancer at the present time." Sixty-seven percent of the doctors in that study dispensed antibiotics "indiscriminately."[13] As recently as 1995, a team from Johns Hopkins and Harvard concluded that primary care physicians in Alabama, Iowa, and Maryland failed to adequately manage the care of elderly diabetics.[14]

As with hospital care, the problem isn't "bad" doctors, but bad systems. Pulled a thousand ways, harried family doctors can't always do everything well all the time. At Family Physicians of Northfield, however, the doctors had some expert assistance in turning the sometimes intimidating accouterments of medicine's information age into something they could use with patients. The expert's name was Nancy Jaeckels.

Jaeckels, an energetic Northfield native, was trained as a laboratory technician. Accustomed to calibrating instruments to be as accurate as possible, Jaeckels gravitated naturally toward quality improvement activities. On her own initiative, she went to the clinic's computer one day to collect the names of women whose age indicated they should be receiving a mammogram and a professional breast exam. Then she looked through each patient's paper medical record to determine whether the proper screening had been done. Even in this small-town practice, Jaeckels discovered that preventive care often fell between the cracks. Only 40 percent of the women who needed a mammogram or a breast exam had received one. Jaeckels's response was inexpensive, low-tech, and effective. When an eligible woman came to the clinic for any reason, the receptionist at the front desk stamped her chart in red ink: "Last mammogram; last breast exam." If the patient could not provide dates, or if the dates were too far in the past, the mammogram was immediately scheduled and the breast exam performed by the doctor on that visit. Within two years, 70 to 80 percent of women were getting the right preventive treatment.

David Larson, one of the clinic's four physicians, took special notice of Jaeckels's success. Although Family Physicians was tiny, Larson sat on ICSI's influential planning committee. Soon Jaeckels found herself answering phone calls and running off to suburban Minneapolis meetings as part of this or that ICSI committee. At Family Physicians, meanwhile, she turned guideline implementation into a personal cause. When ICSI drafted a guideline, it was Jaeckels who asked clinic doctors and nurses to review it for hidden problems. When the revised guideline appeared, Jaeckels took responsibility for setting up training sessions for the doctors, nurses, and support staff and organizing the scientific support material in a neat three-ring binder. Most important of all, it was Jaeckels who came up with the idea of drawing up flowcharts on five-by-eight-inch reference cards—she called them "shingles"—to take nurses and doctors step by step through the different decision points in a guideline algorithm. ("If the patient answers the question yes, do A; if the answer is no, ask the following.") Jaeckels broke down each guideline into simple steps that could be followed with a minimum of fuss. In other words, she moved CQI out of the realm of theory and philosophy and turned it into a tool that busy people caring for patients could quickly understand and follow.

Take, for example, the treatment of women with urinary tract infections (UTI), the subject of one of ICSI's first guidelines. As related in the introduction to this book, this common problem gives rise to an uncommonly large number of treatment approaches: ICSI's members reported an almost unbelievable 180 different therapies. A typical treatment sequence included asking the woman to come to the physician's office for an examination; performing a complete urinalysis and urine culture; doing sensitivity studies for antibiotics; prescribing an antibiotic for ten days; and finally, doing a follow-up urine culture. The average total cost was $133. After studying the medical literature, the UTI guideline committee found ample evidence that the same results could be achieved by a phone consultation with a doctor (or a visit to a registered nurse); a complete urinalysis (with a urine sample held for a culture if symptoms did not disappear); and a prescription for three days of antibiotics. The cost of this alternative was $39, a savings of nearly 70 percent.

At Family Physicians, the system to implement the UTI guideline was triggered as soon as the receptionist picked up the phone. One Monday morning, a woman patient who called complaining of burning during urination was immediately transferred to Edie Mickelson, a licensed practical nurse. Mickelson, in turn, took out one of Jaeckels's shingles and began asking the woman the questions printed on it. The shingle was labeled: "UTI in Women (Age >18 or <65): Nursing Triage Guidelines." Was there pain on urination? Frequent urination? Were there complicating factors like blood in the urine or pain in the side? ("If yes: see M.D.," the shingle advised, then added in boldface type: "[Schedule] same day visit to on call M.D.")

After a few moments, it became clear that this infection was routine. Mickelson told the woman her doctor would call in a prescription to the pharmacy for a three-day course of antibiotics. The patient was more than happy to forgo a trip to the doctor's office. Explained Mickelson: "She was at work and didn't want to leave."

The clinic staff also understood the shingle could not be followed blindly. For instance, a patient might not state her true motives for wanting to see a doctor. A complaint about a urinary tract infection could signal the start of sexual activity by an adolescent or could be a symptom of the spread of a sexually transmitted disease. A patient who wants to see the doctor is never turned down. Says Mickelson: "If they want to come in, we'll let them come in."

As simple as what Jaeckels was doing might seem, it succeeded because she had instinctively grasped that changing patient care is complex. Change required the cooperation of all parts of the Family Physicians of Northfield clinic staff. At the Kasson Clinic, a small family practice group owned by the Mayo Clinic, family practitioner Greg Angstman admits he learned that same lesson the hard way. Angstman, an active member of ICSI's policy committees, was perplexed that Kasson's initial rate of implementing the UTI guideline was low. Even more disturbing was the discovery that his own rate of compliance was no better than that of less well informed colleagues. Since Angstman was personally involved with developing the UTI measure and similar protocols, "I thought I would end up being better [at complying] all of the time," he said.

A little detective work soon confirmed a truth asserted by CQI advocates like Berwick: all doctors, whether they know it or not, depend on systems. When patients with a possible UTI called the Kasson Clinic, the nurses were telling them to come in for a urine culture even before a doctor was notified about the problem. Educating doctors about the guideline was only one piece of the puzzle. "It was a process problem, not a knowledge problem," said Angstman.

Unfortunately, successful implementation of practice guidelines by ICSI members exposed a hidden but critical system problem that had not been anticipated. Family Physicians of Northfield noticed it first. The better the clinic got at practicing cost-efficient medicine, the emptier its waiting room became. Patients with a urinary tract infection could often be handled over the phone by a nurse; the patient paid nothing but the cost of the drug prescription. The guideline for viral upper respiratory infections like the common cold also encouraged doctors to discourage office visits; patients were counseled to be patient. (Contrary to popular wisdom, a cold can remain "common" and still linger for weeks.) Back pain patients who pressed for expensive CT or MRI scans were shown the guideline's conclusion that bed rest for six weeks (without expensive tests) was the first treatment choice; most often, the pain would go away on its on. On and on the list went. The guidelines encouraged doctors to spend time in person with patients most likely to benefit from the physician's expensive training. Complaints that could be handled over the telephone were.

After just a year and a half of work, a clear consensus emerged among ICSI members who were most diligent in following guidelines. Thanks to the way the BHCAG contract was structured, efficient and effective medicine was costing guideline-conscious medical groups thousands of dollars.

The problem wasn't just in Northfield. The big groups in the Twin Cities were losing bigger dollars. At Park Nicollet, James Reinertsen had told his doctors that guidelines promised better care for patients and a more satisfying work life for physicians. Why spend hours looking at colds when you could spend that time counseling elderly diabetics or helping children with asthma? Moreover, guideline implementation and measurement helped physicians link their care processes to outcomes so they could know whether a therapy was effective. "We are what we measure," Reinertsen repeatedly told the staff.

What the measures showed was that a cost-effective Park Nicollet was losing its shirt. In early 1994, the clinic made a terse presentation to BHCAG. One bulleted slide read:

- BHCAG winner
- Park Nicollet loser
- U.T.I. as an example

Take away the lab tests, X rays, and other routine diagnostic work from a medical office, and its bottom line will quickly atrophy. The doctor's time in the office (or a hospital's daily room charge) may be the main course, but it is the extra tests for "dessert" that often make the difference between black and red ink at the end of the month.

The physician groups participating in the BHCAG contract increasingly found themselves in the position of a restaurant owner who offers free drinks and dessert to lure new customers but finds himself profitlessly serving the same old dinner crowd. BHCAG paid the consortium doctors on a discounted fee for service basis. When the volume of medical services went down, so did doctors' income. But instead of high quality bringing in new patients—the kind of reward Walt McClure saw as critical to the success of his Buy Right program—the BHCAG employers mostly just shifted doctors' previous patients to this new insurance plan. Patients kept their doctors but got a cheaper premium. Although that was fine for workers and employers, the doctors got little more than a warm feeling and an empty bank account.

Consider once more the urinary tract infection guideline. It saved the time of hundreds of women who would have had to visit the doctor's office, decreased the chances that they would develop resistance to antibiotics, and reduced the number of irritating vaginal yeast infections many women suffer following a long course of antibiotic therapy. By any measure this was an improvement in the quality of care. As a reward, Park Nicollet lost $100,000 in revenue in 1993 from never-performed lab tests and empty space on doctors' appointment calendars. Mayo, with just a few small clinics participating in the UTI guideline, gave up $55,000 in potential revenue.

The picture got even bleaker when one included the costs involved in getting the clinic staff to comply with the guidelines. In 1993 Park Nicollet took some 6,300 hours of physician time and 12,400 hours of support staff time to implement sixteen guidelines. Had that time been devoted to patient care, it would have generated nearly $500,000 in revenue. As another Park Nicollet slide mournfully put it: "The more Park Nicollet succeeds in fulfilling BHCAG objectives, the closer Park Nicollet moves towards serious financial difficulty."

At Family Physicians of Northfield, senior physician Kenneth Sansome well understood the extent of the financial discomfort. The clinic was a dream come true for Sansome, a pleasant and outgoing man with a bushy brown mustache and square gold-rimmed glasses. He first came to Northfield as an undergraduate at Carleton College in the late 1960s and met his wife, Connie, at school. He studied medicine in the Twin Cities and did his family practice residency in Oregon, then "looked all over the Pacific Northwest for a town like Northfield." Disappointed with imitations, the couple came back to the original.

Ken Sansome found a position at one of the two small clinics in town, but he soon grew dissatisfied with their outmoded facilities and old-fashioned ways. He struck out on his own in 1983 and took on Dave Larson as a similarly minded partner just six months later. In 1985 the clinic added Mark Mellstrom, followed by Jeff Meland in 1991. Not long afterward, the four family practitioners moved to a modern one-story brick clinic building that Ken Sansome designed and whose examining rooms he decorated with the works of local artists. Sansome grumbled about the time Jaeckels spent away from the clinic working with ICSI, but he ultimately supported her efforts as right for the doctors and right for their patients.

"Paradigm pioneers," wrote Joel Arthur Barker in *Future Edge,* "risk their reputations, their positions, even their economic situations, on a non-rational decision." They change "not as an act of the head but as an act of the heart."[15] Near the end of a long day, sitting in an office filled with photos of family and of Minnesota geological formations, Sansome wrestled with the different messages his head and heart were sending him about the future of American health care.

"There's a need for leadership and setting an example," Sansome said. "We like to be at the forefront. We realize this is cutting edge. The future of medicine is involved with this."

And yet, if "improvement requires a system to nurture [it]," as Donald Berwick had told the Mayo Clinic, the improvement efforts of Family Physicians of Northfield were being starved. The clinic had little financial margin. It brought in about the same revenues as an average McDonald's hamburger franchise, but the manager and staff of a McDonald's aren't on call twenty-four hours a day every day of the year. In one twelve-month period, the four Northfield doctors saw some 3,600 people who made 11,384 visits to the clinic. They visited patients at Northfield Hospital 784 times, answered 219 calls to the emergency room, and made 52 critical care visits (Larson heads up the critical care unit). There were also 400 nursing home visits (the hospital has a twenty-seven-bed nursing unit attached) and 138 house calls. Since the doctors routinely work fifty-hour weeks, the easiest way for them to see some patients is to drop by their houses on the way to or from the clinic.

Paradigm pioneers can gain "substantial advantage" over competitors, goes the theory. But sometimes the pioneer may not survive long enough to reap those rewards. Sansome's main competitor in Northfield—a bigger clinic financed by a rich out of state company—was also affiliated with the BHCAG consortium and ICSI. Although the competing clinic was not as successful in implementing guidelines, potential patients didn't see that. What they did see was that the bigger competitor could offer a lower health plan premium. Nor did BHCAG's members offer any reward for virtue. Yet looking at his financial records, Sansome tallied up some $25,000 for expenses related to ICSI in the previous year. "Doing good work and service to the customer," said Sansome with a touch of bitterness in his voice, "that's not what gets the business to come through the door."

Back in the Twin Cities, BHCAG's Steve Wetzell acknowledged that Sansome had cause for his frustration. The Northfield physicians "are the silver lining in medicine, one tiny practice trying to do the best," Wetzell said. "[But] I'm not sure this kind of sophisticated CQI is economically viable for them. They're not being rewarded in the marketplace." The blunt truth remains that "what [most] employers and government still care most about is next year's premium."

In 1997, BHCAG began to straighten out the skewed system of punishment and rewards. The group started contracting directly with groups of physicians and hospitals—"care systems," they are called. Patients can choose these groups directly, and the groups will be held accountable for meeting quality and cost goals. At the same time, BHCAG altered its payment system from simple, discounted fee for service to a complicated formula that attempts to ensure that care systems that deliver effective and efficient care gain patients and income instead of losing. Meanwhile the health plans, such as the HealthPartners HMO, will contract with the care systems to provide administrative services.

BHCAG has also increased its buying clout. After the state of Minnesota announced it would join the group, substantially increasing the number of employees covered by members, BHCAG changed its name from "*Business* Health Care Action Group" to "*Buyers* Health Care Action Group." And just as BHCAG was a hot media story in 1993 as an example of managed competition, its decision to substantially bypass managed care plans and deal directly with those who provided care made BHCAG a hot media story again in early 1997. The NBC Nightly News, *Business Week,* and others all alerted their audiences to pay attention to the show on display in Minneapolis–St. Paul. By that time, BHCAG had thirty-nine guidelines in at least limited use and another six in development. Meanwhile, 550 doctors were working directly on guideline development teams. Mosser acknowledged that ICSI could not yet claim to be "an example of what is right in American medicine"; that kind of inflated expectation, he sighed, was "unfortunate." But ICSI was successful enough that two cities were talking about imitating the BHCAG-ICSI arrangement. ICSI was also setting up a for-profit consulting arm to take the ICSI message across the country.

By the time BHCAG shifted its payment strategy and enjoyed a new round of media attention, however, it was too late for Ken Sansome. A small business with a bottom line that is hemorrhaging today cannot wait for a cure too far in the future. Looking forlorn, Sansome one day pointed out to a visitor a long brown envelope containing a dry legal contract. "The papers are in there," he said. After twenty-two years of being a family doctor in a small town, Sansome had learned that the pioneer can get scalped and that the early worm can have an unfortunate encounter with the early bird. Clinics and health plans with hundreds of doctors can absorb a temporary financial setback. These four family physicians, two of whom still carry large medical school debts, could not.

Perhaps the financial competition from the town's other clinic would have doomed Sansome's group even had it not been so eager to practice more cost-effective medicine. No one will ever know for sure. Family Physicians of Northfield was sold in June 1995 to HealthSystem Minnesota and became one of its "regional health services." ICSI stopped reporting the small clinic's guideline results separately, but Nancy Jaeckels remained active in the organization. Within a short time, she moved to HealthSystem Minnesota and became its coordinator of guideline measurement.

Jaeckels's new job is in the Twin Cities, but she still visits the Northfield clinic on business at least once a week. Family Physicians now employs several part-time midwives and a full-time pediatrician, and HealthSystem Minnesota was planning on expanding the building. This time, though, Ken Sansome won't be there to give tips on decoration. At the end of January 1997, he resigned. At his going-away party, he didn't make clear his future plans.

PART 4

The Promise and Perils of Managed Care

CHAPTER FOURTEEN

Money, Managed Care, and Mom

> Some people believe that when health care is involved, any reference to cost is repugnant, even immoral. It is doubtful such a belief was ever defensible. But the rising cost of medical care, in our opinion, has made that belief untenable. . . . As soon as one determines in some way, other than by caprice or lottery, not to provide all care that is expected to yield [any] benefits, the value of care is being weighed against its costs, explicitly or implicitly. Care actually given is implicitly judged to be worth more than it costs; care not given is worth less. . . .
>
> The problem that all developed nations face is how to alter the behavior of providers and patients so that expenditures are curtailed on care that, in some sense, is worth less than it costs.[1]

The quotation above has nothing to do with managed care. It comes from *The Painful Prescription: Rationing Hospital Care,* a book by Brookings Institution economist Henry Aaron and Tufts University professor of medicine William Schwartz. In 1984 *The Painful Prescription* helped fuel a national debate over how the United States should deal with rapidly rising medical costs. What made the book provocative was its examination of the way the British National Health Service controlled costs. Explicit rationing of care in Great Britain had led to a level of medical spending per person that was only one-third as high as in the United States. In discussing the American system, *The Painful Prescription* mentions HMOs only in passing, in a few paragraphs. They simply were not very important.

The Painful Prescription appeared at a time when there was a widespread feeling that the United States was about to reach an upper limit on health care spending. Almost seven of ten Americans said the cost or care was the biggest problem with our system.[2] Within that context, the British experience was seen as possibly foreshadowing the grim choices we would soon face. As Schwartz cautioned in the 12 November 1984 issue of *Newsweek:* "Either we will accept the continued rise of hospital costs that results from full exploitation of technological advances or we will start to ration hospital care."

Today the rationing obsession of the mid-1980s is rarely if ever mentioned. Although rationing worries are back in vogue, hospitals are no longer the potential villains: the managed care companies are. In the 1997 State of the Union Address, the president of the United States publicly recognized a Connecticut surgeon who brought to national attention that some HMOs denied an overnight hospital stay to women who had just undergone a mastectomy. Many of the elite of medicine and journalism have also taken to regular attacks on managed care.

During 1995 and 1996, the nation's most prestigious publications routinely warned about such dangers as managed care "rationing" (an opinion piece in the *Wall Street Journal*) or "torture by HMO" (a columnist for the *New York Times*).[3] A *Time* cover story promised, "What your doctor can't tell you: An in-depth look at managed care—and one woman's fight to survive."[4] "Beware your HMO," cautioned *Newsweek.*[5] An investigative series on HMOs by the flamboyant *New York Post* included the headline, "Ex–New Yorker Is Told: Get Castrated So We Can $ave." A seventy-six-year-old man with prostate cancer reportedly was told by his HMO that it would rather pay for castration to halt the cancer's growth than continue making monthly payments for his costly anticancer medication.[6]

"The quality of health care is now seriously threatened by our rapid shift to managed care as the way to contain costs," declared a 1996 editorial in the *New England Journal of Medicine* that appeared over the signatures of both the managing editor and executive editor. "We have embraced a financing and delivery method that rewards doctors, sometimes quite directly, for doing less for their patients."[7]

The central focus of this book has been the ways medical treatment can be improved. But if cost containment reduces access to needed treatment in the first place, then the struggle to improve care will have little meaning. Are HMOs "health maintenance organizations" or more like "horrifying medical ogres"? Are the tales of HMO misdeeds a warning about "managed profiteering" or are they isolated anecdotes? There are few questions that are so important to the future of American medicine and that have also been the subject of so much misleading information.

Before coming to any conclusions about managed care, we should understand where HMOs originated and how and why they have come to be so successful today.

WORKING-CLASS MEDICINE

In the days when "health maintenance" meant trying not to die from an infection or in childbirth, the insurance arrangement we now call a health maintenance organization was known as a prepaid group practice. The mission of these first prepaid plans was to treat sick or injured workers who might not otherwise be able to afford the medical care that would help them return to their jobs. Prepaid plans sprung up during the 1800s in places as diverse as the iron mines of northern Minnesota and the pineapple plantations of Hawaii, but the direct ancestors of today's HMOs emerged out of the lumber camps surrounding Tacoma, Washington. Between 1910 and 1916, physicians Thomas Curran and James Yocum converted their Western Clinic into a prepaid plan that received a retainer of fifty cents per worker per month from mill owners who wanted to ensure that a doctor would be available to treat injured employees. A Seattle branch of the Western Clinic evolved into the present-day Group Health of Puget Sound.

Curran said he was motivated by idealism: he had seen too many injured workers forced to rely on the charity of friends to pay for medical treatment. As would be true decades later, however, other physicians saw prepaid care as a straightforward business opportunity. A "Dr. Bridge" in Tacoma established a chain of some twenty clinics across Washington and Oregon in what we might call the "industrialization of medicine." Private practice physicians responded by organizing medical service bureaus that tried to limit the gains of prepaid care. Those bureaus were the forerunners of the county medical societies that would later oppose HMOs at every turn.[8]

Physicians of the era were not very well paid, and they were sensitive to any threat to their livelihood. For example, in 1895 a large United States life insurance company attempted to reduce the fees it paid for physical exams to screen would-be policyholders. The company reasoned that it should get a discount because it sent the doctors so many cases. This line of thinking—similar to arrangements now common in managed care—quickly brought an editorial rebuke from the *Journal of the American Medical Association.* Reducing the doctor's fee, warned *JAMA,* invited reduced medical vigilance.

> The examination of the present policy holders involves the exercise of professional skill and ability, not too highly paid for even by a five dollar fee. How will [present policyholders] relish seeing the value of their policies and their prospective profits impaired by the accession of lives admitted on a scrutiny 40 percent less thorough—measured by the fee—than that to which they were subjected?[9]

This theme of "you get what you pay for" would continue to be one of the strongest leitmotifs of American medicine.

Prepaid groups, meanwhile, continued to reach out to the working class. In 1929 the Ross-Loos Clinic offered prepaid care to the two thousand employees of the Los Angeles Department of Water and Power, the first inroads made by the prepaid concept into a major city. Northern California's giant Kaiser Permanente plan arose out of industrialist Henry J. Kaiser's need to provide health care for his army of workers: first those building the Grand Coulee Dam in the California desert in the 1930s and later shipyard workers in Oakland during World War II. In Washington, D.C., the Home Owner's Loan Corporation provided start-up assistance for the Group Health Association health plan after noticing that customers who incurred large medical expenses often defaulted on their mortgage loans. And in New York City, populist mayor Fiorello La Guardia worked with the labor movement to launch what became the Health Insurance Plan of Greater New York.

The fierce opposition to prepaid care by many fee for service physicians did not lessen with the passage of time. Local medical societies often denied membership to any doctor who worked in a prepaid group. Since doctors needed society membership to obtain malpractice insurance and hospital privileges, the sanction had serious consequences. This type of intimidation did not stop until the U.S. Supreme Court ruled in 1943 that the Washington, D.C., medical society and the American Medical Association (which backed the society) were guilty of violating antitrust laws in their attempts to prevent Group Health doctors from obtaining hospital privileges. Still, it wasn't until 1959 that the AMA conceded that giving a patient "free choice of *policy or plan,*" not just "free choice of *doctor*" was ethical behavior (emphasis added).[10]

Although prepaid practice was viewed the most suspiciously, the solo practitioners who dominated fee for service disliked *any* kind of group. In 1952 a presidential Commission on the Health Needs of the

Nation concluded that physicians working in groups could provide higher-quality care at lower cost by pooling their scientific knowledge and sharing overhead. Organized medicine vociferously disagreed.

Ironically from today's vantage point, prepaid groups were criticized for making it *too easy* to use a doctor's services. That same argument was also brought against conventional health insurance. As a 1949 commentary from the New York State medical society protested:

> Any experienced general practitioner will agree that what keeps the great majority of people well is the fact that they can't afford to be ill. This is a harsh, stern dictum, and we readily admit that under it a certain number of cases of early tuberculosis and cancer, for example, may go undetected. Is it not better that a few such should perish rather than that the majority of the population should be encouraged on every occasion to run sniveling to the doctor?[11]

Yet despite the easy access offered by prepaid care plans, they largely remained limited to the West Coast. Whether because of physicians' opposition or patients' concern about the restricted choice of doctors, only about 2 percent of the United States population belonged to prepaid health plans by 1969. And a mere 85 physician groups out of a total of nearly 6,400 nationwide had a patient load where more than half the patients were prepaid.[12] When packaged as moderately priced health insurance for the working class, prepaid care failed to make much of an impression on the American health care system. When the concept was repackaged as something-for-nothing "health maintenance," however, the impact was quite different.

A FREE LUNCH

By the late 1960s, about 90 percent of the United States population had private or public health insurance that reimbursed on a fee for service basis just about any care doctors and hospitals deemed necessary. This did not, however, lead to a period of national good health and good cheer. Instead, it was a time of unprecedented anger and dissatisfaction with American medicine. The epidemic of unneeded surgeries and the growing number of treatment-related injuries and deaths had finally led to widespread public outrage. Public disillusionment with unfettered physician autonomy was so complete that Congress came very close to passing national health insurance. Instead the Republicans, as related in chapter 8, got Congress to support HMOs.

Prepaid care had been tried out in only a very few locations when President Nixon blithely endorsed it in 1971 as the solution to America's health care woes. The concept seemed to offer an economic "free lunch." HMOs would provide more services than traditional insurance—such as access to preventive care—for less cost. HMOs were also billed as a private sector solution to health care reform, even though the Nixon administration promptly redirected $26 million in federal funds to underwrite 155 HMO projects.[13] The Health Maintenance Organization Act later authorized another $375 million.

In 1970 there were just 33 HMOs serving three million people, but optimistic HMO boosters were speaking of 1,700 plans providing care to forty million Americans by the end of the decade. The HMO Act preempted laws in thirty-eight states that restricted prepaid care, laws typically passed at the behest of organized medicine. (Some states specifically prohibited ownership of prepaid group practices by consumer-oriented organizations.) The HMO Act also required companies with at least twenty-five employees to offer their workers a "federally qualified" HMO if such an HMO asked to be offered.[14] Multinational conglomerates like Litton Industries, Texas Instruments, and Westinghouse Electric considered getting into the HMO business but decided it was still too risky. Nonetheless, as the number of new HMOs jumped upward, an announcement that the Wharton Business School was starting a course to train HMO managers drew eight hundred applicants for ten spots.[15] A short while later, reality set in.

Federal qualification was supposed to force corporate customers to open their doors to HMOs. But federal qualification also required plans to offer a long list of mandated benefits, such as mental health and vision coverage. This rich package increased premiums and discouraged workers from joining. By early 1975, the bubble had burst. HMOs are "an idea whose time has not yet come," a senior vice president of Aetna Life and Casualty Company told the *Wall Street Journal*. By mid-1980, HMO enrollment had tripled from its 1970 level, but the 9.1 million people in 236 plans still amounted to only 4 percent of the United States population.[16]

Still, the HMO Act represented a turning point for the United States health care system. Government endorsement—particularly by a conservative Republican president—gave prepaid plans crucial legitimacy. Government backing also prompted researchers to scrutinize HMO quality more closely. A landmark 1978 article in the *New England Journal of Medicine* by researcher Harold Luft, "How Do Health Maintenance Organizations Achieve Their 'Savings'?" concluded that prepaid groups were able to reduce hospital stays by about a third without harming the quality of care. This meant that medical costs at HMOs were from 10 to 40 percent less than in comparable indemnity (fee for service) plans.[17] Luft's conclusions were buttressed a few years later by an analysis of twenty-seven separate studies published from 1958 to 1979, comparing prepaid care and fee for service. "There is little question that facility-based HMO care is at least comparable to care in other health care facilities, if not superior," concluded Frances Cunningham and John Williamson of the Johns Hopkins School of Hygiene and Public Health.[18]

By the end of the 1970s, even the AMA was forced to acknowledge that "the medical care delivered by HMOs appears to be of a generally high quality."[19] Nonetheless, it was not until 1992 that the AMA's executive vice president attended a meeting of the chief HMO trade association and formally acknowledged the equal legitimacy of prepaid care and fee for service practice. For his trouble, Dr. James Todd received a torrent of letters from AMA members calling on him to resign.

HMOs had now been certified as a legitimate alternative to fee for service by the politicians, the profession, and some consumer advocates. However, apart from the success of Kaiser Permanente in California, they had not won over the general public. HMOs were like a sugarless, salt-free breakfast cereal—good for you, no doubt, but nothing most people wanted to eat unless they had to. The Nixon administration had taken prepaid care off the farm and out of the factory, but it was left to the Reagan administration to infuse the HMO movement with the ethos of marketplace capitalism. As for many other businesses, the 1980s were the "go-go years" for HMOs. It was also the time when the structure of the industry underwent a fundamental change whose ramifications are today being felt more strongly than ever.

RATIONING, RATIONALIZATION, AND REFORM

The term rationing conjures up images of children begging for food or of medics deciding which wounded soldier gets the last dose of painkiller. To economists, however, rationing is simply the allocation of resources we all perform every day. We budget a certain amount for necessities and a certain amount for everything else. We might want to spend more in some areas than we do, but the knowledge that our bank account is limited forces us to make decisions.

Prepaid group practices—HMOs—have confronted the problem of resource limitations since their inception. In fact, the very act of making medical choices within financial limits seemed inherently suspicious to many. After all, if unrestricted fee for service provided "the best medical care in the world," how could care that came with restrictions possibly be as good? It was only in the 1980s that the country as a whole had to grapple with the idea that denying—rationing—some care might be justified allocation. On the other hand, the 1980s were also the first time a provider of care could make extra money by *not* doing something. The rationing the public feared, as we saw at the beginning of this chapter, had nothing to do with HMOs. The villain was the hospital, and the reason was that the federal government had changed the rules governing Medicare.

As discussed earlier in this book, the Reagan administration decided to wean Medicare away from the traditional "do more, get paid more" method of reimbursement. Starting 1 October 1983, the "prospective payment" system began paying hospitals a fixed amount, set in advance (prospectively), for each Medicare patient treated. The precise amount paid was based on each patient's diagnosis.[20]

In some respects the switch to prospective payment was a brilliant political step. There are only two ways to reduce the money spent on any good or service: by controlling the supply or by controlling the demand. The prospective payment system cleverly invoked the laws of economics at one remove from the elderly (voter) on Medicare. Hospitals could supply as much care as they wanted—but the government was going to pay only a preset price. If the hospital spent more than that, it lost money. If it spent less, it made money. When it came to inpatient treatment, hospitals were functionally transformed into HMOs: the hospital assumed responsibility both for providing care and for the financial risk of paying for that care.

Prospective payment also avoided the practical problem of directly affecting doctors. But since doctors' orders controlled the demand for care, the hospital would go out of business if every patient got a couple of extra X rays "just to be sure," received a full laboratory workup "because that's how we do things," and stayed over the weekend "until she feels better."

"[Doctors] are really worried that they're not going to be allowed to practice medicine as they know it . . . based on their own judgment," fumed the AMA's outspoken executive vice president, James Sammons, to the *New York Times* in 1984. He added: "Financial restraints have led to the rationing of health care, and this rationing is going to increase."[21]

In fact, Medicare's initial payments were based on hospitals' bloated historical costs. Calling that rationing was a bit like describing the monthly expenditures of the British royal family as an allowance. Nonetheless, prospective payment clearly represented a break from the past, and soon enough, Sammons's warnings seemed to be realized. The tale one elderly couple told the House Aging Committee rivaled anything written about profit-driven HMOs a decade later. As related by *American Medical News,* the story went this way:

> Sixty-eight miles from home, still recovering from a collapsed lung after open-heart surgery and clad only in his pajamas, George Price was unexpectedly dismissed from an Oklahoma hospital and had to be driven home in a cold December rain.
>
> That was only the beginning, his wife told a congressional panel looking at the impact of Medicare's new prospective pricing. . . . By the next afternoon, chest pains and breathing difficulties had brought her husband to the emergency room of their local hospital, where he was stabilized and then sent home. Price still was not admitted to the local hospital even after a second trip to its emergency room, and the Prices spent an "anxious weekend" before he finally began to recover.
>
> Based on conversations with her husband's physicians and nurses, Mrs. Price blames Medicare for what she views as a premature discharge at the first hospital and for the second hospital's "unjustified" failure to admit her husband.
>
> She said nurses had told her that the facility "had no choice but to send him home with Medicare being the way it is."[22]

Senator John Heinz (R-Pa.), chairman of the Senate Special Committee on Aging, also held hearings on prospective payment and charged that patients "are being sent to a no-care zone." Separately, the Reagan administration announced that it was investigating "hundreds of doctors" who allegedly discharged patients too early or violated other Medicare standards.[23]

Small wonder a majority of physicians answering a 1985 AMA survey on the new payment system believed that "quality had [deteriorated] or would deteriorate."[24] Or that a little under half the doctors in a 1986 poll felt "unduly pressured" to discharge Medicare patients early.[25] The American Society of Internal Medicine said it received "over 200 specific reports of incidents in which the internists believed the quality of care had been compromised." The Federation of American Health Systems, the trade group representing for-profit hospitals, produced a short video called "Protecting Our Health Care System." It began: "We're on the brink of a potentially disastrous period in our health care system, a period when the quality of care we and our elders have come to expect is seriously threatened." The video ended by accusing the government of breaking its promise to fund Medicare adequately, and it warned that the health care system could become a "shambles."[26]

However unhappy prospective payment made some hospitals and doctors, the new system turned out to be one of the best things that ever happened to HMOs. Prospective payment forced community doctors to reconsider the reasons for admitting patients to the hospital and to reassess how long they needed to remain. As a result, the gap narrowed between the practice "styles" of the fee for service community and HMOs. Simultaneously, the long years of a doctor shortage were giving way to a doctor surplus. Between 1970 and 1982, the number of potential patients per doctor tumbled by 25 percent.[27] In a 1978 survey, four out of ten doctors said they were not practicing at full capacity.[28] Affiliating with an HMO started to look like a reasonable way for community physicians to keep their waiting rooms full, even if it meant discounting fees. Hospitals, facing a sea of empty beds once occupied by Medicare patients, were more amenable to HMO contracts as well.

Another economic side effect of prospective payment also boosted HMOs. Medicare accounted for about 40 percent of the average hospital's revenues. When the government cut payments, many hospitals raised their charges to privately insured patients. This cost shifting, combined with looser HMO regulations, finally let HMOs price themselves at or below the level of indemnity competitors while simultaneously offering a richer package of benefits.

The stage was set for an HMO boom. HMOs were now reasonably priced and, with their new contracts, could offer prospective members a choice of doctors and hospitals that were familiar names in the community. HMO membership, steady for several years, rose 15 percent in 1983, another 21 percent in 1984, and yet another 25 percent in both 1985 and 1986.[29] By 1986, each of the nation's thirty-eight major metropolitan areas had at least one HMO, and most had several. Medicare and Medicaid were also told by Congress in 1982 to test out HMO care for the elderly and the poor.

In the first part of this century, a few HMOs had contracted with community physicians, even while most HMOs used a group of doctors working for them full time. But the new HMOs that sprang to life in the 1980s were very different. Their owners and managers often regarded health care as just another business opportunity. Nurtured on the art of the deal, their expertise lay in writing lucrative risk-sharing contracts with doctors and hospitals. It didn't take them long to conclude that a contract that succeeded in one city might do equally well elsewhere. To obtain the money needed to grow, the onetime health care delivery system of the working class entered the thickly carpeted offices of Wall Street's investment bankers.[30] Philadelphia-based U.S. Health Care Systems, founded in 1974 as a not-for-profit plan, went public in February 1983. The HMO eventually raising $25 million in two stock offerings. HealthAmerica and Maxicare Health Plans followed later that year. A "decade of doubt" about HMOs gave way to "euphoria" on Wall Street, said *Barron's.* "The future's in for-profit HMOs," gushed *Venture.*[31]

"Prepaid health plans will ultimately be the dominant form of health care delivery in the United States," predicted Douglas Sherlock, an analyst for the investment banking firm of Salomon Brothers, in 1985.[32] Sanford Bernstein and Company's Kenneth Abramowitz agreed the next year: "The HMO industry is now poised to take control of health care delivery in America over the next five to ten years."[33]

The medical community saw itself as beleaguered on all sides. A physician correspondent for the *British Medical Journal* wrote after a 1986 visit to this country:

> Medical care in America is in the middle of a revolution. The cost of care has rocketed. Doctors are complaining of loss of power, au-

> tonomy, patients and pay. Hospitals are fighting for survival. Academic institutions are under threat. And in the midst of this unrest, a controversial form of delivery of health care—the HMO—is gaining momentum. HMOs are unlikely to be the answer to all America's complex health care problems, but they have attracted tremendous interest, not to mention near vitriolic polemic.[34]

This statement (and many similar ones of that period) eerily echoes today's complaints. Why didn't all the shrill predictions of a system meltdown come true? And what does that mean about predictions made today by some of the same organizations and individuals? And how, in the intervening decade, did the hospitals and doctors get to be the good guys and the HMOs the bad guys?

A FACT MEANS WHAT I WANT IT TO MEAN

> When managers in any field raise the specter of deteriorating quality, it is usually because they can't think of any better argument at the moment.
>
> —Phillip Crosby, *Quality Is Free*

Whose opinion about the quality of medical care could be more reliable than that of the physicians who work within the health care system every day? The answer, as we saw in chapter 7's discussion of paradigm shifts, is that the experts are often the most unshakably convinced that what is constitutes all that can be: witness the scientists who said that machines heavier than air could never fly.

Prospective payment was profoundly disorienting for doctors and hospitals, just as managed care is today. Between 1982 and 1988, the total number of days Medicare patients spent in the hospital decreased by a little over 20 percent—an extraordinary drop in such a short period. If one takes into account that hospital use by the elderly was increasing before prospective payment came on the scene, then the reduction from what hospital days would otherwise have been was more like 40 percent, according to a 1991 analysis by William Schwartz and Daniel Mendelson.[35] Before prospective payment, talk of that much waste in the system was largely confined to the theoretical.[36] Practicing physicians "knew" better. After all, they were the ones taking care of patients, and they did not see themselves as egregiously wasteful. Yet study after study of prospective payment found no significant evidence of patient harm from the new practices. In fact there was even some evidence of benefit.

Among the studies giving the new system a clean bill of health were one from the nonprofit Commission on Professional and Hospital Activities (the group traced its origins to Paul Lembcke's "medical audit" work), the Massachusetts Department of Public Health (liberal regulators), and *JAMA*.[37]

As the studies accumulated, one initially vocal PPS opponent conceded:

> Some hospital administrators considered any constriction of the revenues available from third parties a threat to their ability to provide high quality services, while others used PPS [the prospective payment system] as an all-purpose excuse to defend any action employees or attending physicians might not like. . . . There may, in other words, be less here than meets the eye. . . . Unless one believes that every dollar reimbursed to hospitals by Medicare before the implementation of PPS was used optimally to promote quality and efficiency, it is hard to make a convincing argument against some kind of prospective limitation on payments to hospitals.[38]

The politicians were not as easily persuaded. When I asked Pennsylvania's Heinz in 1988 about the accumulating scholarly evidence in favor of prospective payment, he gave an answer that made perfect sense for the world of politics, where perceptions are often as important as facts: "The issue is not whether, in retrospect, the number of victims of premature discharge meets some researcher's definition of statistical significance. *We know that thousands of people have been harmed,* and in some cases have died, as a result of being released too soon from a hospital" (emphasis added).[39]

Heinz's response is interesting to consider today, in the midst of the present managed care backlash. There is no doubt that the introduction of prospective payment led to some genuinely harmful treatment of patients by hospitals, particularly in the beginning. And I certainly believe that publicity about abuses and the threat of legal action against the hospitals and doctors responsible for them helped prevent more problems. But widespread harm is something else again. The prosaic truth was that prospective payment went through a shakedown period. Some minor modifications were made legislatively, and Medicare patients were sent a bill of rights telling them that hospitals could not summarily discharge them without their consent—a reminder that could well be made again to HMO members. The most important change of all, however, was that the doctors and hospitals began to get used to the new system. They started to figure out how they could effectively provide more and better care inside the hospital in a shorter time and provide other care outside it. Similarly, patients began to adjust their own expectations of how sick they could be and still "safely" go home. By itself, however, prospective payment was not enough to control rising health care costs for long. There were simply too many other areas where controls were lax. Once more, it is important to remember that it was the problem of rising costs that led to the ascendancy of managed care—costs that were not necessarily related to better patient care.

Modern Healthcare examined hospitals' claims of financial distress throughout the 1980s in a six-part series that culminated in its 12 November 1990 issue. The hospital trade magazine found that hospitals were using Medicare and Medicaid reimbursement as an excuse to pad their bottom lines; were spending millions of dollars on giveaways to doctors to maintain the loyalty of heavy admitters; were wasting millions on bloated corporate management structures; and were buying expensive new technology with little real assessment of need. This is a part of the past hospitals would just as soon forget.

Similarly, in 1993 *Modern Healthcare* ran a gimlet-eyed review of the first ten years of prospective payment. "Hospitals tend to cry poor," concluded reporter David Burda, "[but] look at hard numbers." Hospitals had learned how to "upcode" a Medicare patient's diagnosis to one paying the maximum revenue, how to boost prices to payers other than Medicare, and how to find other sources of revenue to make up for Medicare cuts.[40] In early 1997, American Hospital Association statistics on hospital profits during the mid-1990s showed that profitability steadily increased even while the whining about managed care reached a peak.

And what about doctors? "We loved the old way," acknowledged Dr. James Silverman, chief of staff at Stanford University Medical Center, in the 10 February 1986 issue of *Forbes.* "There was no shortage of work, and everyone was happy. At the beginning of the year, doctors would target their income and reach it in a number of ways. You could always charge for lab tests you didn't do." The good old days did not die easily, however. An investigative story on managed care in the March–April 1995 issue of the liberal muckraking magazine *Mother Jones* straightfacedly quoted Alan Stone, a professor of law and medicine at Harvard, as blaming greed in medicine on managed care. Said Stone: "When you introduced the profit motive into health care, the whole industry became permeated with greed." In fact the truth is precisely the opposite, as difficult as it is for physicians to acknowledge: uncontrolled greed in medicine is what enabled managed care to take power in the first place.

To quote just a few examples: "Increasingly, physicians have found a profit center and a marketing tool in selling the drugs they prescribe," reported the 25 May 1987 issue of *Newsweek.* A 1989 investigation by the Department of Health and Human Services confirmed that Medicare patients whose doctors owned or invested in clinical laboratories received 45 percent more clinical services than other Medicare patients. And, of course there were always the patients with private insurance. By the late 1980s, wrote one scholar, there were "more patients in the hospital for hemorrhoids than heart disease, for hernia repair than cancer." Then there was the fifty-seven-year-old Florida man who went to see his physician because of a splinter in his big toe. One thing led to another, and the man ended up with an operation by an orthopedic surgeon after undergoing a presurgical chest X ray, electrocardiogram, blood tests, and urinalysis. The hospital bill amounted to over $3,000, the pathologist's and anesthesiologist's fees came to about $600, and the surgeon's bill was still pending. An indignant Ann Landers, relating the splinter incident in a 1990 column, called it "a perfect argument for hospital—and physician—cost containment."[41]

Prospective payment provided two critical insights into cost control. First, it showed that substantial waste could be eliminated without harming patient care, even if community physicians and hospitals complained bitterly all the while. Second, it showed that putting the providers of care "at risk" for the financial consequences of their actions could produce dramatic results. Neither of those key lessons was lost on the HMO industry. What HMOs did not fully understand, however, was the lesson about the short-term perils and turmoil that accompany rapid change.

"Managed care" was the perfect phrase for the business-oriented 1980s. Interestingly, I could not find anyone in the HMO industry, in the Medicare program, or among the prominent policy analysts I asked who knew exactly how or when the term was first used. (It seems to have originally referred only to Medicaid.) The appeal of managed care was that it offered a way to control both the price of medical services and what resources were used. It would encompass all aspects of care, including the doctor's office, diagnostic tests, outpatient surgery, and inpatient care. Managed care was unapologetically about managed cost—specifically, controlling the excesses of the health care providers. The do-gooder promise of "health maintenance" was shelved in favor of businesslike efficiency.

After all, the health care "crisis" was about cost, not quality. Whether the managed care organization was an HMO, PPO (preferred provider organization), or some other alphabet soup variant of a modern health insurer, the bottom line remained the bottom line. Unfortunately, without the benefit of any systematic measurement of medical quality, it remained a matter of subjective opinion just where benign capitalistic efficiency ended and ruthless capitalistic profit maximization began.

IMAGES VERSUS REALITY

In 1986 I took a one-year leave of absence from the *Chicago Tribune* and, with an Alicia Patterson Foundation Fellowship, set out to examine "the deregulation of the American health care system." The effort to introduce competition and economic discipline into health care was in full flower. As a Patterson fellow, I quickly discovered that what experts told me as a reporter did not always reflect what I learned by spending time with doctors, nurses, hospital administrators, and patients. The best example was managed care.

I grew up in an HMO, the Group Health Association of Washington, D.C., during the 1950s and 1960s. My father had a white-collar job, but with a modest salary to support a wife and three children. Although I had a personal pediatrician at Group Health, she (one of the few women doctors of the time) was a salaried physician working in a cliniclike environment. In researching this book, I came across a study comparing the care of children at Group Health with the care in fee for service practices during part of my childhood. The study told me my parents had made a smart decision. "The prepaid system . . . maximized patient access [for children] and did not appear to inhibit physician initiated care," the study concluded. "In addition, services were less equitably distributed in the fee for service system than in the prepaid system relative to both income and medical needs."[42]

The HMOs I saw as a reporter, both on my fellowship and afterward, were different from Group Health. Kaiser Permanente was (and remains) unique, owning its own hospitals in California and operating on a vast scale. Elsewhere, though, most HMOs were of the type that contracted with local physicians and hospitals. Often,

HMO managers seemed oblivious to the effect blunt incentives could have. As Indiana University professor Marc Rodwin points out in *Medicine, Money, and Morals,* eliminating the fee for service incentive to do more doesn't guarantee that the care that remains will be appropriate. "Rewarding physicians for using resources frugally does not eliminate financial conflicts of interest," notes Rodwin. "It creates new conflicts with different effects.[43]

In Minneapolis, Houston, Miami, and a few other cities, newspapers and television stations were starting to report allegations that HMOs were denying needed care in order to save money. It wasn't hard for me to find similar cases: some ended up in articles I wrote for the Patterson Foundation,[44] and some later became part of a front-page series for the *Chicago Tribune.*[45] I wrote about a woman whose son lost an eye because the family's HMO delayed authorizing surgery. And I published a transcript of emergency room doctors pleading by phone with an HMO reviewer for approval to treat a patient with chest pain who might have had a heart attack.

At the time, HMOs were starting to compete with each other, not just with indemnity insurers, and many HMOs were finding it difficult to make money. Even nonprofit health plans started looking for ways to keep expenses down. In Minnesota, for-profit companies can't own HMOs (although management contracts help bypass the spirit of that prohibition). Yet in St. Paul an anesthesiologist told me a disturbing story about an ill-trained orthopedic surgeon sent to his hospital by one local health plan. The surgeon worked to implant an artificial hip while consulting an open book that told him where to place the screws! The hospital, afraid of alienating a plan that supplied a large number of its patients, said nothing.

HMOs were not yet big news in the national media centers of New York and Washington, so anecdotes like these received only a flurry of attention. The only scandal that attracted any national notice occurred in Florida, where one of the first big Medicare HMOs turned out to be run by scam artists. A 1987 General Accounting Office investigation of HMO financial incentives, sparked by the Florida embarrassment, concluded that incentives to withhold care could cause undertreatment, but that there was no conclusive evidence they were doing so.

I was surprised by the variety of financial incentives HMOs employed. If fee for service doctors are small businessmen, then nonsalaried HMO doctors have become miniature insurance companies, both providing care and assuming financial risk. I was troubled that most patients had no idea this was happening, even though the HMO industry clearly knew there were potential problems. At the 1986 meeting of the Group Health Association of America, as the main HMO trade group was then called, one medical director boasted of teaching a lesson to a doctor who had prescribed an expensive drug when the HMO's formulary dictated a cheaper one. The doctor was told to make up the difference in cost by taking another patient off a prescription anti-inflammatory medication and putting him on aspirin instead. A gasp of disbelief went up from the crowd—but nothing happened to the boastful medical director. Trade groups have never been much good at regulating themselves.

I learned about "gatekeepers," the term for a primary care doctor whose approval is needed before the HMO will pay for a visit to a specialist or an emergency room. The catch is that the gatekeeper's own reimbursement is often linked to his patients' use of those services. Unknown to patients, the more care they get, the more money their doctor can lose. I wrote about a Michigan mother of two in her early thirties whose HMO physician neglected to properly treat her vaginal bleeding and pain. By the time the woman took herself to a hospital emergency room—without a referral—she had an advanced case of cervical cancer. She sued her primary care doctor and the HMO, charging that the physician delayed referring her to a gynecologist because the money to pay specialists came out of the gatekeeper doctor's payment from the HMO.

This woman's lawsuit was perhaps the first to challenge the gatekeeper arrangement. After my story on the case appeared, the HMO asked a judge to seal the court records and place a gag order on the woman and her attorney. Since HMO scandals weren't a big deal then, the judge readily complied. Just before the case went to a jury trial—where evidence would have to be made public and where a ruling might set a precedent—the HMO and the doctors involved paid the woman an undisclosed sum in return for her silence on the case.

In the old prepaid care world, it was easy to analyze the effect of a few financial incentives. Newer HMO payment schemes are so diverse that the academics can find no common thread. "How Do Financial Incentives Affect Physicians' Clinical Decisions and the Financial Performance of Health Maintenance Organizations?" asked a special article in a 1989 issue of the *New England Journal of Medicine.* The conclusion, in essence, was "we have no idea."[46] Similarly, in

1994 Robert Miller and Harold Luft published an article *JAMA* to update Luft's 1978 analysis of the scientific literature on HMO quality. Once again, the researchers acknowledged that they had no reliable measure of how the new incentives were affecting quality.[47]

In any event, the world was changing too rapidly for the academic rearview mirror to be much use. HMOs merged, altered their payment methods, or switched from not-for-profit to for-profit status. In 1981 more than 40 percent of all HMO members in the country belonged to one plan, the nonprofit Kaiser Permanente. By the end of 1991, more than half of all HMO enrollees belonged to for-profit plans. Teams of actuaries and accountants designed finely calibrated reimbursement contracts, but they often ignored the warning sign flashed by prospective payment: as important as the way an incentive really works is the way doctors *perceive* the incentive to work. Medicare's payment for each diagnosis was an average—some patients were expected to cost more, some less—but some physicians still wrote in the patient's hospital chart, "Have to be discharged because out of money."[48]

The kind of careful guideline development and educational effort characteristic of Minnesota's Buyers Health Care Action Group and the Institute for Clinical Systems Integration, discussed in the previous chapter, has been largely absent from the approach taken by the financial types. Whether from trust in the doctor or from a cynical attempt to avoid legal responsibility, the standard procedure has been to give doctors a set pot of money and trust they will know which care to cut out and which to keep.

There was another lesson the HMOs failed to garner from prospective payment. Medicare made its rules in public view, and the public, through the political system, eventually came to grips with those new rules. HMOs preferred secrecy. They traded on members' ignorance. In the early 1990s, most Chicagoans were still so new to managed care that it was common for someone to say, "I belong to HMO," as if the particular plan were irrelevant. That experience is undoubtedly being repeated in other parts of the country now experiencing managed care for the first time.

"HMOs are commonly marketed with the rhetoric that they keep people healthy and contain costs by avoiding serious illness," observed Rutgers University professor David Mechanic. "A more accurate, but less common, representation is that HMOs offer a more comprehensive benefit package without additional out-of-pocket expenditures in exchange for the patient's acceptance of the primary physician as gatekeeper and some rationing consistent with the physician's best judgment."[49]

In other words, HMOs did not offer a "free lunch." The richer benefit package and lower cost of HMOs involved trade-offs. Whether restricted access was better for members (the HMO protected them from unnecessary surgery and uncoordinated treatment) or worse (the HMO blocked their ability to get needed treatment) is a separate argument. The cold reality remains that many HMOs have tried to disguise their true functioning from members. Worse, even knowledgeable members who directly ask for explanations have not always gotten straight answers.

The public rightly began to feel uneasy as HMOs became mainstream medicine. With recalcitrant doctors and hospitals finally stampeded into HMO contracts by the 1993 threat of national health reform, and with corporate benefits managers giving HMOs their strong support, HMOs added more than seven million new members between 1 July 1994 and 1 July 1995. By the middle of 1996, more than sixty million Americans, or one-quarter of the population, belonged to nearly six hundred HMOs.[50] Among Americans working for an organization with at least ten employees, seven out of ten were covered by an HMO or other "managed care" plan in 1995.[51] Considering that as recently as 1983 fewer than half of all employers even admitted to having a "positive feeling" toward the "HMO concept," it was a breathtaking turnaround.[52] Similarly, Medicare HMO membership, long stagnant, topped four million in early 1996 and was growing rapidly. The same trend held true for Medicaid, where more than twelve million people were enrolled in managed care programs.[53]

But rapid and unanticipated change provides a fertile environment for backlash, particularly when confusion goes along with it. Neither HMO supporters nor critics really understood the link between the new financial incentives and quality of care. "The crucial question is not whether financial incentives *affect* physicians' decisions, but whether some financial incentives *distort* physicians' judgment," wrote the University of Pennsylvania's Alan Hillman, a physician with a master's degree in business administration, in a 1990 editorial in the *Annals of Internal Medicine.* "The effect of these financial incentives may be most important in cases where the correct [medical] decision is not obvious."[54]

Newspaper columnists, television reporters, and cartoonists did not wait for the research community to make up its mind. Anecdote became conventional wisdom, with a 1995 *New Yorker* cartoon aptly summarizing the public mood. "I wish I could help you," a physician tells his perplexed patient. "The problem is that you're too sick for managed care."

But the worst news for HMOs was symbolized by a *Boston Globe* cartoon showing two startled women in a maternity ward. Next to them, the initials "HMO" were written to stand for "Heave Mom Out." The "quicker and sicker" controversy involving Medicare patients in the mid-1980s was being replicated in the mid-1990s by a new phrase that referred to HMOs: "drive-through deliveries."

WOMEN AND CHILDREN FIRST

> I gather, young man, that you wish to be a Member of Parliament. The first lesson that you must learn is, when I call for statistics about the rate of infant mortality, what I want is proof that fewer babies died when I was Prime Minister than when anyone else was Prime Minister. That is a political statistic.
> —Winston Churchill

In the early 1970s Kaiser Permanente established a special family-centered birthing program in the San Francisco area. At a time of insurgent feminism, more and more couples were demanding an alternative to the overmedicalization of childbirth. The new program enabled many mothers and babies to go home from the hospital within twenty-four hours—sometimes in as little as twelve hours. The secret to success was careful prenatal care, extensive follow-up visits by home nurses, and a joint decision by mothers and doctors that the discharge was medically appropriate. Kaiser also tracked its patient outcomes and published the results in a peer-reviewed journal.[55]

Some twenty years later, a spokesman for the Travelers Insurance Company explained to me how the insurer's Pennsylvania HMO decided to mandate a twenty-four-hour hospital stay after normal vaginal births. First the HMO tried offering women who agreed to go home within one day a certificate good for four hours of free housekeeping services, plus the normal home nursing visits. This deal doubled the number of voluntary one-day discharges, but the HMO remained dissatisfied. "It wasn't up to our expectations," said the spokesman. "Now it's a mandatory one-day coverage."[56] By the mid-1990s a similar one-day stay was being recommended to a long list of managed care companies by the Seattle-based consulting firm of Milliman and Robertson, an influential commercial developer of guidelines.

There is no evidence that the Travelers Insurance directive or the Milliman and Robertson guidelines have been any better or any worse for the health of mothers and their babies than the program at Kaiser. But the difference in how the decision was reached and implemented is important. It's not just that the shorter stay mandated by the HMOs was at odds with most professional opinion. For instance, joint guidelines issued in 1992 by the American College of Obstetricians and Gynecologists (ACOG) and the American Academy of Pediatrics recommended a minimum forty-eight-hour stay after normal vaginal deliveries unless a long series of preconditions were met. The expert opinion could have been wrong. The real problem was that many HMOs were pushing the limits of good medicine without studies to assure them in advance or retrospectively that they were causing no harm. It was just opinion against opinion, with the HMOs' opinion perhaps influenced by monetary considerations.

Moreover, the short-stay limits did not apply to selected patients or even to the "average" patient, as with prospective payment. In other words, discharging one new mother in twelve hours didn't build up enough monetary savings to justify keeping another woman for thirty-six hours. The new rules covered all new mothers unless the physician could convince the HMO reviewer they should not. But many doctors feared, rightly or wrongly, that they would be dropped from a plan's contracting list if they regularly argued with its reviewers.

It was inevitable that some mother or baby would come to harm and that the blame would be placed on this early discharge policy. It was also inevitable that politicians and the news media would find out. On 24 September 1995, New Jersey residents Michelle and Steve Bauman told a United States Senate hearing room packed with reporters how their daughter Michelina died from a streptococcus B infection two days after she was born. If mother and baby hadn't been discharged after only twenty-eight hours, the couple averred in heartbreaking testimony, "her symptoms would have surfaced and professional trained staff would have taken the proper steps, so that we could have planned a christening instead of a funeral."

The couple added: "Her death certificate listed the cause of death as meningitis when it should have read, 'death by the system.' A law needs to be passed to make sure that no other babies, anywhere in the country, ever die because their HMO made them leave the hospital too soon. . . . We are here today for all future babies. Life must be the consideration, not the dollar sign that our HMO carriers have placed before anything."

The legislation the Baumans were advocating would have been hard to oppose based on its name alone: the Newborns' and Mothers' Health Protection Act. Sponsored in a bipartisan show of support by Senators Bill Bradley (D-N.J.) and Nancy Kassebaum (R-Kan.), it mandated a minimum hospital stay of forty-eight hours after a normal vaginal birth and ninety-six hours after a cesarean section, unless mother and doctor agreed on an earlier discharge. At the same hearing where the Baumans spoke, an ACOG representative replied that some insurers who were beginning to require hospital stays of as little as twelve or eight hours after a normal delivery.

"I have . . . generally resisted government micromanagement of the private health-care market," said Kassebaum, chairman of the Senate Labor and Human Resources Committee. "We cannot, however, allow our zeal to control health spending to outweigh the need to protect the most vulnerable and fragile in our society."

The Senate passed the federal act ninety-eight to zero with President Bill Clinton's strong support, and the House soon followed suit. The federal law applied to situations where states did not have jurisdiction, such as the health plans of self-insured corporations, and it marked the first time the government had ever intervened in the details of a specific medical treatment.[57] By the time Congress acted, more than two dozen states had also passed some sort of minimum-stay legislation for new mothers.

Were drive-through deliveries a manifestation of dangerous HMO greed? Or, as with prospective payment, was emotion driving the process? I do not know the answer, but I do know that the Baumans' written testimony raised questions I never saw addressed in any of the news accounts I read. For instance, the Baumans indicated that their HMO did not immediately find out about their baby's birth, so the plan did not send a home nurse within twenty-four hours of mother and baby's going home. Moreover, when the baby fell sick, there was some confusion when the parents called the hospital about whether they needed to take their child to the emergency room. Might the twenty-four-hour discharge have been safe without these administrative foul-ups? No politician (or reporter) seemed to pursue that sensitive line of questioning.

Even more touchy is whether the outcome of treatment would

have been different had the baby's illness been detected during a longer hospital stay. Obviously the Baumans genuinely believed their baby would have been saved, but what did the physicians who worked on the child think? Again, these were not questions any sane politician was going to ask a grieving parent in public. And maybe the questions were unanswerable. But shouldn't the "new Democrat" Clinton administration and the "conservative revolution" Republican Congress have quietly tried to find the answers before so eagerly endorsing federal micromanagement of medicine?

In August 1996, *Pediatrics* published the largest controlled study ever done of neonatal deaths with known hospital discharge times. It reviewed the outcome of care of some 109,000 babies and included a detailed examination of the medical records of 115 who died in the neonatal period. Lead author Susan A. Beebe and her University of Utah colleagues found no significant association between neonatal death and discharge home. They concluded:

> Although we cannot conclude that no infant would benefit from a longer hospital observation time, certainly the majority of infants who die in the neonatal period have signs or symptoms present within the first 18 hours of birth. . . . A careful prospective study might reveal that the infants were actually symptomatic at even earlier times. . . .
>
> It does seem that if a prolonged hospital stay were to have a protective effect on neonatal mortality, it would affect very few infants.[58]

The article had no effect on the politics of "drive-through" deliveries, of course. Still, four million babies are born in the United States every year, and several foreign countries have routine maternity stays of twenty-four hours or less. One would think that any large-scale danger from the practice would have produced more than one or two often repeated anecdotes. On the other hand, even if a twenty-four-hour maternity stay was not ordinarily hazardous—and the evidence might yet show that it is—the HMOs pushing the short stay were no better informed than their critics. Too many of them were racing blindly to manage costs, unconcerned that they had nary a clue as to when they might cross the line between efficient medical practice and being a party to involuntary homicide.

"In the Navy, it is traditional to fire a shot across the bow of a ship before taking more aggressive action," wrote Boston University ethicist George Annas in a 1995 article in the *New England Journal of*

Medicine. "The symbolic initiatives on the length of hospital stays after childbirth . . . are a shot across the bow of marketplace medicine. The signal can be ignored only at the peril of the new health care industry; politicians will not remain their captives forever. The message is that patients are patients, not customers."[59]

Since then, presidential and congressional initiatives on "drive-through" mastectomies and other alleged violations of patient rights have continued to reinforce that message. The message is a necessary one, even if some of the individual justifications for sending it are questionable. For instance, it turns out that outpatient mastectomies may be safe, and in any event, they are more common in fee for service practice than in managed care. Meanwhile, the managed care industry, like any other industry caught violating the public trust, is ardently promising better self-control. HMOs may even be scared enough of government intervention to follow through. At year end 1996 the American Association of Health Plans (an HMO trade group that studiously avoids the term "managed care") rolled out a series of principles called "Patients First." They included open disclosure of financial incentives and of the basis for utilization review decisions and "more research on the outcomes of care provided in health plans."

MARCUS WELBY DOESN'T LIVE HERE ANYMORE

Can limits on access to care be dangerous to health? Of course they can, which is why it is odd that the debate over access seems to have gotten stuck on questions about how many days well-insured middle-class women spend in the hospital. There are plenty of good studies showing that large numbers of poor and minority women—and men and children—die every year because they have no access to preventive or acute medical care.

The managed care backlash may have crested. Knee-jerk criticism is starting to be replaced by more thoughtful critiques. For example, the 2 October 1996 issue of *JAMA* was entirely devoted to managed care, and its lead article cast doubt on how well HMOs care for the elderly and poor who are chronically ill.[60] Nonetheless, an editorial written jointly by Paul Ellwood and *JAMA* editor George Lundberg was carefully titled, "Managed Care: A Work in Progress." It argued, "The new American health system works. It has contained costs, it provides easily accessible comprehensive health care to its insured members, and, on the whole, it has not yet jeopardized quality. But patients, physicians, the uninsured and the country deserve better. The American health system is a work in progress; it can and, we believe, will get better."[61]

In the general news media, references to "Marcus Welby–style" medicine—the presumed alternative to managed care—have begun to diminish. After all, despite the kindly Welby's enduring stature, he suffered from one severe flaw: he was not real. This hero of television medicine never existed, nor—most important—was there ever a time when most real doctors were like the fictional Welby. What *is* real is that the resources to pay for medical care remain limited. That is why Medicare prospective payment stayed in place, despite the horror stories, and that is why managed care will remain in some form. We will never return to an uncontrolled, doctor-run, fee for service system. The success of HMOs in controlling medical costs is why employers offer them and why most individuals, seeking to limit their personal medical expenses, continue to join them.

That leaves us with the question posed by *The Painful Prescription* at the beginning of this chapter: "how to alter the behavior of providers and patients so that expenditures are curtailed on care that, in some sense, is worth less than it costs." I believe that question is best answered if posed from a different perspective than that of the economist or even the physician. Joseph Cardinal Bernardin, the late archbishop of Chicago, was a man who thought long and hard about the ethical implications of managed care. Bernardin announced in late 1996 that he had terminal cancer, but even before then he spoke eloquently about medical issues. In Bernardin's view, we can neither turn away from the hard decisions nor ignore the effect of those decisions on real people.

"If we accept, as we must, that our resources are finite, then we must address this issue openly and clearly," Bernardin said. "The very concept of rationing is explosive. I prefer the concept of 'stewardship.' How do we best protect human life and enhance human dignity in a situation of limited health resources?"[62]

Our national debate over managed care is part of a very American attempt to grapple with the issue of stewardship. Unlike the British, we do not trust the government to make these decisions. On the other hand, we do not wholly trust the marketplace either.

Although I am personally sympathetic to Bernardin's views, I decided to telephone a few people I trusted to speak authoritatively about managed care. They were not academic experts or health care executives. Instead, I tracked down the HMO "horror story" participants I mentioned earlier in this chapter: the anesthesiologist who had watched the open-book surgery by an orthopedic surgeon, the mother whose son lost an eye because the HMO did not authorize an operation quickly enough, and the woman whose cervical cancer went undiagnosed. All of them continued to be associated with managed care plans. All had thoughtful criticisms about cost cutting they saw as overdone, but none was as vituperative as the journalists and physicians who were shocked (shocked!) to discover financial factors affected the practice of medicine. They were realists, not idealogues—and in two of the cases they had paid dearly for that realism.

Bush, the woman who received a delayed diagnosis of cervical cancer, was particularly eloquent in her comments. Bush, in her early forties, had defied the pessimistic predictions about her life expectancy. When I called her, she immediately remembered our conversations of a decade ago and told me her son was now fourteen and her daughter twenty. We avoided discussing topics she was still legally barred from, but we caught up on how her very difficult life (five surgeries, chemotherapy, radiation, a shortened bowel, an ostomy bag) had gone since her diagnosis.

"What it comes down to is the doctor paying attention to the patient," said Bush, when I asked her to tell me what she would say to someone considering an HMO versus fee for service. "No matter where you go to the doctor, you really have to be your own health advocate. [You must] really not just be trusting that they're doing the right thing."

The keys to medical excellence, in other words, are information and accountability.

CHAPTER FIFTEEN

Medicine in the Information Age

Despite its bombastic title, a World Wide Web site called "Empower! The Managed Care *Patient* Advocate" offers intelligent and informed commentary. The site's editor, Mark Braly, is a longtime member of California's Kaiser Permanente health plan. He sees managed care not as a usurper of fee for service medicine, but as a legitimate delivery system whose flaws, though serious, are fixable.

"The problem of making medicine accountable to patients is not new," writes Braly. "It is just more urgent because of managed care. Although no one likes to talk about it, managed care is basically about rationing care. That is not necessarily a bad thing. We'd be better off without some of the care we sometimes get. . . . But is that the part that's being rationed?"[1]

Managed care has brought to a head the insistent question that has been one of this book's central themes: If more care isn't always better, then what is? Although Americans who have generous fee for service insurance still receive deficient and even dangerous treatment every day, the public attention to the financial incentives of managed care has highlighted our ignorance about quality of care. The relative responsibilities of health plan, hospital, and doctor are ambiguous. We are not sure either what information we really need to know or what to do with the information we have. We are presented with choices in black and white when what we need are subtle shades of color. Intimidated by data, we end up choosing hospitals or physicians because they are nearby or maybe because they were used by a friend.

Yet for all the confusion, the transition toward genuine accountability in health care is inexorably under way. A system that has blithely accepted wide variations in medical practice is beginning to demand measurable medical consistency. A system that has unhesitatingly deferred to the preferences of physicians is beginning to listen to the preferences of patients. And a system that has defined quality by what doctors do is starting to assess care by how clinical interventions affect patients' lives. Managed care does not have to doom our medical system to austerity and parsimony. We have been given a historic opportunity to embrace, instead, the late Joseph Cardinal Bernardin's gentler ideal of stewardship: "How do we best protect human life and enhance human dignity in a situation of limited health resources?"

Such an ambitious goal for information age medicine, however, demands much more than merely digitizing data. Plugging numbers into a computer is an easy trick. Changing people's expectations and behavior is something else again. True stewardship requires a relationship among doctors, patients, health plans, and employers that rests on a foundation of shared information. The outline of what that new relationship will look like is now beginning to emerge.

WHOSE LIFE IS IT ANYWAY?

> Physicians . . . should unite tenderness with firmness, and condescension with authority, [so] as to inspire the minds of their patients with gratitude, respect and confidence. . . . The obedience of a patient to the prescriptions of his physician should be prompt and implicit. He should never permit his own crude opinions as to their fitness to influence his attention to them.
>
> —First code of ethics of the American Medical Association, 1847

Tracey Campbell was just six years old when she fired one of her doctors. Campbell, who is now in her middle thirties, was diagnosed with epilepsy at a time when the disease was thought to consist only of grand mal seizures. She had difficulty finding a physician who took seriously the small seizure she suffered in her foot or her experiencing a sudden strong aura of burning rubber. When a neuropsychiatrist finally suggested she was just looking for attention, young Tracey decided she had had enough of experts.

"I walked out [of the doctor's office] to my parents and said, 'He's supposed to make the seizures stop, and he didn't. So I'm leaving.' My mom said, 'Should we pay the bill, dear?' And I said, 'He did teach me to stop the hiccups, so let's pay half of his bill and leave now.' "

These days Campbell's doctors "view our relationship as a team effort, not a dictatorship." Her seizures are being treated with an amino acid she found out about while researching the medical literature on her own. Her primary care doctor was skeptical, but after the therapy proved effective for her, he began prescribing it for other patients. Campbell also writes a regular self-help column, "Tracers' X-Files," that provides tips about medications and lifestyle changes. Like Mark Braly's writings on managed care, Tracers' X-Files appears on an independent Web site, in this case one dedicated to those with epilepsy. Other Web sites offer free access to databases such as Medline, which contains more than seven million article abstracts and references taken from more than four thousand medical journals at the National Library of Medicine.

The belief that patients can or should be partners with their physicians is relatively new. "Physicians have always maintained that patients are only in need of caring custody," observed Jay Katz, himself a physician, in *The Silent World of Doctor and Patient.* Doctors acted as "rational agents" on the patient's behalf. They intuitively believed that sharing information with patients was "inimical to good patient care."[2]

In part, doctors understood that the very mysteriousness of their art constituted a powerful therapeutic tool. "Some patients, though conscious that their condition is perilous, recover their health simply through their contentment with the goodness of the physician," is the way Hippocrates put it. Yet this "goodness"—what physicians call "beneficence"—somehow got distorted over the years. It required a decision by the U.S. Supreme Court to establish a patient's simple right to know in advance of an operation exactly what surgical procedure the doctor was planning to do.

The case involved forty-year-old Parmelia Davis, a woman with epilepsy who went to a renowned surgeon considered an authority on the disease. Without informing Davis of his intentions, the surgeon removed her uterus and ovaries. The surgeon later explained that he had deceived his patient so that she would not resist having the procedure. Unless the patient expressly limits what the doctor can do, contended the legal brief for the surgeon, "she thereby in law consents that he may perform such operation as in his best judgment is proper and essential to her welfare."[3]

The Supreme Court emphatically disagreed. In a 1905 opinion, the Court declared that an American's rights as a free citizen prohibited "a physician or surgeon, however skillful or eminent . . . to violate without permission the bodily integrity of his patient . . . and [to operate] on him without his consent or knowledge." In a Court decision involving a similar case in 1914, Justice Benjamin Cardozo added: "A surgeon who performs an operation without his patient's consent commits an assault."

Despite these rulings, it was not until the late 1950s that patients acquired the legal right to an answer to the next logical question about treatment: not only what the doctor was going to do, but the possible effects of those actions. The requirement for a patient to give "informed consent" to a treatment resulted from a lawsuit filed by a fifty-five-year-old man named Martin Salgo. What the doctors of the time called the "hazards of modern diagnosis and therapy" had left Salgo with paralyzed legs following a hospital diagnostic procedure. He claimed that his doctors were legally liable for not warning him of that risk. On 22 October 1957, the California Court of Appeals agreed. Wrote the court: "A physician violates his duty to his patient and subjects himself to liability if he withholds any facts which are necessary to form the basis of an intelligent consent by the patient to the proposed treatment." That ruling was subsequently broadened in other cases elsewhere.

By the early 1970s, physicians for the first time had a clear obligation to disclose to the patient not just what they were going to do (the process of care), but also the evidence about its likely effect on the patient's life (the outcome). The disclosure also had to be in simple language that a layman could understand.

These court rulings obligating doctors to share information paralleled a new assertiveness on the part of the public. Long before anyone dreamed of the Internet, a book by a California pediatrician started the dismantling of the paternalistic model of medicine. The *Common Sense Book of Baby and Child Care* was Dr. Benjamin Spock's guide to the perplexed parents of Baby Boomers. From its very first edition in 1946, a time when doctors were still perceived as gods, the book straightforwardly advised parents to trust their own instincts. Parents could decide when to feed their baby, for example, rather than having to adhere to the rigid feeding schedules set by many pediatricians. Over the next half century, Spock's baby book sold forty-three million copies in thirty-nine languages.[4]

Spock, though, was still a doctor granting permission to patients. By contrast, *Our Bodies, Ourselves,* published in 1969 by a collective of Boston feminists, demanded to be heard. The book brought the sensibilities of the civil rights movement to medicine. Feminists began to force the profession to confront unneeded hysterectomies, cesarean sections, and other grossly inappropriate procedures. Feminists and the broader consumerism movement also gave grassroots political punch to discussions about the patient-doctor relationship. Now, instead of one individual meekly asking his doctor for information, groups of patients were successfully pressuring the entire medical community to publicly acknowledge patients' rights.

In 1978 an activist involved in *Our Bodies, Ourselves* founded an alternative birthing center. It was an omen of a shift in the childbirth experience that would demonstrate the enormous power of consumer preferences. In the typical postwar hospital, a doctor delivered the baby out of an unconscious, anesthetized mother in a sterile operating room. The nervous father waited somewhere outside. By the 1980s, when the children raised on Dr. Spock began to produce children of their own, that venerable model of doctor omnipotence had been discarded forever. In response to patients' demands, the conscious mother shared responsibility with the doctor for decisions such as whether to continue natural breathing exercises or accept an injection to dull the pain. The solicitous father typically remained by his wife's side in a labor and delivery suite decorated like a bedroom. It was by any measure an unusual scene. Hospitals that had always focused on making themselves attractive to doctors were forced by the marketplace to invest millions of dollars to make themselves attractive to patients. Today's "patient-centered care" movement, embodied by Boston's Picker Institute, continues in that same tradition of reminding hospitals that people do not lose their humanity when they become patients.

In a completely different way, the deadly AIDS pandemic prompted gay activists to take patient empowerment to a more sophisticated level. Outraged over what they saw as complacency in the straight medical community, gay activists immersed themselves in the clinical details of AIDS research and treatment. Nonphysicians became the acknowledged information equals (or more) of many doctors. The gay community also showed shrewd insight into language's power to shape the patient-doctor relationship. Just as feminists rejected the word girl in favor of woman, the dependency implicit in the terms AIDS sufferer and AIDS victim was discarded in favor of the designation PWA, or person with AIDS. The phrase unmistakably asserted that the disease, no matter how deadly, was less important than the individual harboring it, and that the individual, however sick, remained a person whose voice deserved to be heard.

Other advocacy groups were quick to adopt the AIDS groups' tactics, both in heightened patient education efforts and in terminology. The Web site where Tracey Campbell's column is found, for example, does not use the word epileptic. It appeals to PWEs: people with epilepsy. The precedent set by AIDS activists in their insistence on access to outcomes information about the disease gradually changed the cultural context of the doctor-patient interaction. Although the torrent of medical information (and sometimes misinformation) available on the Internet owes its existence to technology, the necessary first step was to change the cultural context so that it felt natural to provide patients with access to a wealth of clinical detail.

Stewardship, however, cannot be built solely on a base of patients' demands. Doctors' expectations about their own professional role must change too. Patients' preferences need to be incorporated directly into medical decision making. To do that, patient and physician both have to evaluate the available scientific evidence. A true patient-physician partnership will help push medical practice away from the old capriciousness of subjective physician judgment and toward a better-informed and ultimately more caring model for the future.

QUALITY OF CARE IS WHAT I RECEIVE

> Each patient carries his own doctor inside him. They come to us not knowing that truth. We are at our best when we give the doctor who resides within each patient a chance to go to work.
> —Albert Schweitzer, M.D.

One moment Albert G. Mulley Jr. was brushing his teeth. The next, the nerves in his back were urgently broadcasting a message of intense pain. Not the strained muscle, "take two aspirin" kind of pain, but the searing "my nerve endings are on fire" kind that accompanies a herniated disk. Since Mulley is director of the division of general internal medicine at Massachusetts General Hospital, he quickly obtained an examination by a respected Harvard Medical School neurosurgeon. Then he got a second opinion. And a third.

His case was not particularly complicated. According to an MRI scan, Mulley was an excellent candidate for an operation to fuse the vertebrae. Yet he hesitated. Maybe it was because he knew that research showed an eightfold difference between the rate of back surgery on the West and East Coasts. That wide swing was a tip-off to a procedure whose value was suspect. Or maybe the problem was the scientific evidence justifying surgery. It was based on a twenty-year-old randomized trial involving a total of sixty-six nonsurgical patients and sixty surgical patients at a hospital in Norway. "Does that make sense?" asked Mulley. "[That] what we can say confidently about the natural history of this condition is based on sixty-six patients in Oslo, Norway?" Whatever the reason for his reluctance, Mulley decided to wait and see whether his back pain would subside on its own, as it does for nine out of ten people. Mulley was fortunate. After bed rest and careful exercise, his pain went away.[5]

The movement to provide outcomes information to patients is rooted as much in experiences like Mulley's as in the history of informed consent. The "best" treatment for a bad back or other condition might be a matter of intense medical debate, but that is often kept from the person who is sick. Whatever the legal requirement for informed consent, doctors routinely seek to influence the patient's choice so that it coincides with the doctor's. If a patient resists the hint, the doctor may well respond "by repeating in rote fashion all the information previously given (perhaps in a louder voice), or may simply shrug her shoulders and allow the patient to do without the treatment," writes internist and medical ethicist Howard Brody in *The Healer's Power.* "Talking *with* patients about medical facts remains rare." Concludes Brody: "The central ethical problem in medicine is the responsible use of power."[6]

The degree to which even the most sophisticated patients are left feeling powerless and uninformed can be seen in the experience of Andy Grove, the brilliant and hard-driving chief executive officer of silicone chip maker Intel Corporation. In a candid confessional that put him on the cover of the 13 May 1996 issue of *Fortune,* Grove told of finding out at age fifty-eight that he had prostate cancer. Although more than 300,000 men are diagnosed with prostate cancer annually—and 41,000 die of it—good comparative treatment information was nearly impossible to obtain. Wrote Grove of his frustration:

> When I was doing semiconductor device research, it was expected that I would compare my results with other people's previously published results and that I would comment on any differences. But it seemed to be different in medicine. Medical practitioners primarily tended to publish their own data; they often didn't compare their data with the data of other practitioners, even in their own field, let alone with the results of other types of treatments for the same condition.

Grove also discovered that the doctor's-eye view of a therapy did not always mesh with the patient's experience. His urologist, for example, confidently recommended surgery while downplaying unpleasant surgical side effects. Grove found himself staring at examining room walls that "were covered with posters of contraptions like penile implants and vacuum pumps. I knew that they were devices meant to restore potency, but they evoked images of medieval torture."[7]

After many twists and turns—including participating in on-line chat groups of prostate cancer survivors—Grove ultimately chose an experimental treatment that promised results almost comparable to those of surgery but without the side effects. Some months later, he told the *Washington Post* that his cancer had been controlled and that the chances of a recurrence "are mathematically smaller than the average person getting it in the first place." On 24 February 1997 Grove again graced the cover of *Fortune*, but this time the topic was how much money Intel was making.

The problem with the Andy Grove model of shared medical decision making, of course, is that the average patient does not possess anything remotely close to Grove's technical education and financial resources. The average person who falls sick needs other sources of information. One of those sources might be the Foundation for Informed Medical Decision Making, created in 1989 by Mulley and Dartmouth's John Wennberg. The foundation's mission is to develop and disseminate video programs that enable patients to become partners in their care. Emile Kunz, a seventy-four-year-old retired machinist from Quechee, Vermont, was one of the first people to put this hypothesis to the test.

Kunz did not have prostate cancer, but he did have a condition even more common among older men: benign prostate enlargement. In the early 1980s, Wennberg and his colleagues at the Maine Medical Assessment Foundation began to examine why doctors varied in their use of three common surgical procedures, including transurethral resection of the prostate (removal of part of the prostate) as a treatment for enlargement.[8] The researchers were unable to find a single prospective clinical trial comparing surgical and nonsurgical treatments for prostatectomy, even though "TURP" is the second most common surgery for men over sixty-five and costs billions of dollars annually. Not only that, the urologists who recommended surgery didn't even agree on the reason. One group believed the operation was needed because benign prostatic hyperplasia (BPH), the technical term for prostate enlargement, could lead to life-threatening complications if surgery was delayed until the patient was older and more frail. Another group of urologists was equally certain that BPH would not get worse as the patient aged, but they felt the operation was a good way to reduce unpleasant symptoms and improve the quality of life.

Wennberg and his colleagues took an unusual step to resolve the controversy. They designed a special questionnaire asking BPH patients how their lives had been affected either by surgery to relieve symptoms or by "watchful waiting." In 1985 the group published its findings. Based on the patients' own evaluation of their health status, "watchful waiting" was as legitimate a therapeutic response to BPH as was surgery. The surgery did not prolong life, so the decision whether to have it depended on how badly the symptoms bothered the individual patient. Thanks to that research, the American Urological Association agreed to a standardized questionnaire that used patients' responses to characterize the severity of BPH symptoms.

In effect, Wennberg's work flip-flopped the definition of good quality care from the physician's view ("Quality of care is what *I* provide") to the patient's perspective ("Quality of care is what *I* receive"). And the answer to the crucial question Wennberg had posed years before about practice variation ("Which rate is right?") acquired a new dimension that changed the frame of reference for clinical problems.

"Inevitably, once you start down the variation path and ask which rate is right, you come up against who's making the decision and whose preferences are being reflected," Wennberg said. "That's where the revolutionary aspects of what we're doing really are." And, in fact, "watchful waiting" is now routinely presented in scientific articles on a number of conditions as a legitimate therapeutic alternative to intervention.

In the interactive version of the video programs produced by the Foundation for Informed Medical Decision Making, the patient begins by filling out a health questionnaire. A computer then uses the medical literature to generate customized statistics that show this particular patient's likely outcomes from different treatments. Patients don't need computer skills; all they have to do is watch the video, which blends general and customized content. (As of early 1997, the videos were still shown only on special laser disk equipment that a hospital or group practice had to purchase.) What makes the videos so immediately compelling is that they present striking personal narratives. These patient testimonials on breast cancer, heart disease, and other conditions are edited only for length and to make certain they reflect the scientific evidence on likely outcomes. In the BPH video, two Dartmouth professors shared their intimate and very different reactions to treating their problem by surgery.

One professor was distinctly unhappy about his decision to have an operation. He was particularly displeased with the sensation of retrograde ejaculation, a frequent complication of prostate surgery. "I thought [a prostatectomy] was like getting your hair cut," this academic said dryly. "A prostatectomy is not like getting your hair cut."[9] His colleague, on the other hand, was delighted with the results of surgery and cited an earthy rationale missing from any medical textbook. The increased urine flow after surgery, exclaimed this professor, restored his ability to "put my initials in the snow."

Emile Kunz was leaning in favor of prostate surgery after talking to his urologist, but he tentatively turned against it after speaking further with his family doctor. The BPH video, which Kunz called "a little more graphic than reading about [surgery] in a brochure," confirmed his decision to stay with "watchful waiting" a while longer.

Shared decision making has limits: it applies only to decisions where the patient's opinion is appropriate. Mulley compares it to traveling by air. "If I get on an airplane, and the guy with four stripes on his sleeve says, 'Do you want to fly this thing?' I'm going to say no. There is certain technical knowledge that I don't have. But if he asks me if I care where the airplane lands, I feel very strongly about that."

Moreover, a partnership is just that: as a partner, the physician still has an obligation to express his or her professional judgment about the best course of action. The difference is that this opinion is given openly rather than being disguised as objectivity. As Doctors Howard Brody and Timothy Quill wrote in an article exploring the balance between physician power and patient choice, the model doctor-patient relationship involves "an intense collaboration between patient and physician . . . [that is] informed by both the medical facts and the physician's experience."[10]

Perhaps the ultimate test of that collaboration involves the most painful and difficult medical decision of all, the decision to cease treatment and let a patient die. From 1989 through 1994, a group of clinicians around the country worked on the Study to Understand

Prognoses and Preferences for Outcomes and Risks of Treatments (SUPPORT). Part of the project included giving sophisticated outcomes information to patients, families, and doctors. Another part was having special nurses give more attention to patients' and families' emotional needs. At Wisconsin's Marshfield Clinic, deep in the rural heart of the state, a young farming couple were early and tragic SUPPORT participants. Most SUPPORT patients were elderly. But Mary Lou Wolosek, just thirty-four years old, had mysteriously developed lung cancer despite being a nonsmoker. By the time she came to Marshfield, after futile treatment elsewhere, the cancer had metastasized throughout her body. She and her husband, Conrad, age forty-two, agreed to enroll her in SUPPORT.[11]

"I could see this program was directed at that need for the patient not to be just an object to be treated," Conrad recalled. Besides, Conrad was ready to grasp at any opportunity to get more information about his wife's disease. "I would go along [to Mary Lou's doctor appointments] and literally walk in with a notebook of questions," he said, and then paused: "I had a wonderful wife, and I wanted her to have the best that was possible, at least what[ever] I could give her."

Shortly after the couple's arrival, a nurse entered information about Mary Lou's cancer into a specialized software package called APACHE. Drawing on fourteen data elements, APACHE was designed to predict the likelihood of death or serious disability in critically ill patients over a six-month period—much as other software analyzed the chances of a patient's dying on the operating table from bypass surgery. With Mary Lou Wolosek, the computer drew a curve that plunged swiftly downward over a very short time. Nurse Sue Kronenwetter, after talking over this prognosis with Mary Lou's physician, came with the doctor's permission to speak with Conrad about what he wanted to do next.

"She helped me to understand and accept," Conrad recalled, the ache of the loss still etched in his voice. Although he never gave up hope, he did decide not to insist on painful and expensive "heroic measures" to try to restart Mary Lou's heart if it stopped. One week later, Conrad held Mary Lou's hand as she died.

The SUPPORT results, which appeared in major scholarly articles in early 1995 and early 1997, found that the Woloseks' experience was unfortunately atypical. Patients too often died alone, in pain, or unnecessarily hooked up to machines. Two-thirds of the doctors who received a patient's advance directive didn't even look at it.

Moreover, patients and families alike were often shocked to find that real-world outcomes information rudely conflicted with the routine medical miracles presented on television. Researcher Joanne Lynn and her colleagues made clear their belief that end-of-life care would change only when doctors and hospitals were held accountable for their actions. Their 1997 article concluded: "It is likely that quality of care at the end of life will have to be routinely measured and that the public and other health care purchasers will have to demand and pay for adequate performance before lasting and sustained improvements are possible."[12]

Evaluating the effect of medical treatment for those with chronic diseases that do not threaten their lives is certainly as important as evaluating what happens to those who are at the end of life. Just as critically ill patients and their families want to know whether a treatment will make a real difference in how the patient *feels,* so too do millions suffering from asthma, arthritis, or other ills crave the same kind of information. That measurement of health status provides one of the most striking changes in the practice of medicine in the information age.

A QUESTION OF STATUS

Every few months, Margaret Doyle's dialysis sessions at Boston's New England Medical Center are punctuated by a request to fill out a thirty-six-question form. The questionnaire asks her to rate on a scale of one to five the way she feels physically and mentally compared with a few weeks or months ago. It asks about her ability to get through her daily activities at home and on the job (Doyle works at a public school cafeteria). It asks about pain, sleeping habits, and "general vitality." Doyle, fifty-eight, sees nothing remarkable about the inquiry. "If you don't feel good about yourself, how can you get better?" she demands. Besides, she figures that the dialysis center's director, Dr. Klemens Meyer, "has so many patients, he can't keep track of everybody. If [the form] will help him to help us, what's a few minutes?"

Not every patient being treated at the center agrees with Doyle. Some younger patients with renal failure caused by AIDS or drug or alcohol abuse complained that the questionnaire only reminded them how much worse off they were than when they were healthy. But the "SF-36" (for short form thirty-six, referring to the number of questions) is not supposed to be a medical mood ring. Its questions, which have been carefully validated in different patient populations, are designed to evaluate the effect of medical treatment on the life of someone with a chronic disease. Meyer has been collecting quarterly health status reports at the dialysis clinic since October 1990, a longer track record than anyone. He candidly acknowledges that the questionnaires have caused him to change patients' therapies and to explore problems that would otherwise have gone unrecognized.

"My role as a physician is to try to understand my fellow human beings," says Meyer simply, but the implications of regular health status assessment are more radical than that modest statement suggests. The use of the SF-36 and similar measures effectively makes the patient's own experience of illness a part of the medical record that is on a par with the assessments of the physician. As modern as this "empowered patient" approach may feel, it fits precisely the recommendation made some four decades ago by medical audit originator Paul Lembcke. "The best measure of quality is not how well or how frequently a medical service is given," wrote Lembcke, as described in chapter 7, "but how closely the result approaches the fundamental objectives of prolonging life, relieving distress, restoring function and preventing disability."

To Meyer, the health status questionnaire has a very practical application. It levels the playing field for doctor and patient, providing patients who may find it difficult to express their feelings with a way to convey their direct experience of illness and therapy. "By quantifying the patient's subjective experience, health status assessment makes that experience more consistently accessible to the [clinical] staff," wrote Meyer and his colleagues in the *American Journal of Kidney Diseases.* "It puts the patient's experience on their agenda."[13]

The "patients' rights" movement of the 1970s gave rise to a very visible medical consumerism. The mirror image of patients' asking better questions of doctors, however, was some doctors' new sensitivity to asking better questions of patients. For instance, one of the earliest attempts to collect systematic and comparable information on patients' health status was the Sickness Impact Profile. It listed over three hundred items of sickness-related behavioral change and grouped them into fourteen categories of daily activities.[14] But a breakthrough in developing an easy-to-use health status measure did not come until the 1980s. The Medical Outcomes Study produced three articles in the 18 August 1989 issue of the *Journal of the American Medical Association.* Researchers collaborated in a two-year examination of the functional status and well-being of thousands of patients with chronic conditions. In the process, they gave unprecedented attention to how patients' and physicians' perceptions of outcomes can differ. An instrument to measure that difference, predicted an accompanying editorial, "will help us to practice what we and those who taught us have always preached: 'Treat the patient, not the disease.'"[15] The Medical Outcomes Survey instrument was the SF-36.

Sheldon Greenfield, a physician who helped develop the survey with his RAND Corporation colleague John Ware Jr., said it forced physicians to treat patients as "more than a bundle of lab symptoms."[16] Paul Ellwood, the popularizer of HMOs, again found a catchy phrase to summarize the opportunities. The health care system, wrote Ellwood in an influential 1988 article in the *New England Journal of Medicine,* needed "*a technology of patient experience* designed to help patients, payers, and providers make rational medical care–related choices based on better insight into the effect of these choices on the patient's life" (emphasis added).

Building a database that showed how a particular treatment affected a patient's functioning in the real world, continued Ellwood, opened up the possibility of "*outcomes management* . . . that estimates as best we can the relation between medical interventions and health outcomes, as well as the relation between health outcomes and money"[17] (emphasis added).

Some hospitals and individual physicians have adopted the SF-36 on their own initiative. One of the more aggressive has been St. Vincent Hospital and Medical Center in Portland, Oregon. Spine doctors Frederick Waller and Thomas Lorish started screening patients with injured backs. Based on their data correlating health status and return to work, the physicians were able to direct some new patients away from a gradual rehabilitation program and send them directly to more intensive therapy. Jay B. V. Butler Jr., a St. Vincent orthopedic surgeon, used the questionnaire to evaluate the effectiveness of two artificial hip implants. Butler wanted to know whether his patients could walk as freely and painlessly with the more expensive implant as with the less expensive one. And a St. Vincent cardiology practice used the questionnaire as an aid in evaluating the appropriateness of angioplasty and bypass surgery. One heart patient, retired accountant Theodore Graham, said he had already applied an informal health status check to himself before seeking care. The eighty-eight-year-old Graham, an enthusiastic golfer, said he hadn't wanted to interrupt his golf outings to go to the hospital. He reluctantly changed his mind only after increasing chest pain started to affect his swing. It was time to see a doctor, he said, "when my handicap went up some, to twenty from fourteen."[18]

The growing popularity of the SF-36 and other health status measures, however, is not due to individual doctors earnestly pursuing a better method to "treat the patient, not the disease," as the high-minded editorial in *JAMA* urged. Instead, it is a by-product of health plans and physician groups seeking a practical and inexpensive way to demonstrate the value of the care they provide. At the same time, an increasing number of employers are viewing a health status measuring tool as a critical component in comparing health plans in order to "buy right." In one indication of that trend, a health status instrument developed at Dartmouth Medical School was licensed by a large national consulting firm to provide employers with an easy way of comparing health plans with each other and managed care with fee for service care, both nationally and locally.

In an age of increasing competition among health plans, information that can be used to enhance accountability is becoming a critical component of rational marketplace behavior. Economics is giving a boost to idealism. And though HMO horror stories still hog the headlines, the man-bites-dog news is that health maintenance organizations are finally discovering health maintenance.

CHAPTER SIXTEEN

Power to the Population

> There are only two classes of mankind in the world—doctors and patients.
> —Rudyard Kipling, 1908

In 1835 a Rhode Island textile mill owner named Zachariah Allen formed a mutual insurance company to protect himself and his fellow mill owners against the devastating financial consequences of fire. Rather than simply collecting premiums, Allen methodically searched for ways to minimize the chances of calamity; for example, he ordered a subordinate to investigate whether Thomas Edison's new electric light bulb might replace dangerous kerosene lamps and candles. More than a century and a half later, the successor organization to Allen's company—the Factory Mutual System—continues the same philosophy. Factory Mutual employs a small army of scientists, engineers, and researchers who specialize in "risk management" techniques, and the company ranks among the best in its field at collecting information and using it to accomplish one specific task: minimizing losses.

In its own way, the HMO industry is headed in much the same direction. The reason is not altogether surprising. Despite the unique vocabulary of health care, the basic task of an HMO is still insurance. It is not the absence of health maintenance efforts that has gotten some HMOs into trouble, but their alleged reluctance to pay medical bills for policyholders who fall sick. This is hardly a unique problem in the insurance industry. An HMO's putting up bureaucratic barriers to needed medical care is little different in kind from an auto insurer's mandating that accident damage be repaired with inexpensive replacement parts or a home insurer's paying only for cheaper building materials. The risk management approach of a Factory Mutual stands in stark contrast to this penny pinching. And though there are obvious limits to the similarities between property and health insurance, some clear parallels also apply.

So, for instance, Factory Mutual's consultants help customers design advanced safety features into their new facilities. An HMO would call a similar endeavor "prevention" or "wellness." Factory Mutual's affiliated insurers have for years carefully measured and quantified the customer's risk exposure. An HMO that wanted to do the same thing would ask a new member to undergo a complete physical examination and fill out a health status assessment questionnaire. Perhaps most compelling is the way the Factory Mutual system shares research about loss prevention with its clients and then zealously insists that they put "best practice" to actual use. The insurance companies affiliated with Factory Mutual are self-confessed fanatics about preventing fires. "Our main business is being a loss prevention organization first and an insurance company second," a senior executive with a Chicago-based Factory Mutual affiliate told me earnestly. Said a fellow manager: "We're a loss prevention engineering company with a money-back guarantee. If your building burns down, we'll pay for it."[1]

Until now, no HMO in America can say it has been anywhere near that aggressive about maintaining its members' health. As the managed care backlash shuts off easy cost cutting, however, a rapidly growing number of health plans are turning serious attention to risk management. The process is given a different label. It's called population-based care, meaning an attempt to maximize the health of all a plan's members. Or it's known as demand management (reducing demand for medical services) or disease management (reaching out to HMO members who have chronic diseases). Whatever the name, the common thread is using health maintenance to ameliorate the need for expensive acute care. In plain language, the goal is to prevent the factory from burning down instead of paying to rebuild it.

This is a much more difficult task for HMOs than it might first appear. An individual insuring a car or home fills out an insurance application that discloses risk; for instance, whether a car is driven by a teenager or whether a home is near the fire department. Since most HMO members are covered by an employer's group policy, they don't apply individually. The HMO has no idea which members are chain smokers and which are vegetarian joggers. In any event, health plan managers have not really seen health maintenance as their job. The HMO collected the insurance premiums, but it carefully left anything with a clinical component to doctors. Boston's Harvard Pilgrim Health Plan, New England's oldest HMO, is one of the first health plans to break out of that mold and move toward comprehensive disease management.[2] The health plan initially targeted asthma, a chronic disease characterized by inflammation and narrowing of the air passages to the lungs. For Colleen O'Brien, a suburban Boston teenager, that decision by Harvard Pilgrim may have saved her life.

Asthma has emerged as by far the most prevalent chronic disease of childhood. It affects about five out of every hundred children, compared with just three out of a thousand for the next most frequent chronic ailments. The disease annually causes more than ten million missed school days and some 200,000 hospitalizations of children.[3] Worst of all, deaths of children from asthma have more than doubled since 1980. Once again, the problem is putting research into practice. "There's no reasonable justification for [the increase in deaths]," says the American College of Allergy, Asthma, and Immunology. "Asthma is a disease we know how to control."

On a hot morning in June, Colleen O'Brien, then age fifteen, almost became one of those unreasonable deaths. Colleen had suffered from severe asthma since she was eight, but this attack stood apart in its intensity and duration. As she wheezed and panted for breath, her worried parents brought her to one of the Harvard physician centers. When the doctors there could not bring her breathing under control, she was rushed to the nearby Children's Hospital emergency room. Colleen was quickly admitted to the intensive care unit, where she remained for an entire week. "We almost lost her," said Kathleen O'Brien, Colleen's mother. Gradually, the Harvard disease management program eased much of the family's worry that a similar asthma attack, with a grimmer outcome, could happen at any time.

The Harvard program began by taking a fresh look at its information systems. Data on drug prescriptions, hospital admissions, and emergency room visits had been routinely used to track cost. With disease management, the health plan used the same databases to identify possible asthmatics. After evaluating the medical records of those identified by the computer, the health plan came up with the names of more than three thousand asthmatic adults and children and their doctors in its Boston-area centers.

Next, Harvard educated its physicians for an intensified risk management role. In the case of asthma, the "best practices" for treatment were taken from a consensus panel of the National Institutes of Health and translated into an easy to use clinical pathway. Harvard also reemphasized the big impact of seemingly small actions. For example, asthmatics have typically been taught to use an inhaler by closing their lips over the spout and then spraying. Yet the scientific evidence has shown for more than a decade that this method is an inefficient way of delivering a drug dose. Simply dispersing the medication with a plastic or cardboard "spacer" puts at least 30 percent more of the drug into the lungs, while 60 percent less goes elsewhere in the body (reducing side effects). Harvard took the responsibility for making sure that its doctors and nurses were teaching asthmatics the better spraying method.

Once the doctors were ready, Harvard directly involved children with asthma and their parents. The health plan gave them peak flow meters—a red plastic tube with a little ball inside—and taught them how to administer different medications to prevent asthma flare-ups from mushrooming into debilitating attacks. In essence, the health plan was putting into place the three-part blueprint for good quality of care discussed earlier in this book: structure (giving members the proper equipment), process (teaching them how to use it properly), and outcome (preventing severe asthma attacks).

For Colleen, the lessons of disease management begin anew every morning. When she awakens, the first thing she does is breathe into her meter. If her breath moves the ball above the 300 mark, Colleen figures it's going to be a good day, and she adjusts her medications accordingly. If the ball lingers around the 200 level the prognosis is more guarded, and she chooses a different medication mix. But if the ball doesn't move above 100, Colleen immediately knows she's reached the limits of self-medication. "That's when I have to go to the hospital [emergency room]," she says matter-of-factly.

Harvard also recognized that genuine stewardship—or sophisticated risk management—meant looking at asthma in a broader social context. Asthma attacks are often triggered by stress, and they can lead to depression. The asthma disease management program mobilized pediatricians, social service workers, allergists, and other professionals. Colleen regularly sees Walter Torda, a pediatrician and asthma specialist with a counseling background, and speaks by phone with Patricia Glidden, one of several outreach nurses hired to stay in regular contact with patients.

Not all HMOs are as active as Harvard Pilgrim in reducing risk, and not all asthma sufferers are as interested as Colleen O'Brien in sharing responsibility for their health. Cheryl Monaghan, a Harvard outreach nurse who deals with adult asthmatics, says that most ignore her appeals to participate in managing their disease. Many other asthmatics take home a peak flow meter, only to use it as infrequently as the proverbial exercise bike bought right after Christmas. "People want a quick fix," Monaghan sighs.

Still, when patients do take on responsibility for their care the results are startlingly positive—and not just with asthma. Sharing information with patients not only can reduce the risk of an acute episode of a chronic illness, it can also aid healing. Researchers from the Group Health Cooperative of Puget Sound and the Center for the Advancement of Health who reviewed the medical literature gave a ringing endorsement to "collaborative management" or "self-management" of chronic disease:

> There is now strong evidence that self-management can improve the process and outcomes of care for chronic illness. . . . [A]cross a wide variety of chronic conditions, co-management has repeatedly led to improvements in: daily functioning; adherence to medical treatments; control of pain and other symptoms; disease severity; [patients'] confidence in ability to manage illness; sense of control over illness; emotional well-being; and health care utilization and costs. . . .
>
> [C]o-management interventions do not reliably produce each of these effects in every circumstance or for every patient. Still, the strength of evidence for co-management interventions for chronic illness is comparable to that for [other] widely accepted medical treatments.[4]

A number of major health plans and health systems—among them California's Sutter Health, New Mexico's Lovelace Clinic, and the Mayo Clinic—are investing significant amounts of money and time in disease management. The reason can be found in the changing nature of sickness in America. Chronic disease is now the major cause of illness, disability, and death in the United States, affecting almost 100 million persons and accounting for 70 percent of all medical expenses. Yet according to a Kaiser Family Foundation report, one-third of people with a chronic disease are confused over how to go about getting care.[5] Disease management addresses that need.

At Harvard, for instance, the outreach to pediatric asthmatics cut inpatient admissions for asthma by 86 percent and emergency room visits by 79 percent in the initial pilot phase. By 1995, as more children participated, hospital admissions and emergency room visits continued to plunge. Asthmatic children also reported a significant increase in their ability to function at school or home, as measured by their own reports on the SF-36 questionnaire (see chapter 15).[6] The outreach program is not cheap: it costs more than $1 million annually. But the physicians at Harvard Pilgrim, like the executives at Factory Mutual, aren't calculating the precise monetary benefits. Even in the era of marketplace medicine, keeping kids out of a hospital bed doesn't have to be justified with a calculation of return on investment.

Indeed, new guidelines for asthma care issued by NIH in early 1997 explicitly endorsed a disease management approach, calling for patients and doctors to work together to control what the chairman of an expert panel called "the most underdiagnosed and undertreated chronic disease in the country." "Medicine is a partnership now," added Dr. Shirley Murphy, a professor at the University of New Mexico School of Medicine and chairman of the National Asthma Education and Prevention Program, "[and] patients need to take a greater responsibility for managing their chronic disease."[7]

A few physicians are experimenting with even more customized disease management. In this version, a biological marker of disease severity—such as the blood sugar level in diabetes or blood pressure in hypertension—is viewed as analogous to an industrial process to be brought under control. Larry Staker, an internist at Salt Lake City's Bryner Clinic, was one of the first to try this technique. His inspiration was a course in quality improvement at Intermountain Health Care, parent of medical informatics leader LDS Hospital.

Using the regular desktop computer in his office, Staker began by analyzing a sample of the nondiabetic patients in his practice. They had a median blood sugar concentration of 94. ("Median" means that the same number of patients were above this number as below it.) Staker then manually reviewed the charts of his diabetic patients and entered their blood sugar levels into the computer. Since Staker was seeing these diabetics regularly, he expected their typical reading to be about 130, or the high end of normal. Instead, it was 169. "My reaction was, 'Here is a view of my practice that's a little painful to look at but deserves some attention,' " Staker recalled. "In other words, I'm not taking as good care of my diabetics as I thought I was. There's need for improvement."

"I think doctors basically view themselves as doing everything right," he added. "I don't think they've had the ability to really look at what they're doing by looking at the data. Nor have they wanted to."

In an effort to improve blood sugar control, Staker invited some diabetic patients to a special Saturday morning education session. Each attendee was given a $50 glucometer and taught how to use it. In addition, medical student volunteers (led by Staker's daughter and son-in-law) showed the patients how to plot the blood sugar readings from the glucometer on graph paper. Staker then set individualized upper and lower "control limits" for each patient based on the readings. In effect, this treated the production of glucose in the blood like any other production process. Any variation between the natural "control" boundaries was considered random; anything above or below them was considered significant.

The complications of diabetes can be serious. Brain cells depend on glucose for energy, and too much or too little in the blood can lead to unconsciousness or even death. That's why doctors constantly admonish their diabetic patients to watch their diet. Yet just a few weeks after Staker's diabetic patients began to plot their blood sugar levels, something happened that his lecturing hadn't been able to accomplish. The average glucose reading began declining toward normal. Said Staker: "It basically told me that when the patients know where they're supposed to be, they can do things that will change their sugars."

Doris Clark, a seventy-two-year-old retired laundry worker at the Mormon Temple, is one of those patients. In the past, her blood sugar level has risen to more than 300, sending her to the hospital. Participating in Staker's self-management program helped her descend to a "control" level of about 135. She and her husband, Wilfrid, say they regularly use the "run chart" to stabilize her blood sugar level after a change in diet or some other departure from the normal routine. "To be honest, this tells you what to do," says Wilfrid Clark. "This is a marvelous thing, no doubt about it."

The Clarks are not the only enthusiasts. Other patients talked of having power over their bodies and of being "part of the action." The results reflect that positive sentiment. The median blood sugar level of the diabetics using run charts declined by more than 25 percent, going from 169 (well above normal) to 121 (within the accepted range of normal). Staker would like to reduce that figure even further, since "tight" control of diabetes has been shown to have significant health benefits. Meanwhile, he has been encouraged enough to expand his experiment to some patients with other chronic ills, such as high blood pressure.

Staker thinks that the traditional economics of medicine, and the old-fashioned doctor-patient relationship, have stood in the way of a true partnership that focuses on better outcomes. "Patients go to the doctor for everything, [and] they're not willing or responsible to take care of themselves," he argues. "We [doctors] foster that dependency: you make a lot more money if you see slivers and runny noses. You get those patients through [your office] pretty fast and skim the money from the insurance companies." With self-management, "you return control to the patients and ask them not to come in as often," Staker continues. "The patients are enabled and empowered to be responsible for their own care."

But what happens when accountability for a patient population means doing "less" for some people in order to do "more" for others? Even if that "less" is based on evidence that outcomes are not affected, will patients accept care that "feels" wrong? How we answer that question is of critical importance not just for managed care companies, but for those who hope for a rational—and just—allocation of limited resources in the American health care system.

LOOKING, AND NOT LOOKING, FOR CANCER

The bulletin board and wall adjoining Peggy Shepherd's desk are covered with letters ("You were always there, with helpful words of comfort and care!"), thank-you cards, and snapshots of children. The outpouring of affection is a testimonial to the quarter of a century the energetic nurse-midwife has spent caring for mothers and babies. Although Shepherd coordinates all the nurse-midwives working for the Kaiser Permanente Health Plan in the San Diego area, she still sees patients at a nearby Kaiser office in a working-class neighborhood. On a recent morning, one of those patients was Lisa Farris.

Farris, a tall thirty-two-year-old with short blond hair, drives miles across town each year for her appointment. The nurse-midwife delivered Farris's two small children, and the annual gynecological exam is a chance to catch up socially as well as medically. At the end of the current visit, though, Shepherd deviates from the usual script. She tells Farris she doesn't need to return for a Pap smear for two or even three years. Kaiser has changed its timetable for administering the diagnostic test for cervical cancer to women with no special risk factor. Farris, a schoolteacher whose health is excellent, takes this news in stride. "I like coming in and talking to Peggy," Farris tells a visitor, "so maybe [next year] I'll just come and talk to her, instead."

Shepherd acknowledges that it feels odd to tell a patient she will be getting less frequent cancer screening. And as an ardent women's health advocate, she hesitates to embrace anything that smacks of a cutback in care. Yet the nurse-midwife also recognizes that the resources that would have gone to testing low-risk women like Lisa Farris are being redirected by Kaiser. They're going to an outreach program aimed at getting women who aren't screened regularly to come to their doctor for an exam. Those rarely screened women are the ones whose health is most at risk. "We are trying to look into outcomes, be more scientific," says Shepherd. "It's a really different approach."

Kaiser Permanente's southern California region, with 2.4 million of the national organization's 7.8 million members, is another leader in disease management and population-based care. Historically, Kaiser treated Pap smears the way the fee for service world does. Women who visited their doctor got a screening and were given an appointment for a new screening in a year. Then one day an analysis of the plan's membership rolls uncovered the consequences of that approach: only six out of ten women eligible for the Pap test were receiving it. Kaiser's response was an aggressive outreach program. To make room on the appointment books for the new patients, women who didn't really need an annual screening were tested less frequently. Over a period of several years, Kaiser raised the percentage of eligible women receiving Pap smears to 78 percent. Yet because low-risk women like Lisa Farris were tested only every two to three years, Kaiser actually administered one-third *fewer* tests for each thousand women members.

The outcome of this shift in testing was dramatic. Despite the scheduling changes, the number of cervical cancers detected at an invasive stage did not increase. Instead, the new policy doubled the number of women who were found with precancerous cervical cells. Precancerous cells can be treated easily, effectively, and relatively inexpensively, not to mention with far less worry for the patient. Kaiser's track record of early-rate cancer discovery is also better than the state average, as measured by California's official cancer registry.

"There's no doubt in my mind that these women would have surfaced with late stage cancers [without the outreach program]," declares Joel Hyatt, a Kaiser Southern California medical director specializing in quality issues. "These early-stage cancers are curable. We're saving lives."

The results represented a vindication both for Kaiser and for a prominent consultant who helped guide the new approach. That consultant, David Eddy, has spent his career analyzing clinical policies. A physician, mathematician, and engineer, Eddy approaches the concept of stewardship as a kind of mathematical theorem that warrants careful scrutiny from every possible angle.

"Allocating resources, even optimally, means we will have to withhold *some* things from some people that *might* have benefits," Eddy says. "It's hard from an analytic point of view, it's hard from a political point of view, and it's very hard from an administrative and emotional and ethical point of view."[8]

Since 1990 Eddy has shared his thinking in a periodic column, "Clinical Decision Making: From Theory to Practice," that appears in the *Journal of the American Medical Association.* He has not hesitated to put the intellectual principles he champions in his writing into practice in his personal life. In one 1995 column, Eddy wrote movingly of conversations with his mother about her growing burden of painful illness. The widow of a physician, she had seen too many patients kept alive by medical treatment long past the time when there was a chance for either recovery or a dignified life. Shortly after Mrs. Eddy's eighty-fifth birthday, she entered the hospital with pneumonia. David persuaded her personal physician that it was ethical to take only those actions needed to make her comfortable. Not long afterward, she died peacefully.

The column prompted supportive letters from all over the world. "Virtually everyone who reads it starts crying," Eddy said. Every time he read the draft manuscript, Eddy added, "I started crying [too]."

It is a rare acknowledgment for a man a friend calls "the most . . . data-ridden character on earth." Back in 1840 Jules Gavarret, a French military engineer turned physician, wrote a book instructing doctors on applying probability calculations to the problems of medicine. The concept was far ahead of its time, and it was ignored. Eddy, working in that same tradition, has been much more influential. As discussed in chapter 2, Eddy became interested in medicine's scientific basis in the mid-1970s while investigating the steps doctors took in treating breast cancer. Within just a few years, the regular papers he wrote about the scientific basis of clinical decisions attracted the attention of the prestigious American Cancer Society. The society appointed him to oversee a comprehensive review of its screening guidelines. Those revisions, announced in March 1980, included a new policy on Pap smears. Sexually active women needed a Pap smear not annually, but "at least once every three years."

Eddy's recommendations were controversial, but they were also solidly grounded in science. He calculates risks carefully, even obsessively. (After he completed his doctorate in engineering, a major airline offered him a job helping to design the optimum maintenance schedule for its planes.) In developing the policy on Pap smears, for example, Eddy analyzed a series of scientific studies showing the extra life expectancy associated with annual Pap testing and with testing every two, three, four, five, or six years. Since cervical cancer is extremely slow growing, the changes detected by a yearly test almost always involve precancerous or early-growth cells. The average woman could get 99 percent of the benefit of annual screening with a test every three years, Eddy concluded, "and she would be spared the cost, the chances of a false positive result, and any risks or complications."[9]

Not surprisingly, a recommendation to reduce the frequency of a cancer test caused an uproar. Getting doctors to administer regular Pap smears had been the American Cancer Society's first big success. The test, developed by the Greek American physician George Nicholas Papanicolaou in 1928, was not endorsed for regular use by the medical community until 1943. By that time cervical cancer was the number one killer of American women. To promote the test, the American Cancer Society took the unprecedented step of advertising in women's magazines.

Yet though the test's effectiveness was studied in depth, the relative benefit of different screening intervals was a question that received scant analysis. "The concept was, 'What's good against cancer is good,'" remembers Edward Scanlon, a former American Cancer Society president who trained as a gynecologist in the 1940s. "Nobody ever thought much about the cost of things. Everything written was to promote frequent screening."[10]

Given that history, Kaiser Southern California knew that stretching out the testing interval would not be easy. After all, the prestige of the American Cancer Society had not been enough to win widespread acceptance for the guideline Eddy wrote. Still, Kaiser pressed ahead. Health plans in California are under such intense financial pressure that Kaiser had to cut its premiums several years in a row. Population-based care, in addition to being attractive in terms of fundamental public health, represented a way to make informed choices about limited resources.

"I don't believe it's possible to overstate the potential savings that lie in our future through the application of clinical improvement techniques," says David Lawrence, a physician who is Kaiser's president and chief executive officer. "The pathway to efficient health care is . . . improving quality."[11]

As part of its clinical improvement initiative, Kaiser also revised its guideline on screening for breast cancer. Women with no extra risk factor would not receive a routine annual mammogram until age fifty. As with cervical cancer, the science behind the decision was solid. Repeated randomized clinical trials have generally shown no statistically significant reduction in breast cancer deaths among women aged forty to forty-nine who received regular screening mammograms.[12]

The public perception about mammograms, however, is quite different. The National Cancer Institute discovered that in 1994, after it announced that routine annual mammograms were unnecessary for women under fifty. Despite the institute's prestige, it immediately found itself on the defensive. Colorado representative Patricia Schroeder, one of the most senior women members of Congress, called the policy an "insult" and charged the institute with playing "very fast and loose with women's health." The American Cancer Society, long past the boldness of its David Eddy days, opined that women would be "too confused" if the society changed its screening criteria.

In fact, more than four out of ten cases of breast cancer occur in women over sixty-five. Screening rates for these women, however, lag well behind those of younger women for whom the risk is less.[13] What is confusing to women is the media's portrayal of breast cancer, noted Susan Love, director of the UCLA Breast Center and author of *Dr. Susan Love's Breast Book.* "We are obsessed," she wrote in the *Los Angeles Times,* "with cancer risks faced by *younger* women." She added:

> Almost every woman's magazine article about breast cancer is illustrated with a photograph of a twenty-five-year-old. The public-service announcements on television all feature a thirty-year-old discovering cancer. The older women most likely to develop breast cancer simply don't identify with these women. The message is lost on them—and will continue to be unless we change the way information about mammography is delivered. . . .
>
> [The NCI's] change in policy was not prompted by a desire to save money. . . . Nor was it an "insult" to women. Nor was it intended to deny younger women their God-given right to radiation. Rather, it was about telling the truth. . . .

> Mammography can detect small or early cancers in some women. But that is not the issue. Rather, it is whether finding such lesions early can actually save lives. The answer is consistently no. In some women, cancer is so slow that it doesn't matter whether it is found this year or next; they will live, either way. In others, the cancer is so aggressive they will die no matter when diagnosed.[14]

Love might have added that those younger women tend to be white and middle-class. The screening rates of low-income, black, and Hispanic women lag behind the national average.

In late 1996 several new studies suggested that women in their forties might indeed benefit from regular mammograms. However, an expert panel convened by NIH concluded that the new evidence was not strong enough to change the basic formula. Although extra mammograms could uncover some cancers that would otherwise be missed, that benefit had costs. For instance, the radiation from extra screening might slightly increase the cancer rate, and unneeded biopsies could lead to injury. The panel concluded that insurers should pay for mammograms for women who felt they needed them—but that NIH would not definitively recommend that women in their forties be screened. That Solomonic decision in January 1997 immediately caused a firestorm of controversy.

Many Americans probably wondered what harm there might be in extra screening. David Eddy addressed the economic and ethical basis for targeted screening in a managed care environment in 1994. His *JAMA* article was titled "Rationing Resources While Improving Quality: How to Get More for Less." At the time, Kaiser performed about 300,000 screening mammograms annually, half of them on women between fifty and seventy-five. Using the health plan as an example, Eddy calculated that Kaiser could expect to prevent 909 women from dying of breast cancer from 1995 to 2010. The cumulative fifteen-year cost would be $707 million.

On the other hand, if Kaiser focused on the group of women most at risk and screened 95 percent of older women during that fifteen-year period, it would increase the number of breast cancer deaths it prevented from 909 to about 1,206. The cost was some $497 million. Concluded Eddy: "Thus, making the switch from the low-value mammograms in women younger than 50 years and older than 75 . . . would simultaneously decrease the number of breast cancer deaths by about 33 percent (preventing an additional 297 deaths) and reduce costs by about 30 percent (saving about $150 million)."[15]

Doing "less" really amounted to doing more. It is important to note that Kaiser doctors can always override the guideline, which applies to younger women with no obvious risk factor for the disease.

Can the public ever accept doing less? In the most recent mammogram controversy, there were signs that the dangers of always doing more are finally becoming a legitimate part of the public debate. A *Washington Post* story on the NIH panel quoted outraged surgeons who said the decision represented a death sentence for many women, but the *Post* story gave equal prominence to a warning about overtesting sounded by Maryann Napoli, an executive of a medical consumer group. Napoli, associate director of New York's Center for Medical Consumers, also wrote an opinion piece for the *New York Times* that was paired with another opinion piece by a woman in her forties who said that a mammogram had saved her life. However, an editorial by the *Times* clearly supported the NIH panel's recommendations. Still, outraged politicians continued to protest. A National Cancer Institute advisory board, prodded by NIH, voted in March 1997 to override the consensus panel. The board urged regular screening even for those women in their forties with an "average" risk of cancer.

Whatever science may say, the fear of any type of cancer can be overwhelming. That fear is certainly understandable. In the obstetrics and gynecology waiting room of the Kaiser Permanente offices in San Diego, Aili Hiltunen, sixty-four, insists that "once a year is not too often" for her Pap smear, especially when "there seems to be so much cancer related to that area."

"I'll be coming in next year, and I would like to have a Pap smear," Hiltunen says firmly. Her ninety-seven-year-old mother, adds Hiltunen, will be getting her annual Pap smear too.

THE VOLUNTEER COPS

Early on a muggy Monday, three physicians and two nurses are huddled over a quick breakfast at the Holiday Inn in a medium-sized midwestern city. They have flown here from all over the country for a task that will consume virtually all their waking moments for the next seventy-two hours. Working on behalf of an organization called the National Committee for Quality Assurance (NCQA), their mission is to assess the quality of care that a local HMO provides to its 350,000 members.

It is all well and good to say that doctors have decided to ally themselves with newly empowered patients, or that health plans, newly respectful of the dangers of blind cost cutting, are reaching out to become partners with their members. But if the information age means anything, it means that trusting in good intentions will not be the patient's only recourse. Nowhere is the extent of the change more evident than in the efforts of the NCQA.

The Washington-based NCQA is a private, nonprofit organization that has evolved into the leading source of quality-related information on HMOs. It both accredits health plans and develops performance standards that constitute a health plan report card. The accreditation part of NCQA's work involves reviewing how a health plan manages its delivery system—physicians, hospitals, other health care providers—and its administrative services. Performance measures, on the other hand, involve specific indicators of quality—for example, the percentage of children under age two who receive required immunizations. Another difference is that the performance measures are gathered and reported by the plans themselves. Accreditation requires a thorough inspection by a survey team. At this midwestern HMO, a previous survey team that visited three years ago recommended against accreditation. However, the HMO discovered a technical violation of the survey procedure that prevented NCQA from issuing a formal denial. (NCQA and the HMO agreed to let me observe and write about this survey on condition I not identify the plan or its exact location.)[16] Even though the HMO got to start the process over, the near miss had consequences. "You flunk an NCQA exam, you get a new medical director and new CEO," summarized the HMO's present medical director.

Given NCQA's origins, its present clout is astonishing. Following the passage of the 1973 Health Maintenance Organization Act, there was talk of federal oversight of this new form of health care delivery. To head off government policing, two HMO trade groups set up NCQA as a self-policing agency. For years, however, the organization was more like a rent-a-cop (as low-paid security guards are derisively nicknamed) than a real one. It had an impressive name, no full-time staff, and precious little work. When it did inspect an HMO on behalf of the federal government or one of the states, the HMO always passed muster. No one took standards seriously. "Most of the health-care community still believed that it was not possible to define—let alone measure and report on—quality in a way that would really matter anywhere outside the world of academics," recalled Susan Pisano, a communications official for one of the trade groups that founded NCQA.[17]

In truth, HMO quality was a nonissue until very recently. Consider: by 1988, thirty-three million Americans belonged to HMOs. Yet HMOs weren't even mentioned in an influential report, *The Quality of Medical Care: Information for Consumers,* issued that year by the federal Office of Technology Assessment. Given the burgeoning nature of the HMO industry, the Joint Commission on Accreditation of Healthcare Organizations decided in 1988 to accredit HMOs as well as hospitals. Just two years later, the commission gave up because of a lack of interest in the results.

By coincidence, NCQA received a $400,000 Robert Wood Johnson Foundation grant in 1990 to help it become an independent group serving the needs of corporate purchasers. The Joint Commission gave NCQA its files and wished it luck, and NCQA needed the good wishes.

"There really is no advantage to an HMO to being accredited unless someone asks them to," admitted Margaret O'Kane, NCQA's founding (and current) executive director, in a 1991 interview. "So HMOs wonder why they should do it."[18] Indeed, even though hospital accreditation goes back to 1918, it did not become fully accepted until it was linked to a financial incentive. The Medicare program refused to pay for treatment of elderly patients at hospitals without either Joint Commission accreditation or state certification.

In the case of HMOs, it was corporate America that stepped in to create a demand for information on quality, with a particularly critical role played by Xerox Corporation. Although Xerox invented the photocopying process known as xerography, its share of the domestic copier market had plunged from 85 percent in 1976 to just 13 percent by 1982 as Japanese competitors produced copiers that cost less and worked better. With its survival at stake, the company made "benchmarking" and continuous quality improvement part of its core business strategy.[19] By slashing costs and improving the quality of its copiers, the company slowly beat back the Japanese. So when the cost of health care benefits at Xerox rose steeply during the 1980s, company managers quickly decided that the HMO industry could benefit from the same "quality or else" motivation they had experienced. Said Patricia Nazemetz, Xerox's director of benefits, "The threat of extinction [for the HMOs] was not there."[20]

Xerox helped provide that crucial "or else" message. In 1990 Nazemetz gave an ultimatum to the two hundred HMOs that served its 100,000 workers and their families nationwide: Get NCQA accreditation within five years or be kicked out of the Xerox network. The

HMOs tried to forestall a decision, arguing that no one was sure whether the NCQA measures were truly meaningful. Remembered Nazemetz, a member of the NCQA board: "We finally said, 'This is no longer a discussion, it's a decision. You have five years.'"

Separately, Xerox was also trying to develop a set of performance measures that would allow a company to compare health plans with each other. As it happened, a consortium of old-line HMOs known as the HMO Group was thinking along the same lines. Worried that corporations might buy care on price alone, the health plans—which were often higher priced than competitors—agreed to help Xerox and a few other large employers "add intelligence to the employer purchasing process," as Nazemetz put it. What finally emerged was the Health Plan–Employer Data and Information Set, or HEDIS.[21]

HEDIS 1.0, which appeared in 1991, required data about quality of care, members' access to care and patient satisfaction, utilization and membership services, and finances. The indicators within each category were as basic as asking what percentage of pregnant members received prenatal care during their first trimester. Since few health maintenance organizations were organized for maintaining health, however, most of them had trouble answering even the simplest HEDIS questions.

In 1992 the HMO Group and the corporations working with it decided their performance measures should be applied nationally, and they turned the project over to NCQA. The timing was fortuitous. The 1992 presidential campaign had made health care reform into a national issue, and the insurance industry once again was eager to demonstrate its commitment to self-policing. In early 1993, eight large national employers and thirty health plans representing over fifty-five million HMO members endorsed HEDIS 2.0, a revised report card that had grown to include sixty separate performance measures. During this same time, other large corporations joined Xerox in requiring NCQA accreditation from their HMOs. One of those companies was the largest customer of the midwestern HMO that I was visiting.

As much as the midwestern HMO might have preferred not to invite NCQA back, it had no choice; losing its largest customer wasn't an option. But passing NCQA muster wasn't cheap either. The survey itself cost over $50,000, and that paled in comparison with the tens of thousands of dollars spent bringing the plan into conformance with NCQA standards. Over the years, NCQA had acquired some teeth. Its accreditation requirements emphasized population-based quality improvement projects similar to the asthma outreach program at Harvard Pilgrim Health Plan or the Pap smear screening initiative at Kaiser Southern California. To mount these kinds of efforts successfully takes time, money, and expertise: the midwestern HMO decided to hire a Ph.D. epidemiologist to make sure it got things right. NCQA paperwork requirements had also ballooned over the years. In 1992 the HMO had assembled about ten binders relating its efforts. This time it filled a room-length set of shelves with 194 four-inch-thick binders of letters, memos, contracts, and studies. The plan needed them.

NCQA surveyors have generally spent years in the trenches, which makes many of them quite skeptical. For example, the midwestern HMO said it had denied only two appeals during the previous three years from members who wanted the plan to cover care it initially refused to pay for. Surveyor nurses Tricia Stream, a former NCQA executive, and Barbara Ramsey, a former high-ranking U.S. Army officer, asked to see the complete file of the health plan's grievance committee. In one of the two cases, a woman wanted the HMO to pay for an eye operation to cure her nearsightedness, but her employer's contract excluded vision care. In the other, a man wanted a walker that wasn't a covered benefit.

When the HMO said it had a careful "utilization management" program, the surveyors asked for a copy of the specific instructions given utilization review nurses. "Anybody can have a plan," said surveyor Herb Weinman, a physician from a western Pennsylvania HMO, "but are you implementing?" Weinman also asked for evidence that patients who needed referrals to specialists were getting them promptly.

Samuel "Nick" Barol, a retired physician with managed care experience in New Mexico, quizzed the HMO about its disease management and prevention programs. Barol also looked for evidence that the community doctors were active participants. The HMO medical director confessed that one group of doctors wanted extra payment to administer chicken pox shots that cost $40. The medical director replied by confronting them with the economic facts of life. The biggest employer in town was trying to cut its medical expenses by 20 percent, he said, so the doctors' group wasn't getting an extra dime.

Meanwhile surveyor Peter Betjemann, a Massachusetts physician, combed through the HMO's files on physicians' credentials. This is an area whose importance surprises many laymen, but doctors can fall prey to the same temptations as job applicants in the business world. "Physicians present inaccurate clinical credentials more frequently than might be expected," concluded a 1988 study in the *New England Journal of Medicine.* Of the physicians applying for privileges at Humana's outpatient centers, 5 percent were found to have presented false clinical credentials, 3.5 percent gave false information about their residency, and 1.3 percent falsely reported that they were certified by a specialty board.[22]

Before the NCQA survey team left, it held a summary conference with the HMO's managers to discuss the good and bad of what it had found. "This is both an exhaustive and an exhausting process," soothed Barol as the tired managers tried to summon up a smile. The surveyors still had plenty of work awaiting them when they got home. The team had to write up an eighty-some-page report for an advisory committee of physicians at NCQA that makes the final decision about plan accreditation.

NCQA has won credibility with plans and the public by learning to say no. About 40 percent of plans get a full three-year accreditation; 37 percent receive a one-year accreditation; 11 percent are accredited "provisionally"; and another 11 percent are denied accreditation. One large plan that was turned down thought the stakes high enough to sue, but the legal action was subsequently dropped. As demand for accreditation has risen, so has the wait for a final decision. Several months after the survey of the midwestern HMO, it received a mixed verdict: it won a one-year accreditation, good enough to reassure the big corporation that was its customer. But the short time frame meant the HMO had to prepare almost immediately to undergo another survey, this time in hopes of capturing the coveted three-year "full" accreditation.

NCQA president O'Kane does not pretend that her organization has caused big corporations to contract with HMOs solely based on quality. But she does argue that without NCQA, decisions would be made solely on price. By early 1997 about 50 percent of the nation's licensed HMOs had been reviewed by NCQA, and another 25 percent were scheduled. Even more impressive, nearly 90 percent of all HMOs publicly reported the seventeen HEDIS measures of performance. Those range from the member's access to services to the average maternity stay. NCQA has also begun expanding its standards to include targeted HEDIS measures for Medicare, Medicaid, and behavioral health. The group is even edging into disease management, agreeing to a partnership with the American Diabetes Association to recognize physicians who meet eleven specific standards for providing good diabetes care.

Meanwhile, fears about managed care have given NCQA a high public profile. When the group announced in mid-1996 that it would release summaries of accreditation surveys to the public, O'Kane was asked to appear on the Cable News Network and NBC's *Today* show. By early 1997 the group was receiving more than four thousand requests a month for accreditation statistics. The public scrutiny is also leading to more stringent HEDIS measures. HEDIS 3.0, which went into effect in 1997, included seventy-five indicators in eight areas: effectiveness of care, accessibility and availability of care, satisfaction with experience of care, cost of care, stability of the health plan, informed health care choices for patients, use of services, and plan descriptive information. Another thirty measures were issued as "testing" indicators, including a few that focused directly on specific clinical procedures. Separately, NCQA has released a national database of HEDIS information about managed care plans covering twenty-eight million Americans.

The increased demand for information that can be used for HMO accountability has given NCQA some competition too. HEDIS measures are self-reported, and NCQA's on-site surveyors do not, for example, have the power to extensively audit patients' medical records. Private consultants hired by employers do audit records, with the plan's consent. By mid-1996 the nation's three largest benefits consulting firms, whose clients include 75 percent of the Fortune 500 companies, all had systems in place to help corporations measure both the quality and the price of managed care plans. The Joint Commission had jumped back into accreditation of HMOs and of "health systems" that include hospitals, physician groups, managed care plans, and other components. And the American Medical Association, not to be left out, had suggested there should be just one accrediting standard for ambulatory care, a standard that the AMA intended to provide. Its stamp of approval—and perhaps its accreditation reports—will even be public.

Finally, the NCQA is being pushed to mandate even more sophisticated "outcomes" standards. A great deal of that pressure is coming from a not-quite-competing group, the Foundation for Accountability, based in Portland, Oregon. Begun in late 1995 at the initiative of Paul Ellwood (its executive director, David Lansky, worked closely with Ellwood's Jackson Hole Group), FACCT does not accept payment for accreditation. Its purpose is to jawbone consumers and employers into demanding and using more outcomes measures while pressing health plans to voluntarily supply them in an understandable format. The first set of FACCT-endorsed measures, dealing with breast cancer, depression, and diabetes, was released in mid-1996.

TOO MUCH AND TOO LITTLE OF A GOOD THING

Information may be power, but that power can be grasped only when the information is understood and used. Some are far better positioned for the information age than others. Walt Disney Company's newly built town of Celebration, Florida, plans to connect as many as twenty thousand residents through home computers to physicians, hospitals, and other health care providers: "pushing the envelope of health empowerment," one official calls it. Yet at the same time, millions of Americans can't read well enough to decipher the instructions on a prescription bottle. Most Americans still define a high-quality health plan as one their doctor assures them provides good care. And while the *Today* show producers may book Margaret O'Kane to discuss public HEDIS reports, 55 percent of respondents to a national poll either had not heard the term managed care or did not know what it meant. Worse, 77 percent had not heard the term fee for service or did not know its meaning![23]

Moreover, not everyone who is sick wants to be either the empowered patient liberals dream of or the informed consumer beloved by conservatives. A story from early in this century tells of a passionate socialist haranguing a crowd of workers. "Come the revolution," he declares, "every worker will have chocolate ice cream." "But comrade," one timid worker asks, "what if I don't like chocolate ice cream?" "Come the revolution," the socialist responds, "you will have chocolate ice cream and *like it.*" As the British journal the *Lancet* noted, "Uncertainty in the face of disease and death fosters a compelling need for patients to trust someone and a reciprocal authority among doctors. A leap of faith will always be needed. Information does not, and cannot, provide all the answers. Whether consumers can cope with all the new information, with explicit evidence of uncertainty, and then make their own solitary leaps of faith, remains to be seen."[24]

In many ways, that is why the involvement of the employer community and of government remains so important in any real-world discussion of stewardship. Those who provide high-quality care need to be rewarded for it. For example, the Pacific Business Group on Health surveys consumer satisfaction, measures health status results from different medical groups that treat employees of PBGH members, and posts quality data, such as HEDIS reports, on a World Wide Web page. Working in partnership with the state, the San Francisco–based coalition, with more than thirty member companies, has also persuaded hospitals to voluntarily report their bypass mortality rates using a format very similar to that used in New York. On the hospital and physician side, the Magic Valley Health Network of Twin Falls, Idaho, is promoting to employers its expertise in continuous quality improvement and improving the health of those entrusted to its care. There are many, many similar examples in communities large and small.

Information age medicine remains on the doorstep of its greatest accomplishments. Still, what it has achieved so far represents nothing less than a paradigm shift. We have finally gone from a system that fiercely defended the idea that medical accountability must be defined by the opinions of doctors to a system that accepts the principle that doctors can be held accountable by outsiders using objective data. That most of the public is unaware of this quiet revolution in no way detracts from its magnitude. It is the health care equivalent of the fall of the Berlin Wall, and like that wall's crumbling, it is opening up opportunities that once seemed an impossible dream. We have gone from debating whether the patient deserves to be a partner with the physician to discussing the terms of that partnership: How will doctors and patients discuss clinical studies that each learns about over the Internet? How will they deal with patients' preferences? How can the patient's functional status be used as a legitimate measure of a treatment's effectiveness? How, above all, can doctor and patient work together to achieve better health?

If we have not yet reached the elusive goal of stewardship, it may well be because we are still clearing away the debris from the old structure of medicine that stood for so long. We need to look plainly at where we have been and where we are today if we are to build a health care system for the future whose foundation rests on an uncompromising demand for medical excellence.

EPILOGUE

A Celebration of Medicine's Future

The provision of medical care has become one of the largest industries of the country. Within the lives of many now living, revolutionary changes in science have transformed medicine from a comparatively simple field into a complex domain. . . . Until recently, people . . . rested content because medicine is in good hands. But the unprecedented growth of medicine, the enormous expansion of personnel and facilities, the investment of billions of dollars have created issues from which society cannot escape merely through its own optimism or through confidence in the high character of medical practitioners.
—Ray Lyman Wilbur, M.D., chairman of the Committee on the Costs of Medical Care, 1933

In 1970 the American aerospace industry was considering whether to build a fleet of supersonic passenger planes similar to the joint British and French-built Concorde. Since final development required a substantial government subsidy to the aerospace industry, a fierce debate over the project broke out in Congress. Critics warned that emissions from the plane's engines during its flight high in the stratosphere would damage the ozone layer. Advocates of the supersonic transport (SST) stoutly denied the accusation.

At the time, I was researching the SST as a congressional intern, and I asked a well-known conservative senator about the alleged pollution problem. He promptly dismissed it by citing his personal experience as a pilot. He had flown right next to planes at that altitude and gazed directly at the tailpipes. "There was nothing coming out of there," the legislator assured me. Sincere as this eyewitness report was, it was contradicted by objective scientific analysis of the SST. For a combination of environmental and economic reasons, Congress refused to finance the SST, and the project died.

This assumption that side effects you can't easily see don't really exist is a trap that also ensnares observers of American medicine.

Just as the SST's ability to smash through the sound barrier enthralled aviation enthusiasts, American medicine's technological triumphs can overshadow its serious flaws. The pernicious effects of medical "pollution," like the emissions from the tailpipe of a supersonic jet, become clearly visible only when one examines the scientific evidence. The major criticisms of medicine contained in this book have been deliberately anchored in that evidence.

We have seen that only a small percentage of contemporary medical practices have been scientifically validated. At the same time, effective therapies can take years to make their way into common use. Medical textbooks are frequently outdated, and journals go unread or unheeded. Continuing medical education has proved better at providing doctors with memorable meals or vacation snapshots than at changing their behavior. The consensus conferences on "best practices" sponsored by the National Institutes of Health are no more effective at producing behavioral change than the free meals. Meanwhile, when a group of doctors is asked whether the care in a particular case meets the highest professional standards, the "physician agreement regarding quality of care is only slightly better than the level expected by chance."[1]

Research medicine and everyday medicine often seem to exist in separate worlds. The public thrills to stories about a pill that may slow the aging process. But in everyday medicine we are just now examining the best way to perform the hip-replacement surgery that hundreds of thousands of Americans who *are* aging undergo annually at a cost of nearly $3 billion. In biomedicine, research into menopause captivates Baby Boomer women. In everyday medicine we are just beginning to collect reliable information on alternatives to the 560,000 hysterectomies performed each year, most on women who have not yet reached menopause. And while research into the genetic basis of prostate cancer commands headlines, everyday medicine presents a confusing welter of information to any man trying to make an informed decision about treatment for the cancer growing within him.

In illness after illness and disease after disease we have seen almost random variation in how different doctors treat patients with similar clinical symptoms. The variation occurs both in the therapy a doctor chooses and in how that therapy is provided. It shows up across regions of the country, within metropolitan areas, and within small groups of doctors clustered together in one group or at one hospital. A guest lecturer at an East Coast medical school told of discovering that each of four heart surgeons at the school used a different approach to presurgery care, the surgery itself, and postoperative treatment. When the lecturer, also a surgeon, asked why the faculty didn't compare notes, he was told that it was good for the medical students to be exposed to a variety of techniques. One wonders whether it was equally good for the patients.

In the absence of reliable information about the outcome of care, patients and physicians alike accept proxies such as "trying hard," "doing everything," or "caring." Yet the heart surgery team whose patients consistently die at a higher rate than expected may well be trying just as hard as the team whose patients are more likely to live. The intensive care unit in which a greater than expected percentage of patients die may be just as well equipped to do everything as the ICU where many more patients survive. And the physician who is the most caring may not always be the most competent.

What holds true for the individual physician-patient relationship also characterizes our public policy. The United States has argued on and off about health "reform" for most of the twentieth century, but the debate has centered more on insurance arrangements than on the content of care. A prominent American Medical Association member once told me of speaking before a physicians' fraternal organization affiliated with an old East Coast hospital. One of his hosts showed him the minutes of a 1932 meeting where the group's goals for the year were set forth. They read: keep government out of medicine; avoid socialized medicine; promote public health.

These types of "political prejudices . . . have no relation to the provision of medical care," the reform-minded American Foundation argued—back in 1937. "How much government shall have to do with providing medical care . . . is only a part of the larger problem. . . . There is no panacea for the difficulties facing us."[2]

Those words still ring true. And yet the stock villain of "socialized medicine" that dominated the public policy debate for so long has simply been replaced by "greedy capitalists." As in a refurbished Cold War spy movie, the characters have changed while the basic plot remains the same. In the case of health policy the public is cautioned that it faces a choice between medical decisions made by "good" doctors or "bad" decisions dictated by government or managed care bureaucrats. Preserving maximum physician freedom "preserves" high-quality medical care; any other path leads inexorably to ruin.

This constantly repeated formula has evolved into a set of blinders. In late 1996, the revelation that a few health plans were denying an overnight hospital stay for women with mastectomies quickly blossomed into a national scandal. Outpatient mastectomies graphically illustrated the danger of letting bureaucratic "bean counters" override physicians' judgment. Yet an equally worrisome story about breast cancer earlier that same year attracted much more limited attention. A Dartmouth Medical School study showed a nearly thirty-five-fold difference in the frequency with which elderly breast cancer victims received mastectomies versus breast-conserving surgery. The study, discussed in the introduction to this book, deviated sharply from the good guys–bad guys script. Unlimited freedom for physicians produced not reliable excellence, but enormous variation. Requiring physicians to go through a review process before certain treatments might help some patients, not hurt them.

Which is more disturbing, a woman's being treated callously after losing a breast to cancer or her unnecessarily losing that breast in the first place? More to the point, why has the physician community campaigned vigorously to publicize and eliminate only one of these problems? Even posing that question illuminates the shallowness of viewing clinical quality as synonymous with physician freedom. There is no panacea, and there are no easy answers.

One might respond that the critical difference between the two examples is motivation. The health plan is only trying to save money; the surgeon is trying to save a life and did not knowingly recommend an inappropriate treatment. This formulation, while perhaps excusing the individual doctor, begs the larger question of why the profession as a whole tolerates such widespread variation from achievable excellence.

As we have seen throughout this book, the absence of good information systems in medicine is as intentional as any health plan's budget cuts. "Science and Technology revolutionize our lives," wrote the historian Arthur M. Schlesinger Jr., "but memory, tradition and myth frame our response."[3] Medicine's strongest myths, memories, and traditions revolve around the belief that a well-trained doctor instinctively knows the right thing to do and, as a professional, will do it if given the necessary freedom and resources. There has been little effort to systematically examine what treatments work best, little effort to help doctors consistently apply scientific findings to patient care, and little or no effort to hold doctors accountable for improving care. To the contrary, as Samuel Thier, then president of the National Academy of Sciences' Institute of Medicine, acknowledged in a 1991 article, "Defining what does and does not work in medicine is a professional responsibility of the highest order." Thier concluded: "[But it is] one that physicians have resisted."[4]

The lessons the profession might learn from Ernest Amory Codman's "End Result Idea," Paul Lembcke's medical audit, Vergil Slee's Professional Activity Study, and the National Halothane Study have been conspicuously absent from the clinical mainstream.[5] Instead, a large part of the history of quality measurement and management presented in this book was rescued from medicine's memory hole, the Orwellian place where politically inconvenient events of the past vanish as if they had never been.

From ulcers to urinary tract infections, tonsils to organ transplants, back pain to breast cancer, asthma to arteriosclerosis, the evidence is irrefutable. Tens of thousands of patients have died or been injured year after year because readily available information was not used—and is not being used today—to guide their care. If one counts the lives lost to preventable medical mistakes, the toll reaches the hundreds of thousands. The only barrier to saving these lives is the willingness of doctors and hospital administrators to change.

If many well-intentioned physicians cannot perceive the profession's flaws, the public is often afraid to. Whatever the failings of doctors in general, "to distrust one's [own] doctor is to be vulnerable in the most fundamental and undesirable of ways," noted one researcher. "The image of the doctor in America continues in large part to be an idealization that reflects people's hopes rather than their actual experiences."[6] That is one reason why it is far, far easier to blame "health plans" for all bad care.

This book has shown that the practice of medicine can be dramatically improved. The opportunities for consistent excellence are real, and they are within our grasp. We have seen postsurgical infection rates and the incidence of drug errors plunge at a hospital in Salt Lake City. We have seen the tools of quality measurement and management save the lives of pneumonia patients in Pittsburgh and heart attack victims in South Carolina. We have seen them make a difference for children with heart defects in Los Angeles and asthma in Boston. We have seen everyday care improve at a small family practice clinic and at the prestigious Mayo Clinic. We have seen how presenting surgeons with a carefully calculated "report card" led to a drop in the death rate from bypass surgery in New York State, in Pennsylvania, and at a group of hospitals that voluntarily banded together in New England.

We have seen that patients who share responsibility for decisions about their care often enjoy better health than those whose doctors act out a traditional paternalistic role. Their care can cost less, too. We have seen the growing use of health status measurements that gauge the success of treatment based on how well the patient functions afterward in everyday life. And we have seen how population-based medicine can help people who otherwise would fall through the cracks of the health care system. We have also seen that none of these changes happens easily or quickly.

The speed with which any innovation is put to use depends on how the new way of doing things is perceived by those who must adopt it, according to Everett Rogers, author of a classic study on innovations.[7] Five characteristics hold the key to acceptance: relative advantage over what currently exists; compatibility with existing values and behaviors; lack of complexity; the ability to be subjected to experiment ("trialability"); and producing results everyone can see ("observability"). I read the Rogers book some time after I spoke with Gregory Angstman, a Mayo Clinic family practitioner, and heard him tick off the reasons his colleagues commonly give for resisting quality measurement and management techniques. The list meshed almost perfectly with Rogers's findings. Angstman called it "The Rule of Toos": I know too much (no relative advantage); I'm too good for this (incompatible with existing values); it's too hard to do (too complex); there are too many guidelines (can't be subjected to a valid experiment).

The final requirement Rogers lists—that an innovation produce "observable" results—may depend on what one is prepared to see. Emanuel Papper, a world-renowned anesthesiologist, wrote that the ability of ether to dull pain was known for centuries before anyone thought of applying it to making surgery less agonizing. Suffering was associated with nobility of spirit or viewed as a punishment for sin. "It took so long to discover 'anesthesia,' " wrote Papper, "because there was no societal readiness for it nor interest in the prevention of the pain of surgical intervention or really in the relief of pain for the common man."[8] The acceptable had to become unacceptable, and what had been perceived within society as immutable had to be seen instead as a problem in search of a solution. To use Thomas Kuhn's description of a paradigm revolution: "Scientists [can] see new and different things when looking with familiar instruments in places they had looked before."[9]

The movement to measure and manage the quality of medical

care is emerging from that same transformational process. What so recently seemed quixotic has become nothing short of trendy within some medical circles. As one *JAMA* commentary put it in early 1997: "The dream of medicine for the new millennium [is] that the care of patients will be evidence based, supported by carefully designed randomized controlled trials and validated by focused outcomes studies."[10] Thanks to the convergence of three powerful forces, much of American medicine is finally *seeing* these clinical improvement tools as if for the first time.

THE FORCES OF CHANGE

The first and most important motivating factor is economics. The demand for medical care is steadily increasing. In the aging United States population, there are already as many Americans over fifty as under eighteen. At the same time, technological discoveries continue to make expensive treatments, such as organ transplants, a routine part of care. Yet societal resistance to devoting more resources to medical care has never been more formidable. Medicare and Medicaid expenditures are hemmed in by drum-tight federal and state budgets and public antipathy to either deficit spending or higher taxes. In the private sector, low inflation and intense international competition mean that higher worker and retiree medical costs can no longer be tucked unnoticed into a price increase for a product. Changed accounting rules have also forced American companies to reduce today's profits to account for tomorrow's expected retiree medical expenses. This linking of health care costs to the balance sheet, while mostly unnoticed by political commentators, has put the issue of cost containment permanently on the agenda of the most senior managers of America's most powerful corporations.

A nineteenth-century British novelist wrote: "A reform is a correction of abuses; a revolution is a transfer of power."[11] Managed care, corporate purchasing coalitions, and state health data organizations are all weapons of revolution. Their common purpose is to take power away from the suppliers (the providers of care) and give it to the buyers. The sellers' loss of power has, in turn, exposed the results of years of immunity from economic accountability: too many medical specialists, too many hospital beds, too many unnecessary procedures and surgeries.

"Every industry faces all this during its lifetime," commented Philip Crosby, one of the modern fathers of quality improvement.

"The health-care industry just never thought it would happen to it—but neither did steel, automobiles or television."[12]

In 1982, management consultants McKinsey and Company studied the impact of deregulation (meaning increased competition) on industries such as trucking, airlines, and financial services. What they found was increasing variability in the performance and success of competing companies; prices coming under severe pressure; proliferation of new products; cost cutting; and a higher requirement for investment capital because of the greater competition. Each of those effects can be found today in health care.

Also like other industries, health care is undergoing a wrenching consolidation. Over a third of United States physicians belonged to group practices in 1995, and almost a third of those practices had at least one hundred doctors. The total number of medical groups nearly quadrupled from 1965 to 1995, according to the AMA. Even more telling, the proportion of patient care physicians practicing as employees rose from one in four in 1983 to more than four in ten in 1994.[13] In the hospital field, meanwhile, roughly two out of five nonfederal hospitals were involved in a merger or an acquisition between 1994 and 1996, according to *Modern Healthcare*. Similar forces are at work in virtually every other segment of health care as part of the continuing "social transformation of American medicine" chronicled by sociologist Paul Starr in the early 1980s.[14]

Understandably, change of such scope and speed has sown bitterness and fear among many whose livelihoods are threatened. Consider the situation of medical specialists, long at the top of the profession in income and prestige. If the conservative medical practices typical of a large HMO become the standard of American medicine, then some 96 percent of the nation's population live in areas where there are too many specialists. Even by fee for service standards, 60 percent live in areas with surplus specialists.[15] One can hardly expect thousands of doctors to cheerily accept their redundancy. It's no wonder the public is bombarded with shrill warnings about the threat to medical excellence posed by tightened reimbursement, just as we were once warned with equally sincere fervor about the peril of "cheap" foreign steel, autos, and televisions.

When General Motors abandoned its effort to build a small car right after World War II, GM president Harlow Curtice explained: "You can take the value out much more rapidly than you can take the cost out." In retrospect, however, the real lesson of GM's failure was different. Just as a child is not merely a smaller adult, a small car is not just a shrunken version of a big one. Building a high-quality, low-cost automobile required a radically different management approach and technical skills. GM mastered these skills only when it had to, only when forced by economic crisis. First, though, the company (and its customers) had to suffer through the Corvair, the Vega, and the Citation, three cars with reputations for poor quality. Today GM has gotten skilled enough to build a sporty small Cadillac, the Catera, which has received rave reviews.

The American health care system is experiencing a similar and equally painful learning process, prodded in part by the demands of customers like GM. Make no mistake: the Corvair-type horror stories about managed care are worrisome, are real, and require a response. But they no more are a reliable indicator of the final character of our health care system than the Corvair was the last word in American compact cars or the Toyopet was the best that could be expected from Japan's automakers. In 1997 Toyota introduced a Camry LE that had a more powerful engine, roomier cabin, and better seats while costing $1,500 less than the 1996 model. There is no reason the American health care system cannot reach that same level of achievement, and there are many reasons to expect that it will.

Automobiles at least undergo comparative testing; physicians and hospitals have fiercely resisted comparisons. "The great white lie [of American medicine] is a myth holding that hospitals and doctors are equally good and deserving of our complete, unquestioning trust," wrote journalist Walt Bogdanich in a 1991 book.[16] In a competitive marketplace, however, superior performance cannot be rewarded unless it can be identified. The myth of uniformity no longer preserves autonomy. Instead, it encourages the dreaded "commoditization"—socialism via capitalism's back door.

Dwain Harper, an osteopathic doctor who heads Cleveland Health Quality Choice, a corporate coalition, tells of asking area hospitals to participate in a project to examine the mortality rates of a group of procedures. The hospitals declined, assuring Harper that "quality of care in Cleveland in every hospital is excellent." Said Harper, "Fine, we'll buy cheap." Responded the hospitals, "OK, let's talk." The eventual results of the Cleveland effort demonstrate how the combination of accountability and information can encourage excellence. From 1 January 1993, the first year of data reporting, through the end of 1995, the hospitals reduced the risk-adjusted death rate for patients with general medical conditions (such as pneumonia) by 12 percent—meaning that roughly one in eight who would have died did not.

Just as the "sellers" of care are embracing quality measurement from motives that mix self-interest and idealism, so too are the "buyers." Contracting with a health plan that does things right the first time may be less expensive; "Quality is free," is how Crosby memorably phrased it. Better medical care can also result in more productive and more satisfied workers. And it's the "right" thing to do. Finally, considering quality as well as cost may well avoid negative economic consequences such as a lawsuit or, as one manager put it, "a call from the CEO's wife." Whatever the motivation, managers are increasingly treating medical services "like any other important component of production," as a 1993 article in the *Harvard Business Review* recommended.[17]

The demands of this new approach have brought sophisticated benefits managers to major corporations. Charles Buck, who holds a master's degree in industrial engineering, was director of planning for the Johns Hopkins University medical school, hospital, and school of public health. Today he is a high-ranking staff executive for health care programs at General Electric. Twenty years ago, Buck predicted the end of the "trust me" era of medicine, writing: "Norms and standards in high-quality care are in the short run the responsibility of local physicians, but they increasingly will be compared with regional and national norms and standards.[18] At GE, Buck is able to promote the use of norms and standards through his control of a half-billion-dollar corporate budget for medical care.

Health plans are also rushing to grab the quality measurement and management banner. HMOs have been stunned by the magnitude of the backlash against cost-cutting excesses. In self-protection, the industry has endorsed ever more ambitious reporting requirements and accreditation standards from its trade group and from the voluntary National Committee for Quality Assurance. But as one industry wag likes to put it, "Once you've been a pickle, you can never go back to being a cucumber." The HMO industry is now fair game for the scrutiny of federal and state regulators, politicians, and the news media. Pledges by HMOs to behave in an exemplary manner will not bring back the old freedom from oversight.

In 1987 the *New England Journal of Medicine* published a commentary on Codman's "End Result Idea" that examined whether his concept was technically feasible. The article asked, "Outcome Assessment 70

Years Later: Are We Ready?"[19] Another ten years later, the luxury of intellectual agonizing is gone. Ready or not, accountability has arrived. The confrontational Codman would surely have enjoyed the following exchange within an Internet discussion group. Wrote one participant: "I am wondering if anyone has encountered effective mechanisms or methods for persuading physicians and other clinicians to participate in outcomes projects. We are encountering a little resistance with some surgeons." Back came the reply: "Tell them that tracking outcomes will demonstrate what a good job they're doing, it will get them more patients, and if they don't, they'll be out of jobs, since everyone else is, regardless of whether or not they know what outcomes are."[20]

That electronic opinion exchange highlights the impact of technology, the second major force pushing forward the quality measurement and management revolution. The traditional sources of information in medicine are giving way to an "infomedicine" that both incorporates new kinds of information and uses traditional kinds in new ways. The health care industry, accounting for an estimated one-seventh of the United States economy, is finding itself (willingly or unwillingly) swept into the digitalizing of America.

Outcomes studies and "run charts" do not require a computer, but a computer makes it possible to dig far more deeply in a much shorter time. Like much else in quality measurement in medicine, using computers has been technically possible for a long time. A pathbreaking article in a 1959 issue of *Science,* "Reasoning Foundations of Medical Diagnosis," laid out a blueprint for using computers to improve physicians' decisions.[21] By 1965, no less an authority than Thomas J. Watson Jr., the legendary chairman of IBM, predicted: "The widespread use [of computers] . . . in hospitals and physicians' offices will instantaneously give a doctor or a nurse a patient's entire medical history, eliminating both guesswork and bad recollection, and sometimes making a difference between life and death." This would happen, said Watson, in "just a few years."[22]

Watson could have been proved correct. The technology was available, and some research pioneers were using it. But computers were expensive and exotic, and it was easy to ignore their capabilities even as late as the 1980s. Anyway, most doctors didn't much believe in the purported benefits of "uniform medical care" or the alleged hazards of "guesswork and bad recollection," in Watson's words.

Today, computers represent an innovation that is impossible to ignore. They have become ubiquitous ("compatibility with existing values," as Everett Rogers would put it), easy to use ("lack of complexity"), and inexpensive ("trialability"). Their innovative potential is self-evident ("observability"), and economic changes provide the motivation ("comparative advantage") to take action. Twenty years ago, many doctors feared that computers would replace them. Although the present computers are five hundred times more powerful, doctors now know that computers are essential for helping medicine deal with its twenty-first-century version of the Industrial Revolution. Throughout the country, hospitals and physicians are banding together into integrated health systems such as the Twin Cities partnership profiled in chapter 13. These systems require sophisticated clinical data both for internal management, in order to produce a consistent "product," and for external marketing, in order to differentiate themselves from competitors. As health systems begin to evolve toward an "organized system of care" that coordinates sickness care and "wellness" outreach, the need for better information systems will become even more urgent.

Leaders of the physician and hospital communities see the advent of care systems as a chance to preserve autonomy and ward off micromanagement of medical decisions. Indeed, the contracting between the Buyers Health Care Action Group and Twin Cities care systems is being closely watched as a possible prototype for the employer-provider relationship of the future.

"Are we going to manage the care of the sick, or are we going to manage the providers who manage the sick?" demands Mayo Foundation chairman Robert Waller. "By adopting the guidance offered by continuous quality improvement techniques, by focusing on an autonomy guided by an emphasis on the most appropriate, effective and economically efficient care, Mayo hopes to protect the most important aspects of autonomy for the doctors who practice there. . . . What we will all ultimately be accountable for is quality."

It is not only a handful of leading organizations that are adopting this approach. To cite just a few examples, the Iowa Medical Society plans to produce reports on patient clinical outcomes that the society's members can use in marketing. In Maryland and southern California, medical groups and hospitals are testing an automated patient satisfaction and health status survey system. In locations all over the country, physicians are experimenting with electronic-based clinical protocols that spot potential drug reactions as the doctor enters a prescription on a computer (handheld or desktop). In some places the computer alerts the physician to relevant clinical practice guidelines and the evidence they are based on.

Just as managed care has become the mainstream method of financing medical care, the practices of infomedicine will inexorably become the mainstream method of making medical decisions. Our society's shift from centralized control of information to distributed information—symbolized by the Internet—is changing the process of clinical decision making. The prominent AMA member I quoted earlier in this chapter acknowledged that these new ways are unsettling at first to many doctors.

"Physicians are out there saying, 'Don't change my own little microcosm,' which is his office, his hospital, and his country club," the AMA member said. The changes, however, will bring "more predictability, more accountability. It will improve health care."

The third powerful force for change is the zeitgeist, or "spirit of the times." Intellectual and social trends can help an idea flourish or cause it to wither on the vine. In our times the information explosion, the global marketplace economy, and a general acceptance of the principle of accountability are all helping to advance the objectives of the quality measurement and management movement.

For example, education was once considered impervious to objective measures of achievement. Now policy analysts discuss national standards, teacher competency tests, and linking reimbursement to results. Similarly, Vice President Albert Gore Jr. speaks of turning government agencies into "performance-based organizations." In sports, baseball managers turn to laptop computers to tell them where in the strike zone the next batter is most likely to swing at a pitch and the chances that the pitcher can put the ball there.

In the business arena, meanwhile, intense global competition has underscored the importance of systematic measurement and improvement. *Future Edge* author Joel Arthur Barker asserts: "If you do not have the components of excellence—statistic[al] process control, continuous improvement, benchmarking, the constant pursuit of excellence, the capability of knowing how to do the right thing the first time . . . then *you don't even get to play the game*"[23] (emphasis in the original).

In this environment, how long can the local hospital continue to plead ignorance about the appropriateness and effectiveness of treatment in its emergency room? How credible is it for a health plan to be in the dark about which members have diabetes, high blood pressure, or asthma? How believable is it for every surgeon to claim, when asked about outcomes, "*My* patients are sicker"?

Just as HMOs acquired legitimacy in a gradual process involving government, employers, researchers, and practicing doctors, so is the concept of quality measurement and management going through the same integration into the mainstream of medicine. For example, the idea that employers should contract with health plans based on both cost and quality measures has been endorsed by major business organizations such as the Conference Board and featured in national business publications like *Business Week* and *Barron's.* Virtually every medical specialty society has formed a committee to evaluate outcomes measures, and similar endeavors are under way at the American Hospital Association and the American College of Healthcare Executives. The Joint Commission on Accreditation of Healthcare Organizations announced in early 1997 that it will require hospitals seeking accreditation to integrate the use of outcomes and other performance measures into their daily operations.

Scholarly articles about medical quality, appropriateness, and cost effectiveness have become a routine component of the clinical literature. The *New England Journal of Medicine* ran a six-part series of articles in 1996 that explained and implicitly endorsed quality measurement and management techniques. The AMA was scheduled to put out a "quality" theme issue in each of its scientific publications during 1997. Similarly, the widely read health policy journal *Health Affairs* devoted its May–June 1997 issue to quality of care.

Of equal importance is that courses in clinical effectiveness evaluation are beginning to make their way into the medical school curriculum. There are departments of outcomes measurement, institutes of outcomes, and journals of outcomes and medical decision making. The academic community has created terminology that takes industrial concepts of quality improvement and translates them back into the scientific language they originated in. Ongoing quality measurement now becomes part of the "clinical evaluative sciences." It includes "disciplined practice learning" and "real-time science." New scholarly publications have sprung to life, such as the *Journal of Outcomes Management* and *Evidence-Based Medicine,* a publication jointly sponsored by the American College of Physicians and the *British Medical Journal.*

In fact, the forces that have brought the quality improvement movement to prominence are international in scope. The problems of medical practice variation and of care whose cost is unrelated to its results are by no means limited to this country. Nor, of course, are advances in information technology. (The wide variation in accepted medical practices between science-based doctors in different nations was addressed at length by journalist Lynn Payor in her 1988 book *Medicine and Culture.*) Britain's National Health Service has become a leader in evidence-based medicine. Government ministries in Australia and Austria are trying to reduce medical errors. The French are backing development of a medical information infrastructure, and Norway's general practitioners are exploring the use of quality indicators and standards and the development of medical records software. Even China's senior leader, Jiang Zemin, exhorted physicians at a 1996 conference to "work hard to improve their quality."[24]

For all the progress that has been made, however, this remains a young and fragile revolution. Revolutions can be undermined, misdirected, or taken over. If this one is to fulfill its potential, I believe a series of events must occur.

Maintain the Pressure

Systematic quality improvement is not easy, culturally or technically, and it can be expensive. It is only because of intense financial pressure that the medical community is finally confronting the difficult issues involved. Even in the most advanced markets, candid physician leaders acknowledge that the pressure for accountability must continue if a successful transformation is to be completed.

Deeds, Not Words

The employers who demand quality improvement must reward it as much as cost cutting. For instance, health plans that specialize in reaching out to members who have cancer or AIDS worry that more of the sick will join up, thereby causing premiums to rise and making other customers go elsewhere. Another danger to performance-based purchasing is ideology. Some consumer groups denounce capitation (a fixed payment per health plan member) as an invitation to rationing, even though there is a growing body of evidence that properly done capitation may lead to better-quality care. What counts is improving patient care, not an ideologically pure payment system.

Preserve Choice

The Chevrolet Corvair may have been "unsafe at any speed," but no driver was forced to buy one. Some health plans are already responding to public skepticism about the "gatekeeper" model by allowing members to see a specialist without a referral (for an increased price). Having a choice of providers and easy access to needed care does not guarantee the care will be good, but both items are vital components of an overall high-quality system.

Information, Information, Information

For a marketplace to work, consumers must have access to reliable and relevant information on everything from the health plans' rules and procedures to outcomes information from specific hospitals or for specific procedures. Although there is a danger in issuing report cards that are not carefully validated, the principle of public access to information is a cornerstone of accountability.

At the same time, there must be an intensive educational effort to make information about the quality of care usable by the public. Particular attention should be paid to the needs of the elderly, who are most likely to be sick.

Government Needs to Set the Rules and Serve as Referee, but Not Call the Plays

It took the thalidomide tragedy to shock Congress into strengthening the oversight powers of the Food and Drug Administration. We cannot wait for an equivalent disaster in medical services. "Deregulation" demands watchfulness. Managed care horror stories are not much different from the tales of paid-by-the-mile truckers falling asleep at the wheel, discount airlines cutting corners on maintenance, or inexperienced brokers losing their customers' money.

In some instances, state governments can lead. Massachusetts makes available physician on-line reports that include educational background, a list of publications, and malpractice history. A California law that takes effect 1 July 1998 gives terminally ill patients the right to an external, independent appeal of a health plan's decision to deny coverage for a treatment considered experimental or investigational. Other states may follow.

"Legislating by body part"—such as mandating a minimum maternity stay—should be a last resort. To date, it has been a preferred method of political grandstanding. Yet there are modest grounds for optimism that the nation's political leadership will respond to the challenge of information age medicine. Vice President Gore oversaw the National Information Infrastructure project, which included a health care component. Meanwhile, House Speaker Newt Gingrich has spoken publicly about the need for outcomes measurement in medicine, and benchmarking for excellence. Perhaps this sophistication in rhetoric will be translated into sophistication in government policy. As this book went to press, a Presidential Advisory Commission on Consumer Protection and Quality in the Health Care Industry was considering a consumer bill of rights and other measures.

Successful Revolutionaries Take over Television Stations and Newspapers

The news media play a critical role in defining the context of the public and political debate. Publications such as *U.S. News and World Report, Money,* and *Consumer's Report* have begun to search for objective data on which to base their ratings of hospitals and or health plans. They need to improve and expand that effort.

Similarly, the national media must continue to address socioeconomic issues related to quality of health care.[25] For example, an ABC News *Nightline* segment related how GTE Corporation provides employees with quality information about the health plans it offers and gives them incentives to choose the better plans. Front page stories in the *Wall Street Journal* in 1996 included an exploration of practice variation and an investigation of quality problems in a Chicago hospital's heart transplant program.

A New Power Structure Gives Rise to New Institutions

While traditional consumer organizations maintain an important role in the quality revolution, newer groups are also arising whose sole concerns are outcomes measures, patient privacy in the electronic age, or the patient-physician relationship. Indiana University's Marc Rodwin calls for a new breed of consumer information analysts who, like financial analysts, will analyze the dizzying array of technical information about quality of care on behalf of large purchasers, the news media, or individual consumers.

The jury is still out, however, on whether the legal profession will abet or destroy the changes under way. Lawyers could help promote the use of guidelines and protocols as a legally defensible "community standard." (Maine experimented with a limited program in that regard.) On the other hand, plaintiffs' attorneys might well decide to sue any physician or hospital achieving less than "perfect" results. An adversarial legal system may need to be modified if the public is to reap the full fruits of cooperative quality improvement.

Research on Doing Things Right Deserves Financial Support Commensurate with Its Importance

In 1989, Congress responded to a burst of concern about practice variation by setting up the Agency for Health Care Policy and Research. The little known AHCPR was almost killed in 1995 because it alienated several powerful Republicans, who thought its administrator was a cheerleader for the Clinton administration's health reform proposals, and because a group of spine surgeons greatly disliked a back pain guideline that cited medical evidence indicating that surgery was overused. Reprieved at the last minute, in fiscal 1996 AHCPR rejoiced over a budget of $125 million. That amount equals less than half of one day's national expenditures on health care.

The United States has invested tens of billions of dollars in turning out skilled doctors and in equipping medical schools and hospitals. In fiscal 1997 the National Institutes of Health received $12.7 billion; AHCPR got $143 million, or about one-hundredth as much. Systematic measurement and improvement of everyday medical care may not be as glamorous as searching for the next "magic bullet," but it can save tens of thousands of lives right now if we help. Moreover, a host of complex questions must be addressed if this revolution is to continue successfully.[26] These include not just clinical issues, but ethical and economic ones such as a common definition of cost effectiveness and how we define the proper boundaries of population-based medicine. The government, medical organizations, and private foundations all need to dramatically increase their funding in this field.

Some Questions Can't Be Answered, and Other Times We Don't Want to Listen to the Answers We Get

The medical quality revolution has limits. Improving the treatment of the sick will not provide health care for the uninsured, ensure the future of academic medical centers, or solve all the other pressing problems in health care. And some questions have no answers. We may be able to predict the probability that someone will die in surgery, but we cannot know whether that risk is worth taking for the patient whose life is at stake. That kind of decision is a value judgment. David Pryor, a physician researcher formerly at Duke University, constructed a computer generated curve based on which patients' lives were most likely to be extended as a result of bypass surgery. If your chances of survival are slim, should your insurance company still pay for a procedure, or should you have to bear more of the cost if you want to go forward anyway? These are tough policy decisions. Issues of rationality and rationing look different one life at a time.

Things Take Time

Even if managed care was abandoned tomorrow, its place taken by the liberal dream of a Canadian-type health system or the conservative vision of medical savings accounts, an urgent need would remain to address quality problems in everyday medicine. The need would still be there even if all care was free. Nonetheless, revolutions progress at their own pace. An idea catches fire, dies down, then flares up again and spreads permanently. People do not easily revise well-worn habits of thought. The physicist Max Planck wrote: "A new scientific truth does not triumph by convincing its opponents and making them see the light, but rather because its opponents eventually die, and a new generation grows up that is familiar with it."

If you have been conditioned to expect an endless all you can eat buffet from life, then even an expensive meal at a fine restaurant will feel like rationing. Our expectations about the American health care system will take time to change and evolve. Until they do, ethical and rational stewardship of limited medical resources will not take hold.

NEITHER SAINTS NOR SINNERS

> Physicians are neither saints nor sinners. I find that my fellow managers are more easily disillusioned by the inadequacies of physicians than I am. The truth is that doctors are like everyone else.
>
> —Mike Magee, M.D., president, Pride in Medicine Project, 1992

On the cusp of the twenty-first century, the practice of medicine demands more than sympathetic intuition. It will be indelibly shaped by two separate but related challenges: how to do the right thing, and how to do the right thing right.

The first of those challenges can be seen as Jack Wennberg's question about surgical frequency: "Which rate is right?" The question shines a harsh light on the scientific basis of medicine, asking, Where is the evidence for the appropriateness and effectiveness of this procedure? Where is the evidence this procedure helps more than does an alternative therapy or doing nothing? Shouldn't the patient's preferences help determine whether the procedure is performed?

The second challenge is epitomized by Don Berwick's declaration, "How good you are doesn't say how good you could be." This simple statement expresses deference to reputation-based medicine while implicitly pronouncing it inadequate. Some critics worry that continuous improvement techniques encourage bettering the status quo at the expense of innovation: an efficient iron lung instead of a vaccine for polio. That is a legitimate concern, but it has not been the case in other industries. Continuous improvement provides a framework for change. "How good you are doesn't say how good you could be" is a prod to excellence, not an invitation to incrementalism. Nor is continuous improvement a substitute for finding incompetent physicians and removing them outright from medical practice.

Excellence will often demand new ways of thinking. Lanny Johnson, a North Lansing, Michigan, surgeon, videotaped each of his surgeries until he left the active practice of medicine. Johnson studied his tapes constantly to find ways to improve. (At one point he even offered his local HMO a "no complications" guarantee.) Johnson's review of the videos is something college football coaches do all the time. Are athletes less "artists" than surgeons, or does the difference in our expectations come from the mind-set we bring to that question?

The challenge of "how good you could be" should also compel physicians to see themselves as part of a system of care. (It's no coincidence that those U.S. Army ads that urge "Be All You Can Be" show soldiers working as a team.) The emerging emphasis on a systemwide accountability for results is already beginning to persuade some health plans to pay for "alternative" treatments such as vitamin therapy or yoga, as long as the results can be measured. Systems thinking should not discourage individual achievement any more than continuous improvement discriminates against innovation.

If the basis of the outcomes movement is like the column where Ann Landers asked readers to tell her what happened after they took her advice, then the overall quality revolution should be measured against the standard set by Dear Abby (in real life, Ann Landers's twin). When an unhappy wife writes to complain about her flawed mate, Abby invariably replies: "Are you better off with him or without him?"

Will we—patients, medical professionals, citizens—be better off with a health care system based on performance measurement? Certainly there are dangers as well as opportunities. In the examples cited in this book, individual doctors have been allowed to overrule guidelines and computer analyses whenever they feel it is necessary. Unfortunately, not all proponents of these ideas are that sensitive. As Peter Bernstein cautions in *Against the Gods: The Remarkable Story of Risk:* "Our lives teem with numbers, but we sometimes forget that numbers are only tools. They have no soul; they may indeed become fetishes."[27] Consistent excellence will always be a challenge to the human soul, not just the intellect.

Other critics worry that information-based medicine will devalue the human touch. This is no more true of using a computer than of equipping doctors' offices with telephones. In fact, the opposite may well be true. "There is a real possibility that the information highway and reorganization of the health-care system can create an opportunity for the physician, in collaboration with other members of the health-care team, to provide an even more sensitive, caring and compassionate service to their patients and society," asserts Kenneth Shine, president of the Institute of Medicine. "To the extent that data makes the practice of medicine more scientific, health care reform could bring both science and caring to a new high level over the next decade."[28]

The nineteenth-century rationalists who carefully tracked how many of their fellow citizens died from the plague and how many died from the therapy of their physicians knew something about the connection between science and caring. In the spirit of the Enlightenment, they viewed the numbers they collected as "moral statistics" whose implications would compel action. They believed that "science as public knowledge would be a force for reform and renovation . . . [and] that open discussion of relevant information could move men to correct social injustices and further material progress."[29] It is a belief I share, from both rationalist and religious impulses. Numbers are a tool; stewardship is what we should be building.

The destruction of the old ways of medical practice may be an unavoidable source of anxiety, but it should not be a source of despair. Patients and caregivers alike should celebrate better days ahead. Destruction often precedes renewal, and it is in that renewal that the future of American medicine lies.

NOTES

INTRODUCTION: A DIFFERENT KIND OF REVOLUTION

1. Robert H. Brook et al., "Appropriateness of Acute Medical Care for the Elderly: An Analysis of the Literature," *Health Policy* 14 (1990): 225–42. See also D. V. Axene, R. L. Doyle, and A. P. Fere, *Analysis of Medically Unnecessary Health Care Consumption* (Seattle: Milliman and Robertson, 4 October 1991), and Sharon M. Wilcox, David U. Himmelstein, and Steffie Woolhandler, "Inappropriate Drug Prescribing for the Community-Dwelling Elderly," *JAMA* 272, no. 4 (27 July 1994): 292–96.

2. Mark McClellan, Barbara J. McNeil, and Joseph P. Newhouse, "Does More Intensive Treatment of Acute Myocardial Infarction in the Elderly Reduce Mortality?" *JAMA* 272, no. 11 (21 September 1994): 859–66.

3. Office of Technology Assessment of the Congress of the United States, *The Impact of Randomized Clinical Trials on Health Policy and Medical Practice,* Background Paper OTA-BP-H-22 (Washington, D.C.: U.S. Government Printing Office, August 1983).

4. A. O. Berg, "Variations among Family Physicians' Management Strategies for Lower Urinary Tract Infection in Women: A Report from the Washington Physicians Collaborative Research Network," *Journal of the American Board of Family Practice,* September–October 1991, 327–30.

5. David M. Eddy, "Medicine, Money and Mathematics," *American College of Surgeons Bulletin* 77, no. 6 (June 1992): 36–49.

6. Alvan R. Feinstein, "An Additional Basic Science for Clinical Medicine: I. The Constraining Fundamental Paradigms," *Annals of Internal Medicine* 99, no. 3 (September 1983): 393–97.

7. Gerald T. O'Connor et al., "A Regional Intervention to Improve the Hospital Mortality Associated with Coronary Artery Bypass Graft Surgery," *JAMA* 275, no. 11 (20 March 1996): 841–46. An article by William A. Ghali et al., "Statewide Quality Improvement Initiatives and Mortality after Cardiac Surgery," *JAMA* 277, no. 5 (5 February 1997): 379–82, casts doubt on the relative success of the Northern New England Cardiovascular Cooperative's efforts, but a number of questions remain about both the context of the Ghali paper and some of its methodology. See chapter 9, note 43 for more detail.

8. William C. Nugent and William C. Schults, "Playing by the Numbers: How Collecting Outcomes Data Changed My Life," *Annals of Thoracic Surgery* 58 (1994): 1866–70.

9. Peter C. Amadio et al., "Redesigning Patient Care," *Journal of the Society for Health Systems* 4, no. 2 (1993): 65–83.

10. George Bernard Shaw, *The Doctor's Dilemma* (New York: Brentano's, 1913), xiv.

11. Center for the Evaluative Clinical Sciences, Dartmouth Medical School, *The Dartmouth Atlas of Health Care* (Chicago: American Hospital Publishing, 1996).

12. Bernard Gavzer, "Why Some Doctors May Be Hazardous to Your Health," *Parade,* 14 April 1996, 4–6. Cover of magazine reads: "When Doctors Are the Problem."

13. Morton Thompson, *Not as a Stranger* (New York: Charles Scribner's Sons, 1954), 373.

14. "Learn How Savvy Health Care Managers Are Maintaining Their Market Share, Profitability and Reputation DESPITE Rigorous New Demands for Performance Accountability." Undated letter sent in early 1995 to the author from Richard Biehl, publisher, *Accountability News,* published by Atlantic Information Services, Washington, D.C.

15. From presentation by Robert Waller, M.D., to the Mayo Conference on Quality, Rochester, Minnesota, 27 October 1995.

CHAPTER ONE: LEARNING THE TRUTH

1. Maine Medical Assessment Foundation, *Synernet/MMAF Pneumonia Pharmacotherapy Study* (Portland: Maine Medical Assessment Foundation, November 1994).

2. Karl-Ludwig Neuhaus et al., "Improved Thrombolysis in Acute Myocardial Infarction with Front-Loaded Administration of Alteplase: Results of the rt-PA-APSAC Patency Study (TAPS)," *Journal of the American College of Cardiology* 19, no. 5 (April 1992): 885–91; GUSTO Investigators, "An International Randomized Trial Comparing Four Thrombolytic Strategies for Acute Myocardial Infarction," *New England Journal of Medicine* 329, no. 10 (2 September 1993): 673–82; Gruppo Italiano per lo Studio della Streptochinasi nell'Infarto Miocardico (GISSI), "Effectiveness of Intravenous Thrombolytic Treatment in Acute Myocardial Infarction," *Lancet* 1 (22 February 1986): 397–402.

3. Ibid.

4. John Z. Ayanian, "Knowledge and Practices of Generalist and Specialist Physicians regarding Drug Therapy for Acute Myocardial Infarction," *Health Services Research* 19, no. 3 (August 1984): 307–31. See also James G. Jollis et al., "Outcome of Acute Myocardial Infarction according to the Specialty of the Admitting Physician," *New England Journal of Medicine* 335, no. 25 (19 December 1996): 1880–87.

5. In late 1996 Forbes announced that it would merge with the another regional health care system, the Allegheny Health, Education and Research Foundation, and become part of a subsidiary named Allegheny University Medical Centers.

6. Harold S. Luft and Sandra S. Hunt, "Evaluating Individual Hospital Qual-

ity through Outcome Statistics," *JAMA* 255, no. 20 (23–30 May 1986): 2780–2801.

7. Interview by the author with McGarvey's colleague John Harper, M.D., 9 April 1993.

8. Richard N. McGarvey and John J. Harper, "Pneumonia Mortality Reduction and Quality Improvement in a Community Hospital," *Quality Review Bulletin* 19, no. 4 (April 1993): 124–30.

9. Ibid., 125.

10. Interview by the author with Mel Lopata, M.D., professor of medicine and chief of respiratory and crictical care medicine at University of Illinois College of Medicine, 8 May 1995.

11. McGarvey and Harper, "Pneumonia Mortality Reduction and Quality Improvement in a Community Hospital," 126.

12. National Center For Health Statistics.

13. *Vital Statistics of the United States, Mortality Edition,* 2, sec. A (Atlanta: Centers for Disease Control, 1992).

14. Interview by the author with Frederic G. Jones, M.D., 7 March 1995.

15. D. W. Simborg, "DRG Creep: A New Hospital-Acquired Disease." *New England Journal of Medicine* 304, no. 26 (25 June 1981): 1602–4. In late 1995, meanwhile, the Justice Department launched investigations of two physician billing services based on suspicions that the companies were "upcoding" Medicare claims. As of mid-1997, the Columbia/HCA Healthcare Corp. chain was facing a similar probe.

16. Anderson Area Medical Center eventually looked at the U.S. Health Care Financing Administration data for 1986–88 (including readjustment of the 1987 data made in the 1988 release). The second source of data that prompted action, other than the HCFA numbers, came from a cooperative study of 1987 data on fresh, acute myocardial infarctions sponsored by the Hospital Research and Educational Trust, part of the American Hospital Association.

17. *Heart and Stroke Facts: 1995 Statistical Supplement* (New York: American Heart Association, 1995).

18. GUSTO Investigators, "International Randomized Trial."

19. GISSI, "Effectiveness of Intravenous Thrombolytic Treatment."

20. National Heart Attack Alert Program Coordinating Committee 60 Minutes to Treatment Working Group, *Emergency Department: Rapid Identification and Treatment of Patients with Acute Myocardial Infarction,* NIH Publication 93-3278, September (Bethesda, Md.: National Institutes of Health, 1993), vi.

21. Robert W. Dubois and Robert H. Brook, "Preventable Deaths: Who, How Often and Why?" *Annals of Internal Medicine* 109, no. 7 (1 October 1988): 582–89.

22. Interview by the author with Gregory Zaar, M.D., medical director, Mid-South Foundation for Medical Care, Memphis, 21 March 1995. Figures come from an unpublished report by the group.

23. Presentation and handout from Mark Jewell, president, Epi-Q, and former quality official of Evangelical Health Systems, to symposium, "Leading Clinical Quality Improvement: Less Art, More Science," 23–26 August 1994.

Evangelical/EHS Health Care merged with another Chicago system to become Advocate Health.

24. Edward F. Ellerbeck et al., "Quality of Care for Medicare Patients with Acute Myocardial Infarction," *JAMA* 273, no. 19 (17 May 1995): 1509–14.

25. Ibid.

26. "Simple Steps Help Patients with Heart Attacks Get Treatment More Quickly." Mayo Clinic press release, 22 March 1995. The release ties in with a presentation by Stephen Kopecky, M.D., director of the study, to the annual meeting of the American College of Cardiology.

27. Stephen B. Soumerai et al., "Adverse Outcomes of Underuse of β-Blockers in Elderly Survivors of Acute Myocardial Infarction," *JAMA* 277, no. 2 (8 January 1997): 115–21.

28. *Heart and Stroke Facts.*

29. A. Mark Fendrick, Paul M. Ridker, and Bernard S. Bloom, "Improved Health Benefits of Increased Use of Thrombolytic Therapy," *Archives of Internal Medicine* 154, no. 13 (25 July 1994): 1605–9.

30. Fendrick, Ridker, and Bloom, "Improved Health Benefits of Increased Use of Thrombolytic Therapy."

31. M. J. Fine et al., "Prognosis and Outcomes of Patients with Community-Acquired Pneumonia: A Meta-analysis," *JAMA* 275, no. 2 (10 January 1996): 134–41.

32. Helen J. Neikirk, Gary J. Fortune, and Brad Hegemann, "Identification of Excess In-Hospital Deaths from Community-Acquired Pneumonia: Use of Severity-Adjusted Claims Data," *Journal of Outcomes Management* 2, no. 2 (June 1995): 18–22.

CHAPTER TWO: WHAT DOCTORS DON'T KNOW

1. American Child Health Association, *Physical Defects: The Pathway to Correction* (New York: American Child Health Association, 1934), 82.

2. Harry Bakwin, "The Tonsil-Adenoidectomy Dilemma," *Journal of Pediatrics* 52, no. 3 (March 1958): 339–61.

3. Ibid.

4. S. D. Lipton, "On Psychology of Childhood Tonsillectomy," in *Psychoanalytic Study of the Child,* ed. R. S. Eissler et al. (New York: International Universities Press, 1962), 17:363–417.

5. Archibald L. Cochrane, *Effectiveness and Efficiency: Random Reflections on Health Services* (London: Nuffield Provincial Hospitals Trust, 1971), 60–61.

6. Michael L. Millenson, "Many Medical Procedures May Be Unneeded," *Chicago Tribune,* 21 March 1991. The article describes a review performed by Value Health Sciences, Santa Monica, California, under a contract to the national Blue Cross and Blue Shield Association. The review included records of eleven million insured workers and their families belonging to five fee for service Blues plans and one Blues HMO.

In an interview by the author on 11 July 1995, Jacqueline Kosecoff, Value Health's executive vice president, said the conclusions reached in 1991 remained valid: "We still have tonsils [surgery] being enormously inappropriate," she said.

7. Harry Bakwin, "The Tonsil-Adenoidectomy Enigma," in *Health Services Research: An Anthology*, ed. Kerr L. White (Washington, D.C.: Pan American Health Organization, 1992), 116–31. The Bakwin article was originally published in *Journal of Pediatrics* 52, no. 3 (March 1958): 339–61. Children still die from tonsils surgery, although it is rare. A story from the Associated Press on 23 March 1995 reported that a four-year-old girl in New York City recovering from a routine tonsillectomy "bled to death in her mother's arms four days after the surgery." A spokeswoman for the state health department noted that "this area of the body is very rich in blood vessels. . . . Fewer tonsillectomies are being done because the risks outweigh the benefits in general."

8. D. M. Levy, "Psychic Trauma of Operations," *American Journal of Diseases of Children* 69, no. 7 (1945).

9. J. H. P. Paton, in *Quarterly Journal of Medicine* 88, no. 109 (1928). Cited in J. A. Glover, "The Incidence of Tonsillectomy in School Children," *Proceedings of the Royal Society of Medicine* 31 (27 May 1930): 1219–36.

10. Lawrence C. Kleinman et al., "The Medical Appropriateness of Tympanostomy Tubes Proposed for Children Younger Than 16 Years in the United States," *JAMA* 271, no. 16 (27 April 1994): 1250–55. For dissenting views, see also letters to the editor in *JAMA* 273, no. 9 (1 March 1995): 697–701.

11. Preschool children given gum containing the natural sweetener xylitol had 50 percent fewer chronic ear infections than a control group, according to a late 1996 report from researachers at the University of Oulu in Finland.

12. John P. Bunker, Benjamin A. Barnes, and Frederick Mosteller, eds., *Costs, Risks and Benefits of Surgery* (New York: Oxford University Press, 1977), 176–97.

13. David A. Grimes, "Technology Follies: The Uncritical Acceptance of Medical Innovation," *JAMA* 269, no. 23 (16 June 1993): 3030–33.

14. Ibid.

15. Ludwig Edelstein, *The Hippocratic Oath: Text, Translation and Interpretation* (Baltimore: Johns Hopkins University Press, 1943). Although the oath is attributed to Hippocrates, most scholars believe it was written by his disciples.

16. Hippocrates, "Regimen," in *The Medical Works of Hippocrates*, ed. J. Chadwick and W. N. Mann (Springfield, Ill.: Thomas, 1950), 129, 82.

17. Sherwin B. Nuland, *Doctors: The Biography of Medicine* (New York: Vintage, 1989), 35–36.

18. Luke 6:18–19 New Oxford Annotated Bible: "They had come to hear him and to be healed of their diseases; and those with unclean spirits were cured. And all in the crowd were trying to touch him, for power came out of him and healed all of them."

19. Alan Pollack and Mary Evans, *Surgical Audit* (Essex, Eng.: Butterworth, 1989), 10.

20. Richard Gordon, *The Alarming History of Medicine* (New York: St. Martin's Press, 1993), 179. Gordon says the belief about drinking water from the skull of a bishop was reported as late as 1830 in County Cavan in Ireland. Other folk prescriptions for treating whooping cough included sheep droppings boiled in milk and passing the patient under and over a donkey nine times.

21. William A. Silverman, "Doing More Good Than Harm," in "Doing More

Good Than Harm: The Evaluation of Health Care Interventions," ed. Kenneth S. Warren and Frederick Mosteller, *Annals of the New York Academy of Sciences* 703 (31 December 1993): 5–11.

22. Guenter B. Risse, *Hospital Life in Enlightenment Scotland* (Cambridge: Cambridge University Press, 1986), 205. A Scottish infirmary (clinic) of the late eighteenth century recorded the number of cases bled and the average amount bled by its physicians, which during one period was 15.4 ounces.

23. John A. Carroll and Mary W. Ashworth, *First in Peace,* vol. 7 of *George Washington: A Biography,* ed. Douglas Southall Freeman (New York: Scribner's, 1957), 617–34.

24. John Harley Warner, *The Therapeutic Perspective* (Cambridge: Harvard University Press, 1988), 209.

25. Lewis Thomas, *The Youngest Science* (New York: Bantam, 1983), 18.

26. *The People's Chronology* [CD-ROM] Microsoft Bookshelf (New York: Henry Holt, 1992).

27. E. H. G. Lutz, *Men with Golden Hands: A Book of Surgical Miracles,* trans. W. H. Johnson (London: Allen and Unwin, 1955), 5.

28. Bryan H. Bunch, *Timetables of Technology: A Chronology of the Most Important People and Events in the History of Technology* (New York: Simon and Schuster, 1993), 263.

29. Nuland, *Doctors,* 141.

30. Hermann L. Blumgart, citing Lawrence J. Henderson's assertion in *New England Journal of Medicine* 270, no. 9 (27 February 1964): 449–56.

31. Abraham Flexner, "Medical Education in the U.S. and Canada," *Bulletin no. 4,* Carnegie Foundation for the Advancement of Teaching (1910); Alex Gerber, *The Gerber Report: The Shocking State of American Medical Care and What Must Be Done about It* (New York: McKay, 1971).

32. Anne M. Stoline and Jonathan P. Weiner, *The New Medical Marketplace* (Baltimore: Johns Hopkins University Press, 1988), 15.

33. W. Bruce Fye, "The Literature of Internal Medicine," in *Grand Rounds: One Hundred Years of Internal Medicine,* ed. Russell C. Maulitz and Diana E. Long (Philadelphia: University of Pennsylvania Press, 1988), 73. Some commentators have accused Flexner and his supporters of closing off a path to upward mobility to the working class by reducing the number of medical schools and requiring a high-school diploma for admission. These and other changes had the effect of pricing a medical education out of the reach of anyone below the middle class and in effect, critics charge, helped protect physicians' incomes. Although that argument may have merit on the grounds of economic theory, one suspects that few patients would agree that reducing the number of undertrained and undereducated physicians was not worth the price.

34. Midrashic legend cited by the eleventh-century biblical commentator Rashi in his commentary on Gen. 11:28.

35. Jeremiah A. Barondess, "Medicine and Its Mandate: Reasons for Change," paper presented at the Centennial of Johns Hopkins Medical Institutions, "Doctoring America: The Last 100 Years and the Next 100 Years," 23–24 February 1990.

36. Paul Beeson and Russell C. Maulitz, "The Inner History of Internal Medicine," in Maulitz and Long, *Grand Rounds,* 39.

37. H. F. Dowling, *Fighting Infection* (Cambridge: Harvard University Press, 1977).

38. Thomas, *Youngest Science,* 33.

39. *People's Chronology.*

40. John C. Burnham, "American Medicine's Golden Age: What Happened to It?" *Science* 215 (19 March 1982): 1474–79.

41. Shryock, *Development of Modern Medicine,* 354.

42. Richard Carter, *The Doctor Business* (New York: Doubleday, 1958), 224.

43. Burnham, "American Medicine's Golden Age," 1476.

44. Paul Starr, *The Social Transformation of American Medicine* (New York: Basic, 1982), 342–43.

45. Personal communication from James Wyngaarden cited by Beeson and Maulitz, "Inner History of Internal Medicine," 29–30.

46. Alton Blakeslee, "Seems Like a Good Time, Says Retired AP Editor, for an Old-Coot Salute," *Science Writers News,* summer 1994. In the days before local news teams and ubiquitous minicams, recalled Blakeslee, some two hundred reporters packed into a room pushed and shoved each other to get copies of the report of Salk's clinical trials of the vaccine and relay first word over the phone to newspaper and wire editors standing by. Blakeslee covered Salk's press conference at the University of Michigan for the Associated Press.

47. Bunch, *Timetables of Technology,* 401.

48. Paul B. Beeson, "Changes in Medical Therapy during the Past Half Century," *Medicine* 59 (1980): 79–99.

49. The source for the number of people with insurance coverage was *Source Book of Health Insurance Data* (Washington, D.C.: Health Insurance Association of America, 1992), 9. Calculations of the percentage of all Americans covered were made by the author based on government reports.

50. Medicare later added coverage of the disabled.

51. *Changing Times: The Kiplinger Magazine,* quoted in *AMA News,* 16 October 1967, 4.

52. Helen Clapesattle, *The Doctors Mayo* (Rochester, Minn.: Mayo Foundation for Medical Education and Research, 1969), 1993.

53. Goodhart quoted in Glover, "Incidence of Tonsillectomy in School Children," 1219.

54. Clapesattle, *Doctors Mayo,* 193.

55. Ibid.

56. Ibid., and *Encyclopaedia Britannica,* 14th ed., 22:284.

57. Rosemary Stevens, *American Medicine and the Public Interest* (New Haven: Yale University Press, 1971), 159.

58. Bakwin, "Tonsil-Adenoidectomy Enigma," 118.

59. Rosemary Stevens, *In Sickness and in Wealth* (New York: Basic, 1989), 106.

60. Glover, "Incidence of Tonsillectomy in School Children," 1219.

61. John Romano, M.D., as quoted in Sharon R. Kaufman, *The Healer's Tale: Transforming Medicine and Culture* (Madison: University of Wisconsin Press, 1993), 99.

62. Glover, "Incidence of Tonsillectomy in School Children," 1226.

63. Ibid., 1227.

64. Ibid., 1235.

65. W. J. E. McKee, "A Controlled Study of the Effects of Tonsillectomy and Adenoidectomy in Children," *British Journal of Prevention and Social Medicine* 17 (1963): 49; N. Roydhouse, "A Controlled Study of Adenotonsillectomy," *Lancet* 2 (1 November 1969): 931–32; and R. Hinchcliffe, "Prevalence of the Commoner Ear, Nose, and Throat Conditions in the Adult Rural Population," *British Journal of Prevention and Social Medicine* 15, no. 3 (1961): 128.

66. Cochrane, *Effectiveness and Efficiency,* 60.

67. *Cost and Quality of Health Care: Unnecessary Surgery,* report by the Subcommittee on Oversight and Investigations of the Committee on Interstate and Foreign Commerce, 94th Cong., 2d sess. (Washington, D.C.: U.S. Government Printing Office, 1976).

68. Interviews by the author with John E. Wennberg, M.D., July 1994, August 1994, and September 1994; with Alan Gittelsohn, August 1994; and with John Senning, August 1994.

69. Ibid.

70. John E. Wennberg and Alan Gittelsohn, "Small Area Variations in Health Care Delivery," *Science* 182 (14 December 1973): 1102–8.

71. The quotations that follow are based on interviews by the author unless otherwise indicated.

72. John P. Bunker and John E. Wennberg, "Operation Rates, Mortality Statistics and the Quality of Life," *New England Journal of Medicine* 289, no. 23 (6 December 1973): 1249–50.

73. Interview by the author with Judith Miller Jones, 29 November 1995.

74. John E. Wennberg, "Dealing with Medical Practice Variations: A Proposal for Action," *Health Affairs* 3, no. 2 (summer 1984): 6–32.

75. Opening statement of Sen. William Proxmire, Hearing on Medical Practice Variations, Senate Committee on Appropriations, Subcommittee on Labor, Health and Human Services, and Education, 19 November 1984.

76. Testimony of John E. Wennberg, M.D., Dartmouth Medical School, Senate Committee on Appropriations, Subcommittee on Labor, Health and Human Services, and Education, 19 November 1984.

77. John E. Wennberg, John P. Bunker, and Benjamin Barnes, "The Need for Assessing the Outcome of Common Medical Practices," *Annual Review of Public Health* 1 (1980): 277–95.

78. John E. Wennberg et al., "Hospital Use and Mortality among Medicare Beneficiaries in Boston and New Haven," *New England Journal of Medicine* 321, no. 17 (26 October 1989): 1168–73.

79. Interview by the author with David M. Eddy, 24 November 1992.

80. A rule of thumb is formally known as a heuristic. This does not make it any more scientifically valid.

81. Interview by the author with David M. Eddy, 24 November 1992.

82. David M. Eddy, "Quantitative Analysis and the Practice of Medicine," *Stanford Engineer* 3, no. 1 (spring–summer 1980): 21.

83. John W. Williamson, Peter G. Goldschmidt, and Theodore Colton, "The Quality of Medical Literature: An Analysis of Validation Assessment," in *Medical Uses of Statistics*, ed. John C. Bailar III and Frederick Mosteller (Waltham, Mass.: New England Journal of Medicine Books, 1986), 370–91.

84. Robert H. Brook, *Quality of Care Assessment: A Comparison of Five Methods of Peer Review*, DHEW Publication HRA-74-3100 (Washington, D.C.: U.S. Department of Health, Education, and Welfare, July 1973).

CHAPTER THREE: FIRST, DO NO HARM

1. Richard A. Knox, "Doctor's Orders Killed Cancer Patient," *Boston Globe*, 23 March 1995, sec. 1, p. 1.

2. The surviving cancer patient was eventually identified as Maureen Bateman, a first-grade teacher. In an Associated Press story that moved over the wire on 18 December 1995, Bateman said that although she was not happy about the mistake, she forgave those involved. Bateman died on 28 May 1997, reportedly of cancer of the liver, lungs, and heart.

3. Knox, "Doctor's Orders Killed Cancer Patient," 1.

4. Associated Press, "Hospital Mishap: Rare or Rule?" 17 March 1995, from ClariNet Communications. University Community Hospital called in a New York–based public relations firm for advice on how to restore its reputation after employees acknowledged the pain of seeing their hospital joked about on the *Tonight Show* and in local communities.

5. Christine Gorman, "The Disturbing Case of the Cure That Killed the Patient," *Time*, 3 April 1995, 60–61.

6. Robert E. McAfee, "Malpractice System Needs Reform," letter in "Voices of the People," *Chicago Tribune*, 12 May 1995, sec. 1, p. 27. The estimate of two hundred newspapers to which the McAfee letter was sent comes from a personal communication from Daniel Meier, AMA director of news information.

7. Todd's letter, and a quotation from him in the *Time* article, referred to "six million" physician-patient encounters, or 50 percent fewer than the number used by McAfee. An AMA official told me that the group refined its estimate of patient encounters as time went on; the first and higher estimate was done hurriedly in response to media calls. In any event, both officials emphasize the magnitude of "positive" encounters versus the "isolated" mistakes.

8. Lucian L. Leape, "Error in Medicine," *JAMA* 272, no. 23 (21 December 1994): 1851–57.

9. David Blumenthal, "Making Medical Errors into 'Medical Treasures,'" *JAMA* 272, no. 23 (21 December 1994): 1867–68.

10. American Medical Association, "Report of the Board of Trustees on Medication Errors in Hospitals," submitted to the AMA House of Delegates at the AMA annual meeting, Chicago, June 1994. The report is a public document and was contained in the annual meeting handbook given to AMA delegates and the news media. Board reports are automatically accepted; only if a report contains recommendations is it voted on. The reports are filed for information purposes but are not considered official AMA policy.

11. Associated Press, "Top MD at Dana-Farber Quits," 10 May 1995, from ClariNet Communications.

12. Richard Saltus, "Activist Says Risk Growing of Cancer Drug Overdose," *Boston Globe,* 24 March 1995, 1.

13. Interview by the author with Michael R. Cohen, 7 April 1995.

14. CBS News, "Is Your Hospital Safe?" *48 Hours,* 14 September 1995.

15. Lucian L. Leape et al., "Preventing Medical Injury," *Quality Review Bulletin* 19, no. 5 (May 1993): 144 ff.

16. Lori B. Andrews et al., "An Alternative Strategy for Studying Adverse Events in Medical Care," *Lancet* 349, no. 9048 (1 February 1997): 309–13. See also Frank Lefevre et al., "Iatrogenic Complications in High-Risk, Elderly Patients," *Archives of Internal Medicine* 152 (October 1992): 2074–80.

17. David Barr, "Hazards of Modern Diagnosis and Therapy—the Price We Pay," *JAMA* 159, no. 115 (10 December 1955): 1452–56.

18. Louis J. Regan, "Medicine and the Law," *New England Journal of Medicine* 250, no. 11 (18 March 1954): 463.

19. Robert H. Moser, "Diseases of Medical Progress," *New England Journal of Medicine* 255, no. 13 (27 September 1956): 606–14.

20. "More than a third of a billion dollars is spent annually for worthless or harmful drugs and medicines," declared the 1933 report of the blue-ribbon committee on the costs of medical care. "At least one hundred and twenty-five millions pay for the services of blatant quacks and charlatans and of unscientific or inefficiently trained practitioners." I. S. Falk, C. Rufus Rorem, and Martha D. Ring, *The Costs of Medical Care: A Summary of Investigations on the Economic Aspects of the Prevention and Care of Illness* (Chicago: University of Chicago Press, 1933).

21. Elihu M. Schimmel, "The Hazards of Hospitalization," *Annals of Internal Medicine* 60, no. 1 (January 1964): 100–110. Schimmel's estimate correlated with an informal estimate based on his own hospital experience that David Barr made in the 1955 *JAMA* piece.

22. Digitalis-related problems were also mentioned prominently in the hazards listed in Moser's 1956 article in the *New England Journal of Medicine.*

23. *The People's Chronology* [CD-ROM], Microsoft Bookshelf (New York: Henry Holt, 1992).

24. Knight Steel et al., "Iatrogenic Illness on a General Medical Service at a University Hospital," *New England Journal of Medicine* 304, no. 11 (12 March 1981): 638–42. Researchers examined the records of 815 consecutive patients on the general medical service of a large hospital.

25. Henry Maurer, "The M.D.'s Are off Their Pedestal," *Fortune,* February 1954, 139–86.

26. Don Harper Mills, "Medical Insurance Feasibility Study—a Technical Summary," *Western Journal of Medicine* 128 (April 1978): 360–65. The extrapolation to California was made by Mills.

27. Ibid.

28. I applied Mills's results to the number of United States hospital admissions based on American Hospital Association data.

29. *Statistical Abstract of the United States* (Washington, D.C.: U.S. Government Printing Office, 1994), 358. This represents the number of reported deaths associated with United States military involvement from the sending of advisers in 1957 through the withdrawal of troops in 1973. The exact number of deaths continues to be updated from time to time as individuals officially listed as missing are confirmed dead.

30. National Highway Traffic Safety Administration, *Traffic Safety Facts, 1993* (Washington, D.C.: U.S. Department of Transportation, 1993). By 1994, traffic deaths had declined to a still unacceptable 40,676, the NHTSA said in a press release dated 3 July 1995.

31. Mills, "Medical Insurance Feasibility Study," 360–65. "This sample so closely matched a 759,223 sample from data supplied by the California Health Data Corporation for patient discharges in 1974 that the statistics developed in the study can be generalized to the universe of patients (3,001,000) admitted to short-term acute care non-federal, general hospitals in California in 1974."

32. Ibid. "The purpose of this study was to accumulate data about the PCE [potentially compensable event] universe to provide the opportunity to consider alternative compensation plans."

33. Ibid.

34. Rosemary Stevens, *In Sickness and in Wealth* (New York: Basic, 1989), 246.

35. Robert S. Mendelsohn, *Confessions of a Medical Heretic* (Chicago: Contemporary, 1979), 185.

36. Ibid., 46.

37. Jane E. Brody, "Incompetent Surgery Is Found Not Isolated," *New York Times,* 27 January 1976, A1.

38. Statement of Dr. Sidney Wolfe for Health Research Group, Washington, D.C., before the Department of Health, Education, and Welfare Secretary's Commission on Medical Malpractice, 16 December 1971.

39. "Sidney Wolfe, MD—Excising Medicine's Tumors," *American Medical News,* 17 November 1975, 16.

40. R. B. Talley and M. F. Laventurier, "Drug-Induced Illness," *JAMA* 229, no. 8 (19 August 1974): 1043. See also M. Silverman and P. Lee, *Pills, Profits and Politics* (Berkeley: University of California Press, 1974).

41. Boyce Rensberger, "Thousands a Year Killed by Faulty Prescriptions," *New York Times,* 28 January 1976, A1.

42. Ibid.

43. Interviews by the author with Sidney M. Wolfe, M.D., 30 August 1994 and 4 March 1995.

44. Fred E. Karch and Louis Lasagna, "Adverse Drug Reactions: A Critical Review," *JAMA* 234, no. 12 (22 December 1975): 1236–41. The critique went through *JAMA*'s peer reviews for accuracy, but the group sponsoring the study might not have passed a similar examination. Despite its Naderite name, Medicine in the Public Interest was backed by the large pharmaceutical companies.

45. Hugo L. Folli et al., "Medication Error Prevention by Clinical Pharmacists in Two Children's Hospitals," *Pediatrics* 79, no. 5 (May 1987): 718–22.

46. Timothy S. Lesar et al., "Medication Prescribing Errors in a Teaching Hospital," *JAMA* 263, no. 17 (2 May 1990): 2329–34.

47. Timothy S. Lesar et al., "Factors related to Errors in Medication Prescribing," *JAMA* 277, no. 4 (22–29 January 1997): 312–17.

48. Troyen A. Brennan et al., "The Incidence of Adverse Events and Negligence in Hospitalized Patients: Results of the Harvard Medical Practice Study, I," *New England Journal of Medicine* 324, no. 6 (7 February 1991): 370–76. Like Mills, the Harvard researchers reviewed randomly sampled medical charts, in this case 30,121 patient records from fifty-one hospitals in New York State in 1984. Meanwhile, the United States may be doing better than Australia. About 16 percent (or about one in six) of admissions to Australian hospitals include an adverse event, leading to 14,000 preventable deaths each year, according to a study by Australian researchers that was presented to the nation's parliament on 1 June 1995. See Stephen M. Cordner, "Australia's Preventable Hospital Deaths," *Lancet* 345 (17 June 1995): 1562.

49. Richard A. Knox, "Anguish, Inquiry at Dana-Farber," *Boston Globe,* 23 March 1995, 17; Leape et al., "Error in Medicine"; and Leape et al., "Preventing Medical Injury."

50. Brennan et al., "Incidence of Adverse Events and Negligence in Hospitalized Patients."

51. Lucian L. Leape, "Preventability of Medical Injury," address to the American Association for the Advancement of Science, annual meeting, Chicago, 9 February 1992.

52. David W. Bates et al., "Incidence of Adverse Drug Events and Potential Adverse Drug Events," *JAMA* 275, no. 1 (5 July 1995): 29–34.

53. Associated Press, "Hundreds of Errors Are Found at 2 Hospitals," *New York Times,* 6 July 1998, sec. A, p. 8.

54. David Hilfiker, "Mistakes," in *On Doctoring,* ed. Richard Reynolds and John Stone (New York: Simon and Schuster, 1991), 376–87.

55. Charles L. Bosk, *Forgive and Remember: Managing Medical Failure* (Chicago: University of Chicago Press, 1979), 83.

56. John Christensen et al., "The Heart of Darkness: The Impact of Perceived Mistakes on Physicians," *Journal of General Internal Medicine* 7 (July–August 1992): 424–31.

57. Harold van Cott, "Human Errors: Their Causes and Reduction," in *Human Error in Medicine,* ed. Marilyn Sue Bogner (Hillsdale, N.J.: Erlbaum, 1994), 53–65.

58. Jens Rasmussen, "Afterword," in Bogner, *Human Error in Medicine,* 385–93.

59. James Reason, *Human Error* (Cambridge: Cambridge University Press, 1990).

60. Ibid., 17.

61. George Di Domizio and Michael R. Cohen, "Drug Names Can Be a Factor in Medication Errors," *Leader's Product Liability Law and Strategy* 13, no. 7 (January 1995): 1–4.

62. Ruth Bindler and Tina Bayne, "Medication Calculation Ability of Registered Nurses," *Image: Journal of Nursing Scholarship* 23, no. 4 (winter 1991): 221–23.

63. P. H. Perlstein et al., "Errors in Drug Computations during Newborn Intensive Care," *American Journal of the Diseased Child* 133 (1979): 376–79, and G. Koren, Z. Barzilay, and M. Modan, "Errors in Computing Drug Doses," *Canadian Medical Association Journal* 129 (1983): 721–23.

64. Richard Saltus, "Medication Mixups a Growing Concern," *Boston Globe,* 7 April 1995, 1.

65. Oliver Wendell Holmes Sr., *Medical Essays: 1842–1882* (Boston: Houghton, Mifflin, 1883), 203.

66. Knox, "Doctor's Orders Killed Cancer Patient."

67. Saltus, "Medication Mixups a Growing Concern."

68. Knox, "Doctor's Orders Killed Cancer Patient."

69. Andrew Fegelman, "U. of C. Cancer Patient Dies of Chemotherapy Overdose," *Chicago Tribune,* 15 June 1995, sec. 2, p. 12.

70. Michael L. Millenson, "Doctors' Decisions Put under Microscope," *Chicago Tribune,* 17 June 1987, sec. 1, p. 1.

71. Steve Marshall, "Travelers 'Refuse to Get on Planes,' " *USA Today,* 14 December 1994, A3.

72. National Transportation Safety Board, "Airline Fatalities for 1994 Climbed to Five-Year High," news release, 19 January 1995, and Air Transport Association, "The Annual Report of the U.S. Scheduled Airline Industry," news release, 1994.

73. National Transportation Safety Board, "Airline Fatalities for 1994 Climbed to Five-Year High," and personal communication from Deborah McElroy of the Regional Airline Association, 20 July 1995.

74. Calculations by the author.

75. Linda O. Prager, "Safety-Centered Care," *American Medical News,* 13 May 1996, 1.

76. Di Domizio and Cohen, "Drug Names Can Be a Factor in Medication Errors."

77. The information on the *New England Journal of Medicine* editorial and on the National Practitioner Data Bank comes from Jay Greene, "Malpractice Issues Prove Daunting," *Modern Healthcare,* 10 June 1996, 32.

78. Berkeley Rice, "Do Doctors Kill 80,000 Patients a Year?" *Medical Economics* 71, no. 22 (21 November 1994): 46–56.

79. Marilyn Sue Bogner, "Introduction," in Bogner, *Human Error in Medicine,* 1–11.

80. Prager, "Safety-Centered Care," 1.

81. Interview by the author with Martin J. Hatlie, director of the department of professional liability and patient safety at the American Medical Association and executive director of the National Patient Safety Foundation, 17 January 1997.

CHAPTER FOUR: SAVING LIVES, BIT BY BYTE

1. David C. Classen et al., "Computerized Surveillance of Adverse Drug Events in Hospital Patients," *JAMA* 266, no. 20 (27 November 1991): 2847–51.

2. Diane L. Kennedy, Joyce M. Johnson, and Stuart L. Nightingale, "Monitor-

ing of Adverse Drug Events in Hospitals," *JAMA* 266, no. 20 (27 November 1991): 2878.

3. David C. Classen et al., "The Timing of Prophylactic Administration of Antibiotics and the Risk of Surgical-Wound Infection," *New England Journal of Medicine* 326, no. 5 (30 January 1992): 281–86.

4. Charles Rosenberg, *The Care of Strangers* (New York: Basic, 1987), 23.

5. *AHA American Hospital Association Statistics, 1992–93* (Chicago: American Hospital Association, 1993), xxxviii–xxxix, and *Source Book of Health Insurance Data* (Washington, D.C.: Health Insurance Association of America, 1992), 82.

6. Lewin-ICF and the National Committee for Quality Health Care, *Tracking the System: American Health Care, 1992* (Washington, D.C.: National Committee for Quality Health Care, 1992), 11.

7. William O. Robertson, "Errors in Prescribing," *American Journal of Health-System Pharmacy* 52 (15 February 1995): 382–85; quotation on 383.

8. Interview by the author with Henri Manasse Jr., Pharm.D., University of Iowa, 10 May 1995.

9. William N. Kelly, "Pharmacy Contributions to Adverse Medication Events," *American Journal of Health-System Pharmacy* 52 (15 February 1995): 385–90; quotation on 385.

10. Health and Public Policy Committee, American College of Physicians, Philadelphia, "Improving Medical Education in Therapeutics," *Annals of Internal Medicine* 108, no. 1 (January 1988): 145–47.

11. Henri R. Manasse Jr., "Toward Defining and Applying a Higher Standard of Quality for Medication Use in the United States," *American Journal of Health-System Pharmacy* 52 (15 February 1995): 374–79; quotation on 377.

12. Hermann Blumgart, "Caring for the Patient," *New England Journal of Medicine* 270, no. 9 (27 February 1964): 449–56.

13. Classen et al., "Computerized Surveillance of Adverse Drug Events in Hospital Patients," 2849.

14. Michael L. Millenson, "Computer Watchdogs Are Saving Patients' Lives," *Chicago Tribune,* 10 May 1993, sec. 1, p. 1.

15. Details of Warner's life come from several interviews with him by the author, beginning 13 July 1995; from his writings; from Henry P. Plenk, *Medicine in the Beehive State* (Salt Lake City: Utah Medical Association and LDS Hospital–Deseret Foundation and University of Utah Health Sciences Center, 1992); and from Gilad J. Kuperman, Reed M. Gardner, and T. Allan Pryor, *HELP: A Dynamic Hospital Information System* (New York: Springer-Verlag, 1991).

16. Marguerite Zientara, *The History of Computing* (Framingham, Mass.: CW Communications, 1981), 22–25.

17. While helping out with the census, Billings retained his post as assistant surgeon general in the U.S. Army.

18. Plenk, *Medicine in the Beehive State,* 479.

19. Jonathan Spivak, "Electronic Medicine: Scientists Press Work on Advanced Machines to Aid Medical Care," *Wall Street Journal,* 17 August 1959, 1.

20. Plenck, *Medicine in the Beehive State,* 480.

21. Kuperman, Gardner, and Pryor, *HELP,* 7 ff.

22. Plenk, *Medicine in the Beehive State,* 481–82.

23. Kuperman, Gardner, and Pryor, *HELP,* 7.

24. Homer R. Warner, *Computer-Assisted Medical Decision Making* (New York: Academic, 1979), 1–5.

25. Ibid.

26. Richard A. Shaffer, "Doctors' Helpers: Computers Play an Increasing Role in Diagnosing and Recommending Treatment of Medical Problems," *Wall Street Journal,* 9 July 1973, 24.

27. Eugene Stead, "Patient Management Systems: The Early Years," in *A History of Medical Informatics,* ed. Bruce I. Blum and Karen Duncan (New York: ACM, 1990), 377.

28. Kuperman, Gardner, and Pryor, *HELP,* 9.

29. This description is based on interviews by the author with LDS officials and on articles written by them.

30. Presentation by R. Scott Evans to annual meeting of Association of Health Services Researchers, Chicago, 5 June 1995.

31. Ibid.

32. Troyen A. Brennan et al. "The Incidence of Adverse Events and Negligence in Hospitalized Patients: Results of the Harvard Medical Practice Study, I," *New England Journal of Medicine* 324, no. 6 (7 February 1991): 370–76.

33. Stanley L. Pestotnik et al., "Implementing Antibiotic Practice Guidelines through Computer-Assisted Decision Support: Clinical and Financial Outcomes," *Annals of Internal Medicine* 124, no. 10 (15 May 1996): 884–90.

34. Classen et al., "Computerized Surveillance of Adverse Drug Events in Hospital Patients," 2849.

35. Brennan et al., "Incidence of Adverse Events and Negligence in Hospitalized Patients."

36. C. Gregory Elliott, "Computer-Assisted Quality Assurance: Development and Performance of a Respiratory Care Program, *Quality Review Bulletin* 17, no. 3 (March 1991): 86–90.

37. Reed M. Gardner et al., "Computerized Continuous Quality Improvement Methods Used to Optimize Blood Transfusions," *SCAMC* 17 (1993): 166–70.

38. Pestotnik et al., "Implementing Antibiotic Practice Guidelines through Computer-Assisted Decision Support."

39. Millenson, "Computer Watchdogs Are Saving Lives," 1.

40. Marcus J. Smith, *Error and Variation in Diagnostic Radiology* (Springfield, Ill.: Thomas, 1967).

41. Ibid., viii.

42. Presentation by Spencer Borden IV, M.D., to National Imaging Advisory Council of Medicon, Inc., Palm Springs, California, 2 April 1995. Thomas K. P. Egglin and Alvan Feinstein, "Context Bias," *JAMA* 276, no. 21 (4 December 1996): 1752–55, concluded that "radiologists' diagnoses are significantly influenced" by whether they are told before reading an image that the patient likely has disease.

43. D. Pittet et al., "Nosocomial Bloodstream Infection in Critically Ill Patients," *JAMA* 271, no. 20 (25 May 1994): 1598–1602.

44. Interview by the author with Richard Wenzel, M.D., 4 May 1995.

45. Associated Press, "Doctors Urged to Wash Their Hands," 19 June 1995, from ClariNet Communications.

46. Barbara A. Mark, "Measurement of Patient Outcomes: Data Availability and Consistency across Hospitals," *Journal of Nursing Administration* 25, no. 4 (April 1995): 52–59.

47. S. I. Allen and M. Otten, "The Telephone as a Computer Input-Output Terminal for Medical Information," *JAMA* 208, no. 4 (28 April 1969): 673–79.

48. Interview by the author on 29 May 1995 with Kenneth Barker, Ph.D., professor and chairman of Department of Pharmacy Care Systems, School of Pharmacy, Auburn University.

49. Evlin L. Kinney, "Expert System of Drug Interactions: Results in Consecutive Inpatients," *Computers and Biomedical Research* 19 (1986): 462–67.

50. Charles Clark, "Healthcare Info. Systems," *Value Line* report, 7 April 1995, 679.

51. Sheldon Dorenfest Associates data quoted in John Morrissey, "Growth in Information System Expenditures Will Continue, Study Projects," *Modern Healthcare,* 19 June 1995, 74.

52. Associated Press, "Cancer Misreadings Spark Calls," 12 July 1995, from ClariNet Communications.

53. Interview by the author with Evan Rosen, M.D., 24 June 1994.

54. David M. Rind et al., "Effect of Computer-Based Alerts on the Treatment and Outcomes of Hospitalized Patients," *Archives of Internal Medicine,* 154, no. 13 (11 July 1994): 1511–17.

55. Ibid., 1516.

56. David C. Classen et al., "Adverse Drug Events in Hospitalized Patients," *JAMA* 277, no. 4 (22–29 January 1997): 301–6.

57. David W. Bates et al. for the Adverse Drug Events Prevention Study Group, "The Costs of Adverse Drug Events in Hospitalized Patients," *JAMA* 277, no. 4 (22–29 January 1997): 307–11.

58. Millenson, "Computer Watchdogs Are Saving Lives."

59. Note posted to use group sci.med.informatics. The author of the note did not respond to phone messages asking for further comment.

CHAPTER FIVE: STATE OF THE ART

1. Sharon R. Kaufman, *The Healer's Tale: Transforming Medicine and Culture* (Madison: University of Wisconsin Press, 1993).

2. Bernard S. Bloom, "Does It Work? The Outcomes of Medical Interventions," *International Journal of Technology Assessment in Health Care* 6 (1990): 326–32.

3. J. Rosser Matthews, *Quantification and the Quest for Medical Certainty* (Princeton: Princeton University Press, 1995), 11.

4. Interviews by the author with Dennis Heuston and Gypsy Heuston Martinez, 12 August 1995.

5. Richard Gordon, *The Alarming History of Medicine* (New York: St. Martin's Press, 1993), 173.

6. Associated Press, "PDR Goes On-Line," 5 December 1995, from ClariNet Communications. The prescriptions described were listed in the 1947 edition of the *Physicians' Desk Reference.*

7. Matthews, *Quantification and the Quest for Medical Certainty,* 16.

8. Alfredo Morabia, "P. C. A. Louis and the Birth of Clinical Epidemiology," *Journal of Clinical Epidemiology* 49, no. 12 (December 1996): 1327–33.

9. Gordon, *Alarming History of Medicine,* 170.

10. Matthews, *Quantification and the Quest for Medical Certainty,* 16.

11. Bloom, "Does It Work?" 328.

12. Various experiments with randomization and with large-scale clinical trials were under way in the United States at about the same time as the efforts in Britain by Austin Bradford Hill (later Sir Austin Bradford Hill). These included an investigation of the common cold at the University of Minnesota and a series of experiments carried out by the Veterans Administration. However, Bradford Hill's work is generally considered the research that established the randomized clinical trial. See Streptomycin Tuberculosis Trials Committee, "Streptomycin Treatment of Pulmonary Tuberculosis: A Medical Research Council Investigation," *British Medical Journal* 20 (30 October 1948): 769–82.

13. Matthews, *Quantification and the Quest for Medical Certainty,* 127–19, and William A. Silverman, "Doing More Good Than Harm," in "Doing More Good Than Harm: The Evaluation of Health Care Interventions," ed. Kenneth S. Warren and Frederick Mosteller, *Annals of the New York Academy of Sciences* 703 (31 December 1993): 5–11.

14. Ibid., 131–32.

15. Antonio Anzueto et al., "Aerosolized Surfactant in Adults with Sepsis-Induced Acute Respiratory Distress Syndrome," *New England Journal of Medicine* 34, no. 22 (30 May 1996): 1417–21; quotation on 1421.

16. Alan H. Morris and Mary R. Suchyta, "Extracorporeal CO_2 Removal for ARDS and the Evalaution of New Therapy," in *Principles and Practice of Mechanical Ventilation,* ed. Martin J. Tobin (New York: McGraw-Hill, 1994), 490.

17. Matthews, *Quantification and the Quest for Medical Certainty,* 134.

18. Paul Starr, *The Social Transformation of Amercian Medicine* (New York: Basic, 1982), 130.

19. Rosemary Stevens, *In Sickness and in Wealth: American Hospitals in the Twentieth Century* (New York: Basic, 1989), 177.

20. Paul M. Wax, "Elixirs, Dilutents and the Passage of the 1938 Federal Food, Drug and Cosmetic Act," *Annals of Internal Medicine* 122, no. 6 (15 March 1995): 456–61.

21. Morton Mintz, "Remembering Thalidomide: The Proposed FDA Reforms the Republicans Have in Mind Could Have Tragic Consequences," *Washington Post National Weekly Edition,* 22–28 July 1996, 21.

22. Melvin Konner, *Medicine at the Crossroads* (New York: Pantheon, 1993), 129.

23. *The Mosby Medical Encyclopedia,* rev. ed. (New York: Plume, 1992), 469.

24. Owen H. Wangensteen et al., "Achieving 'Physiological Gastrectomy' by Gastric Freezing," *JAMA* 180, no. 6 (12 May 1962): 439–44.

25. James M. Edmonson, "Gastric Freezing: The View a Quarter Century Later," *Journal of Laboratory and Clinical Medicine* 114, no. 5 (November 1989): 613–14.

26. Kenneth Schulz et al., "Empirical Evidence of Bias: Dimensions of Methodological Quality Associated with Estimates of Treatment Effects in Controlled Trials," *JAMA* 273, no. 5 (1 February 1995): 408–12; Frederick Mosteller, John P. Gilbert, and Bucknam McPeek, "Reporting Standards and Research Strategies for Controlled Trials: Agenda for the Editor," *Controlled Clinical Trials* 1 (1980): 37–58; Coronary Drug Project Research Group, "Influence of Adherence to Treatment and Response of Cholesterol on Mortality in the Coronary Drug Project," *New England Journal of Medicine* 303, no. 18 (30 October 1980): 1038–41.

27. D. Moher, C. S. Dulberg, and G. A. Wells, "Statistical Power, Sample Size and Their Reporting in Randomized Controlled Trials," *JAMA* 272, no. 2 (13 July 1994): 122–24. The authors found that some trials were incapable of showing a statistically significant result unless the treatment was 25 to 50 percent better than the alternative.

28. Alan H. Morris et al., "Randomized Clinical Trial of Pressure-Controlled Inverse Ratio Ventilation and Extracorporeal $C0_2$ Removal for Adult Respiratory Distress Syndrome," *American Journal of Respiratory and Critical Care Medicine* 149 (1994): 295–305.

29. Susan Henderson et al., "Performance of Computerized Protocols for the Management of Arterial Oxygenation in an Intensive Care Unit," *International Journal of Clinical Monitoring and Computing* 8 (1992): 271–80.

30. Alan H. Morris and Brent C. James, "CPI and Computerized Protocols: An Example," in *Clinical Practice Improvement: A New Technology for Development Cost-Effective Quality Health Care* (New York: Faulkner and Gray, 1994), 141–49, esp. 144.

31. Interview by the author with Patty Robbins, mother of Tami Robbins, March 1993.

32. The historical survival rate, as Morris cautioned, was not a good comparison. Other trials going on at the same time as the one at LDS have also increased the survival rate, according to one reviewer, perhaps because of similar attention to better management of patients. However, it is almost impossible to make head-to-head comparisons of trials because of differences in patient selection. The LDS protocol is now being tried out in a randomized clinical trial. For background see Michael A. Matthay, "The Acute Respiratory Distress Syndrome," *New England Journal of Medicine* 334, no. 22 (30 May 1996): 1469–70.

33. Morris and Suchyta, "Extracorporeal CO_2 Removal for ARDS and the Evaluation of New Therapy," 489.

34. Morris et al., "Randomized Clinical Trial of Pressure-Controlled Inverse Ratio Ventilation and Extracorporeal $C0_2$ Removal for Adult Respiratory Distress Syndrome."

35. Interview by the author with Marin Kollef, M.D., 25 July 1995.

36. Personal communication from Thomas East, Ph.D., assistant director of medical informatics at LDS Hospital, 29 January 1997.

37. Michael A. Matthay, "The Acute Respiratory Distress Syndrome," *JAMA* 334, no. 22 (30 May 1996): 1469–70.

CHAPTER SIX: STATE OF THE SCIENCE

1. Unless otherwise cited, the quotations from Scott R. Weingarten and the account of the guideline implementation experience at Cedars are based on interviews with him by the author as well as presentations by Weingarten. These presentations were made at the Zitter Group's First Annual Congress on Health Outcomes and Accountability in Washington, D.C., on 12 December 1994 and at a Chicago conference, "Measuring Performance and Implementing Improvement," sponsored by the Hackensack (New Jersey) Medical Center, the Primary Care Outcomes Research Institute of New England Medical Center (Boston), and the University of Medicine and Dentistry in New Brunswick, New Jersey. Weingarten spoke there on 27 April 1995.

2. Lee Goldman, "Changing Physicians' Behavior," *New England Journal of Medicine* 322, no. 21 (24 May 1990): 1524–25.

3. John W. Williamson et al., "Health Science Information Management and Continuing Education of Physicians," *Annals of Internal Medicine* 110, no. 2 (15 January 1989): 151–60. Conclusions similar to those of Williamson et al. were reached by two physicians in a 1979 article that surveyed primary care physicians about their knowledge of a new therapy to treat diabetic retinopathy, a common problem. See Jeffrey K. Stross and William R. Harlan, "The Dissemination of New Medical Information," *JAMA* 241, no. 24 (15 June 1979): 2622–24. See also D. G. Covell, G. C. Uman, and P. R. Manning, "Information Needs in Office Practice: Are They Being Met?" *Annals of Internal Medicine* 103, no. 4 (October 1985): 596–99.

4. Ann Lennarson Greer, "The Two Cultures of Biomedicine: Can There Be Consensus?" *JAMA* 258, no. 19 (20 November 1987): 2739–40.

5. P. G. Ramsey et al., "Changes over Time in the Knowledge Base of Practicing Internists," *JAMA* 266, no. 8 (28 August 1991): 1103–07.

6. Sherwin B. Nuland, "Medical Fads: Bran, Midwives and Leeches," *New York Times,* 25 June 1995, E16.

7. Cynthia D. Mulrow, Stephen B. Thacker, and Jacqueline A. Pugh, "A Proposal for More Informative Abstracts of Review Articles," *Annals of Internal Medicine* 108, no. 4 (April 1988): 613–15.

8. Stuart J. Pocock, Michael D. Hughes, and Robert J. Lee, "Statistical Problems in the Reporting of Clinical Trials," *JAMA* 317 (13 August 1987): 426–32.

9. Robert Rosenthal, "The 'File Drawer Problem' and the Tolerance for Null Results," *Psychological Bulletin* 86, no. 3 (1979): 638–44.

10. Melville H. Hodge, "Direct Use by Physicians of the TDS Medical Information System," in *A History of Medical Informatics,* ed. Bruce I. Blum and Karen Duncan (New York: ACM, 1990), 352.

11. Gervasio A. Lamas et al., "Do the Results of Randomized Clinical Trials of Cardiovascular Drugs Influence Medical Practice?" *New England Journal of Medicine* 327, no. 4 (23 July 1992): 241–47.

12. Ibid.

13. Warren E. Leary, "Aspirin Proposed for Suspected Heart Attacks," *New York Times,* 19 June 1996, B7.

14. Barry J. Marshall, "*Helicobacter pylori:* The Etiologic Agent for Peptic Ulcer," *JAMA* 274, no. 13 (4 October 1995): 1064–66.

15. Barry J. Marshall et al., "A Prospective Double-Blind Trial of Duodenal Ulcer Relapse after Eradication of *Campylobacter pylori,*" *Lancet* 2, no. 8626–27 (24–31 December 1988): 1437–42.

16. Ibid. The history of ulcer treatment is enough to give scientists heartburn. Well before the recent interest in *H. pylori,* researchers in Denmark looked at a decade's worth of clinical trials testing various treatments. To their dismay, they found that medical textbooks in 1974 continued to recommend—and Danish physicians continued to prescribe—treatments that had been proved by careful analysis to have no effect during trials conducted from 1964 to 1973.

17. D. Y. Graham et al., "Effect of Triple Therapy (Antibiotics Plus Bismuth) on Duodenal Ulcer Healing: A Randomized Controlled Trial," *Annals of Internal Medicine* 115, no. 4 (15 August 1991): 266–69.

18. "NIH Consensus Development Panel on *Helicobacter pylori* in Peptic Ulcer Disease," *JAMA* 272, no. 1 (6 July 1994): 65–69.

19. "Lasker Awards Honor Physicians, Scientists, Senator," *American Medical News,* 9 October 1995, 9.

20. Personal communication from Bernard S. Bloom, Ph.D., University of Pennsylvania. Bloom's assertion was based on an unpublished study of proprietary IMS America data on prescriptions written in the United States.

21. Thomas F. Imperiale et al., "A Cost Analysis of Alternative Treatments for Duodenal Ulcer," *Annals of Internal Medicine* 123, no. 9 (1 November 1995): 665–72.

22. Andrew Haines and Roger Jones, "Implementing Findings of Research," *British Medical Journal* 308 (4 June 1994): 1488–92.

23. E. Antman et al., "A Comparison of the Results of Meta-analysis of Randomized Controlled Trials and Recommendations of Clinical Experts," *JAMA* 268, no. 2 (8 July 1992): 240–48.

24. F. A. Hubbell et al., "The Impact of Routine Admission Chest X-Ray Films on Patient Care," *New England Journal of Medicine* 312, no. 4 (24 January 1985): 209–13.

25. Dan W. Blumhagen, "The Doctor's White Coat: The Image of the Physician in Modern America," *Annals of Internal Medicine* 91, no. 1 (July 1979): 111–16; quotation on 113.

26. Jeremiah A. Barondess, "Medicine and Its Mandate: Reasons for Change," keynote address to the Centennial Symposium, Johns Hopkins Medical Institutions, 23–24 February 1990.

27. Eliot Freidson, *Profession of Medicine: A Study of the Sociology of Applied Knowledge* (New York: Dodd, Mead, 1970), 347.

28. Richard B. Warnecke et al., "The Community Clinical Oncology Program: Its Effect on Clinical Practice," *Joint Commission Journal on Quality Improvement* 21, no. 7 (July 1995): 336–39.

29. E. J. Feuer et al., "The Lifetime Risk of Developing Breast Cancer," *Journal of the National Cancer Institute* 85 (1993): 892–99.

30. John H. Ferguson, "Technology Transfer: Consensus and Participation; the NIH Consensus Development Program," *Joint Commission Journal on Quality Improvement* 21, no. 7 (July 1995): 332–36.

31. Jacqueline Kosecoff et al., "Effect of the National Institutes of Health Consensus Development Program on Physician Practice," *JAMA* 258, no. 19 (20 November 1987): 2708–13. The RAND conclusions were buttressed by later studies and are acknowledged by NIH as accurate. It is not that physicians disagreed with the recommendations; they simply did not change their behavior. See Ferguson, "Technology Transfer."

32. David A. Davis et al., "Changing Physician Performance: A Systematic Review of the Effect of Continuing Medical Education Strategies," *JAMA* 274, no. 9 (6 September 1995): 700–705.

33. Ibid. The conclusions of the article were echoed in a later commentary that called for physicians to use computerized protocols to remind them of the best proven practices. See Bruce Slater, "Systematic Practice-Based Interventions Are Better Than Conferences for Improving Professional Practice," *Evidence-Based Medicine* 2, no. 6 (January–February 1996): 60–61.

34. John M. Eisenberg, *Doctors' Decisions and the Cost of Medical Care* (Ann Arbor: Health Administration Press, 1986), 116–17.

35. Ibid.

36. W. Bruce Fye, "The Literature of Internal Medicine," in *Grand Rounds: One Hundred Years of Internal Medicine,* ed. Russell C. Maulitz and Diana E. Long (Philadelphia: University of Pennsylvania Press, 1988), 73.

37. Everett M. Rogers, "Lessons for Guidelines from the Diffusion of Innovations," *Joint Commission Journal on Quality Improvement* 21, no. 7 (July 1995): 324–28. Adapted from presentations to "Effecting Change in Physician Practice: Moraine Institute Diffusion/Dissemination Conference," Kansas City, Missouri, 26–27 September 1994.

38. David L. Sackett and William M. C. Rosenberg, "On the Need for Evidence-Based Medicine," *Health Economics* 4 (1995): 249–54.

39. David L. Sackett and R. Brian Haynes, "On the Need for Evidence-Based Medicine," *Evidence-Based Medicine* 1, no. 1 (November–December 1995): 5–6.

40. Personal communication to author from John W. Williamson, M.D., 17 August 1994. The 85 percent estimate of untested medical practice—see introduction, at note 3—was challenged in C. David Naylor, "Grey Zones of Clinical Practice: Some Limits to Evidence-Based Medicine," *Lancet* 345 (1 April 1995): 840–42. Nonetheless Naylor, using a different definition of clinical practices, still concluded that 50 percent had not been scientifically validated.

41. D. L. Kent et al., "The Clinical Efficacy of Magnetic Resonance Imaging in Neuroimaging," *Annals of Internal Medicine* 120, no. 10 (15 May 1994): 856–71. See also Lawton S. Cooper et al., "The Poor Quality of Early Evaluations of Magnetic Resonance Imaging," *JAMA* 259, no. 2 (10 June 1988): 3277–80.

42. Peter E. Dans, "Credibility, Cookbook Medicine and Common Sense: Guidelines and the College," *Annals of Internal Medicine* 120, no. 11 (1 June 1994): 966–68.

43. H. David Reines et al., "Chest Physiotherapy Fails to Prevent Postopera-

tive Atelectasis in Children after Cardiac Surgery," *Annals of Surgery* 195 (April 1982): 451–55.

44. Weingarten presentations and the following articles: Scott R. Weingarten et al., "Identification of Low-Risk Hospitalized Patients with Pneumonia," *Chest* 105, no. 4 (April 1994): 1109–15, and Scott R. Weingarten et al., "Evaluation of a Pneumonia Practice Guideline in an Interventional Trial," *American Journal of Respiratory Medicine and Critical Care Medicine* 153 (1996): 1110–15.

45. Weingarten et al., "Evaluation of a Pneumonia Practice Guideline in an Interventional Trial."

46. A. Gray Ellrodt et al., "Measuring and Improving Physician Compliance with Clinical Practice Guidelines," *Annals of Internal Medicine* 122, no. 4 (15 February 1995): 277–82.

47. Weingarten et al., "Evaluation of a Pneumonia Practice Guideline in an Interventional Trial."

48. A 1991 study put the use of prophylaxis in high-risk patients undergoing orthopedic surgery at 38.8 percent. It is unclear what the patient mix was at Cedars-Sinai. See Frederick A. Anderson Jr. et al., "Physician Practices in the Prevention of Venous Thromboembolosis," *Annals of Internal Medicine* 115, no. 8 (15 October 1991): 594.

49. Mark Ferguson, dean of the school of biological sciences in Manchester, England, quoted in an editorial in the *British Medical Journal.* See "From Innovation to Evaluation," *BMJ* 311, no. 7011 (14 October 1995): 961.

50. J. M. Grimshaw and I. T. Russell, "Effect of Clinical Guidelines on Medical Practice: A Systematic Review of Rigorous Evaluations," *Lancet* 342, no. 8883 (27 November 1993): 1317–22.

51. James Reason, *Human Error* (Cambridge: Cambridge University Press, 1990).

52. Interview by the author with William Jessee, M.D., vice president for quality and managed care, American Medical Association, 16 January 1997.

53. Stephen B. Soumerai et al., "Adverse Outcomes of Underuse of β-blockers in Elderly Survivors of Acute Myocardial Infarction," *JAMA* 277, no. 2 (8 January 1997): 115–21. The researchers examined care in New Jersey.

54. William Campbell Felch and Donald M. Scanlon, "Bridging the Gap between Research and Practice: The Role of Continuing Medical Education," *JAMA* 277, no. 2 (8 January 1997): 155–56.

55. Kenneth I. Shine, remarks contained in press release of the New York Academy of Sciences for its conference "Beyond the Crisis: Preserving the Capacity for Excellence in Health Care and Medical Science," 14–15 February 1994.

56. Haines and Jones, "Implementing Findings of Research."

CHAPTER SEVEN: TRUST ME, I'M A DOCTOR

1. Elspeth Huxley, *Florence Nightingale* (London: Weidenfeld and Nicolson, 1975), 186.

2. Florence Nightingale quoted in Richard Gordon's *The Alarming History of Medicine* (New York: St. Martin's Press, 1993), 237.

3. Florence Nightingale, *Notes on Hospitals* (London: John W. Parker, 1859).

The physician E. W. Groves made a plea for uniform surgical statistics in the *British Medical Journal* 2 (1908): 1008–9, with no more success than Nightingale.

4. Adam Smith, *Power of the Mind* (New York: Ballantine, 1975), 19.

5. Thomas S. Kuhn, *The Structure of Scientific Revolutions,* 2d ed. (Chicago: University of Chicago Press, 1970), 175.

6. The discussion of paradigms, in addition to drawing directly on Kuhn's book, is informed by the perceptive treatment in Joel Arthur Barker, *Future Edge: Discovering the New Paradigms of Success* (New York: William Morrow, 1992).

7. Kuhn, *Structure of Scientific Revolutions,* 6.

8. Unless otherwise indicated, biographical information on Codman comes from "An Autobiographic Preface," part of his book *The Shoulder* (Boston: Thomas Todd, 1934). Codman paid for his own printing based on subscriptions from friends rather than be pressed by a publisher to leave out the harangues about contemporary medical practice contained in his provocative preface and epilogue.

9. Duncan Neuhauser, "Ernest Amory Codman, M.D., and End Results of Medical Care," *International Journal of Technology Assessment in Health Care* 6 (1990): 307–25. I am grateful to Neuhauser for the guidance provided by both his writings and his personal suggestions in this discussion of Codman and of the rest of the early history of medical quality research. An early Codmanphile, Neuhauser says he measures the strength of the Codman revival by the price of an out-of-print copy of *The Shoulder.*

10. Ibid.

11. Ibid., xii.

12. The description that follows is based largely on Loyal Davis's *Fellowship of Surgeons: A History of the American College of Surgeons* (Springfield, Ill.: Thomas, 1960).

13. Codman, *Shoulder,* xvi.

14. Duncan Neuhauser, *Coming of Age: A 50 Year History of the American College of Hospital Administrators and the Profession It Serves, 1933–1983* (Chicago: Pluribus, 1983), 172.

15. Susan Reverby, "Stealing the Golden Eggs: Ernest Amory Codman and the Science and Management of Medicine," *Bulletin of the History of Medicine* 55 (1981): 156–71; quotations on 160–61.

16. *One Hundredth Annual Report of the Trustees of the Massachusetts General Hospital* (Cambridge: Cambridge University Press, 1913), 107.

17. Davis, *Fellowship of Surgeons,* 117–18.

18. Rosemary Stevens, *In Sickness and in Wealth: American Hospitals in the Twentieth Century* (New York: Basic, 1989), 77.

19. Davis, *Fellowship of Surgeons,* 176.

20. Ernest Amory Codman, *A Study in Hospital Efficiency* (Oakbrook Terrace, Ill.: Joint Commission on the Accreditation of Healthcare Organizations, 1996), 183. Reprint of 1917 text, with extra commentary material added.

21. James Roberts, Jack Coale, and Robert Redman, "A History of the Joint Commission on Accreditation of Hospitals," unpublished paper, 1987 (later version published in *JAMA* 258, no. 7 [21 August 1987]: 936–40).

22. Stevens, *In Sickness and in Wealth,* 123–24.

23. Codman address of 14 May 1913, later reprinted as "The Product of a Hospital" in the April 1914 issue of *Surgery, Gynecology, and Obstetrics.* Quoted by Codman in the preface to *Shoulder,* xviii.

24. David K. Patterson and Gerald F. Pyle, "The Geography and Mortality of the 1918 Influenza Pandemic," *Bulletin of the History of Medicine* 65 (1991): 4–21.

25. *One Hundred and Thirty-seventh Annual Report of the Trustees of the Massachusetts General Hospital* (Boston, 1950), 45.

26. I. S. Falk, C. R. Rorem, and M. D. Ring, *The Costs of Medical Care: A Summary of Investigations on the Economic Aspects of the Prevention and Care of Illness,* Publications of the Committee on the Costs of Medical Care 27 (Chicago: University of Chicago Press, 1933).

27. See *1955–56 Annual Report, W. H. Kellogg Foundation,* for this and following facts, unless otherwise indicated.

28. Richard Carter, *The Doctor Business* (New York: Doubleday, 1958), 74.

29. Ray Vicker, "Medic Merchants: Doctors Treat More Patients Faster; Some Level Fee Schedules," *Wall Street Journal,* 15 June 1956.

30. Cartoon reprinted in John C. Burnham, "American Medicine's Golden Age: What Happened to It?" *Science* 215 (19 March 1982): 1474–79.

31. Greer Williams, "Unjustified Surgery," *Harpers Magazine* 208, no. 1245 (February 1954): 35–41.

32. Lawrence P. Williams, *How to Avoid Unnecessary Surgery* (Los Angeles: Nash, 1971), 431.

33. Norman F. Miller, "Hysterectomy: Therapeutic Necessity or Surgical Racket?" *American Journal of Obstetrics and Gynecology* 51 (June 1946): 804–10.

34. James C. Doyle, "Unnecessary Ovariectomies: Study Based on Removal of 704 Normal Ovaries from 546 Patients," *JAMA* 148, no. 13 (29 March 1952): 1105–11.

35. James C. Doyle, "Unnecessary Hysterectomies: Study of 6,248 Operations in Thirty-five Hospitals during 1948," *JAMA* 151, no. 5 (31 January 1953): 360–65.

36. Williams, *How to Avoid Unnecessary Surgery,* 215.

37. The biographical information that follows, unless otherwise indicated, is excerpted from George A. Silver's article "Paul Anthony Lembcke, MD, MPH: A Pioneer in Medical Care Evaluation," *American Journal of Public Health* 80, no. 3 (March 1990): 342–48.

38. Paul A. Lembcke, "Prevention and Control of Epidemic Diarrhea Is the Administrator's Responsibility," *Modern Hospital* 60 (1943): 98–102.

39. Paul A. Lembcke, "Medical Auditing by Scientific Methods: Illustrated by Major Female Pelvic Surgery," *JAMA* 162, no. 7 (13 October 1956): 646–55.

40. Codman, "Product of a Hospital."

41. Paul A. Lembcke, "Evolution of the Medical Audit," *JAMA* 199, no. 8 (20 February 1967): 543–50.

42. Lembcke, "Medical Auditing by Scientific Methods."

43. Paul A. Lembcke, "Measuring the Quality of Medical Care through Vital

Statistics Based on Hospital Service Areas: 1. Comparative Study of Appendectomy Rates," *American Journal of Public Health* 42 (1952): 276–86.

44. Williams, "Unjustified Surgery."

45. Lembcke, "Measuring the Quality of Medical Care."

46. Bryan Bunch and Alexander Hellemans, *The Timetables of Technology: A Chronology of the Most Important People and Events in the History of Technology* (New York: Simon and Schuster, 1993).

47. Robert S. Myers, Vergil N. Slee, and Robert G. Hoffmann, "The Medical Audit," *Modern Hospital* 85 (September 1955): 77–83.

48. Vergil N. Slee, "Statistics Influence Medical Practice," *Bulletin of the American College of Surgeons* 39 (November–December 1954): 397–402.

49. C. Wesley Eisele, Vergil N. Slee, and Robert G. Hoffmann, "Can the Practice of Internal Medicine Be Evaluated?" *Annals of Internal Medicine* 44, no. 1 (January 1956): 144–61.

50. Response by a past president of the Association of American Physicians in *American Medicine:. Expert Testimony out of Court,* vol. 1 (New York: American Foundation, 1937), 160.

51. Osler L. Peterson et al., "An Analytical Study of North Carolina General Practice," *Journal of Medical Education* 31, no. 2 (December 1956): 1–165.

52. Slee, "Statistics Influence Medical Practice."

53. Walter McNerney and Study Staff, University of Michigan, *Hospital and Medical Economics: A Study of Population, Services, Costs, Methods of Payment and Controls,* vol. 2 (Chicago: Hospital Research and Educational Trust, 1962), 1430.

54. Ibid.

55. John P. Bunker, "Editorial Views: Final Report of the National Halothane Study," *Journal of Anesthesiology* 29, no. 2 (March–April 1968): 231–32.

56. Lincoln E. Moses and Frederick Mosteller, "Institutional Differences in Postoperative Death Rates: Commentary on Some of the Findings of the National Halothane Study," *JAMA* 203, no. 7 (12 February 1968): 150–52.

57. Ibid.

58. That "poverty" is in itself a "natural" cause of a high death rate remains a controversial assertion.

59. This math assumes that the thirty-four hospitals in the original National Halothane Study sample were representative of hosptials as a whole. Because the original participants were teaching hospitals, one could argue that they were providing *better* care than average, making the calculation of excess deaths even more conservative.

60. "'Care Quality' Forum Theme," *AMA News,* 18 December 1967.

61. Staff of the Stanford Center for Health Care Research, "Comparison of Hospitals with Regard to Outcomes of Surgery," *Health Services Research* 11, no. 2 (summer 1976): 112–27.

62. I am aware that the 75,000 is an extrapolation of the halothane study to the nation as a whole, and that the Stanford study did not use a percentage figure for lives saved. On the other hand, the halothane mortality estimate was based on only six surgical conditions, not fifteen surgical categories. And neither study included medical patients. As for the lack of impact on patients, Brown

was satisfied that the Stanford study provided a basis for the mortality rate calculations by the U.S. Health Care Financing Administration. In that sense there was an indirect impact a decade later. But then why not just credit the whole thing to Florence Nightingale?

63. Interview by the author with Byron W. "Bill" Brown, 27 January 1995.

64. Joel Arthur Barker, *Future Edge: Discovering the New Paradigms of Success* (New York: William Morrow, 1992), 69.

65. Interviews by the author with Paul A. Sanazaro, M.D., 31 January 1995 and 1 February 1995.

66. Interview by the author with John Bunker, M.D., 30 January 1995.

CHAPTER EIGHT: THE DOCTOR'S CAR AND THE CAR COMPANIES' DOCTORS

1. Richard A. Wright, *Detroit Inc.* (Detroit: Communications Department of Wayne State University, 1996; on-line book published to mark the one hundredth anniversary of the auto industry). Selection from chapter 12, "Insolent Chariots/Unsafe at Any Speed."

2. See *1955–56 Annual Report, W. H. Kellogg Foundation,* for this and following facts unless otherwise indicated.

3. Rosemary Stevens, *In Sickness and in Wealth: American Hospitals in the Twentieth Century* (New York: Basic, 1989), 291.

4. Joseph A. Califano Jr., *America's Health Care Revolution: Who Lives? Who Dies? Who Pays?* (New York: Random House, 1986), 52.

5. Howard Wolinsky and Tom Brune, *The Serpent and the Staff* (New York: Tarcher/Putnam, 1994), 47.

6. "Finch Sees No End to Health Cost Rise," *American Medical News,* 4 August 1969, 11.

7. "Medicare Cost," *Congressional Quarterly,* 11 July 1969, 1226–27.

8. "Nixon Sees Care Crisis," *AMA News,* 21 July 1969, 1.

9. Paul Starr, *The Social Transformation of American Medicine* (New York: Basic, 1982), 393.

10. Henry Maurer, "The M.D.'s Are off Their Pedestal," *Fortune,* February 1954, 139–86.

11. "It's Time to Operate," *Fortune,* January 1970, 79.

12. Rosemary Stevens, *American Medicine and the Public Interest* (New Haven: Yale University Press, 1971), 461.

13. The section that follows is based on the author's interviews with Paul M. Ellwood Jr., M.D. For a formal discussion of Ellwood's work within the context of public policy entrepreneurship, see the writings of Thomas Oliver, a political scientist at the University of Maryland, Baltimore campus.

14. During the 1972 presidential campaign, White House insiders working on Nixon's reelection campaign joked to one another: "I'll give you $25 if you can name one of the president's domestic accomplishments, and $50 if you can name both of them."

15. Thomas R. Mayer and Gloria Gilbert Mayer, "HMOs: Origins and Development," *Topics in Health Record Management* 6, no. 4 (1986): 5–12.

16. Al Rothenberg, "Garage Calls: Doctors' Support the Right Prescription for Early Auto Industry," *Chicago Tribune,* 19 November 1995, sec. 12, p. 3. The ad copy for a car "dependable as the doctor himself" is noted in the 8 January 1996 *Advertising Age* supplement, "100 Years of Auto Ads," S14.

17. Michael L. Millenson, "Detroit Eyes Health Cost Cuts; UAW May Help," *Chicago Tribune* 28 June 1982, business sec., 1.

18. Califano, *America's Health Care Revolution,* 11–13. The description of Chrysler's actions that follows is predominantly taken from Califano, but portions also come from my own reporting in 1982 on how rising health care costs were affecting Chrysler and the auto industry.

19. Government estimates, quoted in Michael L. Millenson, "'Bargains' May Be Over for Workers' Health Benefits," *Chicago Tribune,* 27 June 1982, business sec., 1.

20. Califano, *America's Health Care Revolution,* 14.

21. Bradford H. Gray and Marilyn J. Field, eds., *Controlling Costs and Changing Patient Care? The Role of Utilization Management* (Washington, D.C.: National Academy Press, 1989), 40.

22. "Council at a Glance," page from World Wide Web site of the Pennsylvania Health Care Cost Containment Council, April 1996.

23. *Health Care Financing Review* and Department of Commerce.

24. Califano, *America's Health Care Revolution,* 17.

25. Michael L. Millenson, "Doctors' Decisions Put under Microscope," *Chicago Tribune,* 17 June 1987, sec. 1, p. 1.

26. Ibid., 26.

27. "Public Citizen's Health Research Group Publishes First Consumer Directory of Doctors and Simultaneously Files Suit in Federal Court to Strike down Anti-consumer Law," 17 January 1974, Public Citizen Document 138-A. The directory was first published, with responses from only a quarter of Prince Georges County physicians, and then a lawsuit was filed in federal district court by Public Citizen to void the Maryland antiadvertising law and the enforcement of it by the Medical and Chirurgical Faculty of the state of Maryland, the formal name at the time of the state medical society.

28. In 1975 the U.S. Supreme Court, in a case involving attorneys, ruled that antiadvertising bans by professional societies violated antitrust law.

29. David Zinman, "Hospital Reveals Mortality Rate," *Newsday,* 30 June 1973. The rates were not adjusted to reflect patients' risk of death, but the magnitude of the differences between hospitals serving similar populations made it clear that the disparity was real.

30. Personal communication to author from Ronald Kotulak, author of the series.

31. Joel Brinkley, "U.S. Releasing Lists of Hospitals with Abnormal Mortality Rates," *New York Times,* 12 March 1986, sec. 1, p. 1.

32. A casual observer at HCFA press conferences might have concluded that a fair number of hospitals discharged their patients directly onto highway entrance ramps. Meanwhile, the protests of the downstate Illinois hospital were contained in the comments section of one report. They are, I admit, one of my favorite responses to the HCFA data.

33. Remarks of HCFA administrator William Roper, M.D., to Conference on Quality in Washington, D.C., 8 September 1986, sponsored by the newsletter division of McGraw-Hill. (The medical newsletters were later sold to Faulkner and Gray, their current publisher.)

34. Michael L. Millenson, "Hospitals' Shortcomings Shown," *Chicago Tribune,* 18 December 1987. Other quotations come from the author's notes at a briefing by Roper in Washington, D.C., on 1 December 1987.

35. Arnold S. Relman, "Assessment and Accountability: The Third Revolution in Medical Care," *New England Journal of Medicine* 319, no. 18 (3 November 1988): 1220–22.

36. Ibid., and also Remarks of William Roper to 8 September 1986 Conference on Quality.

37. Paul M. Ellwood Jr. and Michael E. Herbert, "Health Care: Should Industry Buy It or Sell It?" *Harvard Business Review,* July–August 1973, 99–107.

38. Interview by the author with John Ball, M.D., 31 August 1994.

CHAPTER NINE: A NEW YORK STATE OF MIND

1. Curtis L. Meinert and Susan Tonascia, *Clinical Trials: Design, Conduct and Analysis* (New York: Oxford University Press, 1986), 17.

2. Marcia Millman, *The Unkindest Cut* (New York: Morrow, 1976), 232–33.

3. SMG Marketing Company data for 1994–95. Personal communication from John Henderson, SMG president, 13 June 1996.

4. Michael L. Millenson, "The Wonder Drug of Information Makes Patients Insiders," *Chicago Tribune,* 11 May 1993, 1, 10.

5. David Zinman, "Rating Healers of the Heart," *Newsday,* 12 March 1991. The 1990 New York State figures gave a clue to why Winthrop-University Hospital may have come in twenty-sixth in its survival rate. Four of its cardiac surgeons performed fewer than fifty operations annually, the largest group of such low-volume surgeons at any hospital.

6. William A. Knaus et al., "An Evaluation of Outcomes from Intensive Care in Major Medical Centers," *Annals of Internal Medicine* 104, no. 3 (March 1986): 410–18.

7. Edward L. Hannan et al., "Adult Open Heart Surgery in New York State: An Analysis of Risk Factors and Hospital Mortality Rates," *JAMA* 264, no. 21 (5 December 1990): 2768–74.

8. V. Parsonnet, D. Dean, and A. D. Bernstein, "A Method of Uniform Stratification of Risk for Evaluating the Results of Surgery in Acquired Adult Heart Disease," *Circulation* 79, suppl. 1 (1989): I-3 to I-12.

9. These figures, and the description of the risk adjustment method, come from Hannan et al., "Adult Open Heart Surgery in New York State."

10. New York previously had available some hospital-specific mortality figures for heart surgery, but the numbers represented "crude" rates, unadjusted for the patient's preexisting risk of death, and were used by only some hospitals.

11. Hannan, "Adult Open Heart Surgery in New York State."

12. Zinman, "Rating Healers of the Heart."

13. Edward L. Hannan et al., "Investigations of the Relationship between Volume and Mortality for Surgical Procedures Performed in New York State

Hospitals," *JAMA* 262, no. 4 (28 July 1989): 503–10. These data constituted baseline information based on a preexisting New York State information system called SPARCS (Statewide Planning and Resource Cooperative System). The state medical society initially opposed SPARCS's development.

14. Zinman, "Rating Healers of the Heart."

15. Interview by the author with David Zinman, former *Newsday* reporter, 10 September 1996.

16. Heather Schroeder, "N.Y. Court: Public Has Right to Mortality Data," *HealthWeek,* 18 November 1991, 7. According to Hannan, Axelrod eventually planned to release the surgeon data to the public when the numbers were large enough to be statistically significant. This lack of statistical significance, says Hannan, is why the state fought the release of the surgeon-specific data in court (personal communication to author, March 1996). Although that may be true, Axelrod apparently did not share his intentions with the public. If statistical significance was the problem, why would it be acceptable for cardiologists to use the data to make decisions?

17. Shirley E. Perlman, "Judge: MD Rankings Can Go Public," *Newsday,* 22 October 1991.

18. David Zinman, "Heart Surgeons Rated: State Reveals Patient-Mortality Records," *Newsday,* 18 December 1991.

19. Robert Panzer, M.D., associate medical director for quality improvement at the University of Rochester (New York) Medical Center, spoke at a workshop meeting on 17 February 1994 in Pasadena, California, sponsored by the Healthcare Forum.

20. In February 1991 Axelrod was unexpectedly felled by a tragic stroke. He lingered in an unconscious state for more than a year before dying.

21. Jesse Green and Neil Wintfeld, "Report Cards on Cardiac Surgeons: Assessing New York State's Approach," *New England Journal of Medicine* 332, no. 18 (5 May 1995): 1229–32.

22. See Hannan et al., "Adult Open Heart Surgery in New York State." Also Edward L. Hannan et al., "Improving the Outcomes of Coronary Artery Bypass Surgery in New York State," *JAMA* 271, no. 10 (9 March 1994): 761–66, and Mark R. Chassin, Edward L. Hannan, and Barbara A. DeBuono, "Benefits and Hazards of Reporting Medical Outcomes Publicly," *New England Journal of Medicine* 334, no. 6 (8 February 1996): 394–98.

23. Chassin mentioned his plans at the end of 1992. See Linda Oberman, "Rating Doctors: Penn. Joins Trend in Releasing Physician-Specific Mortality Data," *American Medical News,* 7 December 1992, 1.

24. Speech by Albert Siu, M.D., to workshop on report cards at the annual meeting of Association of Health Services Researchers, Chicago, 5 June 1995.

25. From presentation 30 September 1992 by Joseph Juran, chairman emeritus of the Juran Institute, to a meeting of the Midwest Business Group on Health, in Rosemont, Ilinois.

26. In 1979 New York State began an unprecedented collection of data on every general hospital admission. Included were the patient's name and Social Security number as well as information on the diagnosis, the treatment, the

treating physician, and the outcome of care. This information system—which would eventually alert the department to the large differences in hospital death rates from bypass surgery—was promptly denounced by MSSNY as "a disaster" that would violate patient privacy. See "New York Data Policy Angers MDs," *American Medical News,* 20 July 1979, 1.

27. Board of Trustees of the American Medical Association, "Release of Physician-Specific Health Care Data," Report I-93-9. Officially, the AMA endorses the release of severity-adjusted, physician-specific data "where the data may be deemed accurate, reliable and meaningful to physicians, consumers and purchasers." In case anyone might think that selectivity meant that surgeons knew the limits of their skills, it was later defined as "inhibit[ing] treatment options for patients." The medical society's antipathy comes through even more clearly in a 20 July 1992 article in *American Medical News* titled "N.Y., Pa. to Release Surgeons' Bypass Outcomes." Reporter Harris Meyer wrote: "The Medical Society of the State of New York says the current data are deeply flawed. . . . The society also says physicians' fear of having a bad outcome that could tarnish their record has led some to avoid high-risk patients. Patients could endanger their health by seeking out distant, higher-ranked surgeons who have lengthy case backlogs, it warns."

28. Philip Galewitz, "A Case Study Analysis of Pennsylvania and New York's Methods and Experience in Evaluating Health Care Providers' Performance in Coronary Artery Bypass Surgery" (master's paper submitted to Division of Public Affairs of the Graduate School of Pennsylvania State University, Capital Campus, May 1994), 27.

29. Mindy Byer, "Faint Hearts," *New York Times,* 21 March 1992, A23.

30. Interview by the author with Mindy Byer, 22 March 1993.

31. Lucian L. Leape et al., "The Appropriateness of Use of Coronary Artery Bypass Graft Surgery in New York State," *JAMA* 269, no. 6 (10 February 1993): 753–69. Also Elizabeth A. McGlynn et al., "Comparison of the Appropriateness of Coronary Angiography and Coronary Artery Bypass Graft Surgery between Canada and New York State," *JAMA* 272, no. 12 (28 September 1994): 934–40. Although Mrs. Byer had a valve problem, the articles in question address the effect of regulatory pressure on the supply of overall heart surgery programs. The conclusion, as McGlynn et al. put it, is that "the regionalization of cardiac procedures that characterizes both [the Canadian and New York State] health care systems contributes to better clinical decision making."

32. David Zinman, "Hearts in Need; MDs: Coronary Specialists Avoiding High-Risk Operations," *Newsday,* 11 May 1992, 7.

33. Linda Oberman, "Valuable Input? Risk-Adjusted Data Credited for Better Outcomes," *American Medical News,* 28 December 1992. In the 11 May 1992 *Newsday* article quoted above, Dr. Anthony Tortoloni, chief of surgery at North Shore University, first disclosed the decision not to operate on twenty-three high-risk patients, calling it an effort to improve the hospital's mortality ranking. In 1990, the hospital ranked twenty-eighth out of thirty centers. "Everybody is concerned about these rankings. And I think it is affecting patient care," Tortolani told *Newsday.*

34. Rebecca Blumenstein, "Heart Surgery Ratings, Report: Survival Odds Improved in New York," *Newsday,* 8 January 1993.

35. N. A. Omoigui, Dave P. Miller, Kimberly J. Brown, et al., "Outmigration for Coronary Bypass Surgery in an Era of Public Dissemination of Clinical Outcomes," *Circulation* 93 (1 January 1996): 27–33.

36. Chassin, Hannan, and DeBuono, "Benefits and Hazards of Reporting Medical Outcomes Publicly." The authors note that the New York data on hospitals were public for three years of the Omoigui et al. research, which covered 1 January 1989 to December 1993. Data on individual surgeons, however, did not become public until October 1991. Although Omoigui et al. might suppose that surgeons acted differently as soon as the state started collecting data—suspecting it would become public—there is evidence that the state itself did not start out with the intent of making surgeons' names available. The figures on the Cleveland Clinic's volume of surgery for 1994–95, some 2,500 CABG operations, come from SMG Marketing, cited earlier in this chapter.

37. Green and Wintfeld, "Report Cards on Cardiac Surgeons."

38. Ibid.

39. In addition to Mineola's Winthrop-University Hospital and Rochester's Strong Memorial Hospital, whose experiences were referred to in the chapter text, other hospitals that have reported substantial changes in their heart-surgery procedures include:

- St. Peter's Hospital (Albany): Presentation, 29 June 1994 workshop of Hospital Research and Educational Foundation by Stanley W. Dziuban Jr., M.D., and article by Dziuban et al., "How a New York Cardiac Surgery Program Uses Outcomes Data," *Annals of Thoracic Surgery* 58 (1994): 1871–76.
- St. Vincent Hospital and Medical Center (New York City): Interview by the author with Denis Tyras, M.D., 19 January 1993, and article by Barry S. Bader, "A Customer Requirements Approach to Comparative Hospital Outcome Data," *Quality Letter,* September 1991, 10.
- Long Island Jewish Medical Center—Blumenstein, "Heart Surgery Ratings, Report."
- St. Joseph's Hospital Health Center (Syracuse)—Cindy E. Rodriguez, "State Rates Local Heart Surgeons High, Low on Bypass Operations," *Syracuse Herald-Journal,* 8 January 1993, A1.
- Erie County Medical Center (Buffalo) suspended its program, then restarted it. See Lawrence K. Altman, "Heart-Surgery Death Rates Decline in New York," *New York Times,* 5 December 1990, B10.

40. Chassin, Hannan, and DeBuono, "Benefits and Hazards of Reporting Medical Outcomes Publicly."

41. Interview by the author with O. Wayne Isom, M.D., 23 February 1993.

42. Eric J. Topol and Robert M. Califf, "Scorecard Cardiovascular Medicine: Its Impact and Future Directions," *Annals of Internal Medicine* 120, no. 1 (1 January 1994): 65–70.

43. See William A. Ghali et al., "Statewide Quality Improvement Initiatives

and Mortality after Cardiac Surgery," *JAMA* 277, no. 5 (5 February 1997): 379–82, and accompanying editorial commentary, Stephen F. Jencks, "Can Large-Scale Interventions Improve Care?" *JAMA* 277, no. 5 (5 February 1997): 419–20. The articles cast doubt on the relative success in reducing bypass mortality of the New York State effort and the Northern New England Cardiovascular Cooperative, which includes Dartmouth-Hitchcock Medical Center. Those results were compared with Massachusetts Medicare data as a proxy for the national trend, and the results were similar. However, it is unclear what quality improvement efforts were going on in Massachusetts at the time and to what extent publicity about various report card efforts caused hospitals in Massachusetts and elsewhere to focus on improvement. There are also a whole set of technical questions that remain to be settled on the comparability of data used in the Ghali et al. article (as that article acknowledges) and about statistical significance of various comparisons. (Personal communication to author from Stephen Jencks, M.D., 5 February 1997.)

44. Elisabeth Bumiller, "Death Rate Rankings Shake New York Cardiac Surgeons," *New York Times,* 6 September 1995, 1A.

45. Jim Montague, "Report Card Daze," *Hospitals and Health Networks,* 5 January 1996, 33–36.

CHAPTER TEN: THE EMPIRE STRIKES BACK

1. *Britannica Online* [CD-ROM], 1996.

2. Max Weber, *The Theory of Social and Economic Organization,* ed. with intro. Talcott Parsons (Glencoe, Ill.: Free Press, 1947), 339.

3. The generally accepted figure of a placebo's being effective with about a third of patients may be low in some cases. See Judith A. Turner et al., "The Importance of Placebo Effects in Pain Treatment and Research," *JAMA* 271, no. 20 (25 May 1994): 1609–14.

4. Unless otherwise noted, the section that follows is based on an interview by the author with Walter McClure, 8 June 1988.

5. Walter Bogdanich, *The Great White Lie: How America's Hospitals Betray Our Trust and Endanger Our Lives* (New York: Simon and Schuster, 1991), 263.

6. Institute of Medicine, *Controlling Costs and Changing Patient Care? The Role of Utilization Review,* ed. Bradford J. Gray and Marilyn J. Field (Washington, D.C.: National Academy Press, 1989), 14.

7. Ibid., 59.

8. Walter McClure, "Redesigning Benefits Stimulates Cost Consciousness," *Business and Health,* November 1983, 24–26.

9. The regulatory and legal changes are addressed in Linda Bergthold, *Purchasing Power in Health: Business, the State, and Health Care Politics* (New Brunswick, N.J.: Rutgers University Press, 1990), 20.

10. Ibid.

11. Interview by the author with Mark Baas, 20 September 1993.

12. "Pennsylvania Plans to Release Doctor and Hospital Outcomes Data," *Medical World News,* 14 December 1987, 8–9.

13. Interview by the author with John Bunker, M.D., 30 January 1995.

14. Bergthold, *Purchasing Power in Health,* 47.

15. Ernest J. Sessa, "Information Is Power: The Pennsylvania Experiment," *Journal of Health Care Benefits,* January–February 1992, 44–48.

16. The historical background on medicine in Pennsylvania comes from articles in a special Health Care Hall of Fame section of the 9 September 1988 issue of *Modern Healthcare.* The articles referenced include Clark W. Bell, "Hall of Fame Honors Healthcare's Best" (35–56); Michael L. Millenson, "Healthcare in America" (58–74); and Sandy Lutz, "Nation's First Hospital Preserves Tradition" (76–78). Although there is some argument over which hospital was America's first, the hospital industry generally accepts the claim of Pennsylvania Hospital to be the first true "hospital," as opposed to an almshouse for the poor.

17. The Medicare program's hospital mortality results were not published in a major medical journal, nor were they based on the kind of credible clinical detail that characterized the National Halothane Study and the Philadelphia study.

18. Sankey V. Williams, David B. Nash, and Neil Goldfarb, "Differences in Mortality from Coronary Artery Bypass Graft Surgery at Five Teaching Hospitals," *JAMA* 266, no. 6 (14 August 1991): 81–85.

19. "Which Hospital Is Which? That's Bypassed in Bypass Report," *Philadelphia Daily News,* 15 August 1991.

20. Remarks made by David Nash at meeting, "Publication of Provider-Specific Outcomes Data: How Far Should Accountability Go?" part of Zitter Group's "Congress on Health Outcomes and Accountability," Washington, D.C., 14 December 1994, and interview by the author with Nash, 27 March 1996.

21. "Rating the City's Hospitals: The Agency's Report May Not Be Perfect but It's a Necessary Start," *Philadelphia Inquirer,* 25 August 1991.

22. Ernest J. Sessa, "Public Disclosure: A Response from the Pennsylvania Health Care Cost Containment Council," in *Physician Profiling and Risk Adjustment,* ed. Norbert Goldfield and Peter Boland (Gaithersburg, Md.: Aspen, 1996), 49–54.

23. Excerpt from Hershey, quoted in Milton Moskowitz, Michael Katz, and Robert Levering, eds., *Everybody's Business: The Irreverent Guide to Corporate America* (San Francisco: Harper and Row, 1980), 44.

24. Michael L. Millenson, "Doctors' Decisions Put under Microscope," *Chicago Tribune,* 17 June 1987, sec. 1, p. 1.

25. Kenneth J. Arrow, "Uncertainty and the Welfare Economics of Medical Care," *American Economic Review* 53 (1963).

26. Mark V. Pauly, *Medical Care at Public Expense: A Study in Applied Welfare Economics* (New York: Praeger, 1971).

27. William M. Mercer, Inc., *Retiree Health Benefits in the 1990s* (New York: William M. Mercer, 1991).

28. Much of the description of the details of Hershey's network evaluation are taken from Jim Montague, "Low Fat, Low Cost," *Hospitals and Health Networks,* 5 August 1993, 76–78. Other parts come from a presentation by Hershey Foods vice president Sharon Lambly to the National Management Health Care Con-

gress in Washington, D.C., 31 March 1992, and from interviews by the author with Hershey officials and consultants.

29. Ezekiel J. Emanuel and Linda L. Emanuel, "What Is Accountability in Health Care?" *Annals of Internal Medicine* 124, no. 2 (15 January 1996): 229–39.

30. Eliot Freidson, *Profession of Medicine: A Study of the Sociology of Applied Knowledge* (New York: Dodd, Mead, 1970), 149, 151.

31. Ibid., 366.

32. Eric C. Schneider and Arnold M. Epstein, "Influence of Cardiac-Surgery Performance Reports on Referral Practices and Access to Care," *New England Journal of Medicine* 335, no. 4 (25 July 1996): 251–56.

33. John H. Evans III et al., "Involuntary Benchmarking and Quality Improvement: The Effect of Mandated Public Disclosure on Hospitals," May 1996. Unpublished paper from Katz Graduate School of Business, University of Pittsburgh.

34. Philip Galewitz, "A Case Study Analysis of Pennsylvania and New York's Methods and Experience in Evaluating Health Care Providers' Performance in Coronary Artery Bypass Surgery" (master's paper submitted to Division of Public Affairs of the Graduate School of Pennsylvania State University, Capital campus, May 1994), 17–18.

35. Because of technical differences in the way New York and Pennsylvania calculate their CABG mortality rates, it is difficult to compare the results of the two states directly.

CHAPTER ELEVEN: SHOW TIME

1. Institute of Medicine, *Controlling Costs and Changing Patient Care? The Role of Utilization Review,* ed. Bradford J. Gray and Marilyn J. Field (Washington, D.C.: National Academy, 1989), 45.

2. The innovations pioneered by Joseph Hudson, according to *Hoover's Handbook of American Business,* included putting a set price on clothing, rather than bargaining, and letting a dissatisfied customer bring the merchandise back for a refund.

3. Thomas R. Oliver, "Ideas, Entrepreneurship, and the Politics of Health Care Reform," *Stanford Law and Policy Review* 3 (fall 1991): 160–80. The 1973 Minnesota bill passed a few months ahead of the similar federal HMO Act.

4. Ibid.

5. Jon Christianson et al., "Managed Care in the Twin Cities: What Can We Learn?" *Health Affairs* 14, no. 2 (summer 1995): 114–30.

6. Oliver, "Ideas, Entrepreneurship, and the Politics of Health Care Reform"; InterStudy; and *Source Book of Health Insurance Data* (Washington, D.C.: Health Insurance Association of America, 1992). Figures quoted by HIAA are for 1991 enrollment reported to the Group Health Association of America.

7. Oliver, "Ideas, Entrepreneurship, and the Politics of Health Care Reform," and Christianson et al., "Managed Care in the Twin Cities." The percentage impact of HMOs on cost depended in part on how much credit HMOs were given for setting a community standard that influenced fee for service practitioners. Although hospital use was declining everywhere during that period

because of the introduction of prospective payment, researchers credit HMOs for bringing a particularly sharp decline in hospital usage to Minneapolis–St. Paul.

8. Information on the RFP comes from "The Quality of Care Partnership" and associated request for proposal materials dated May 1992, from benefits consultants Towers Perrin, and from a September 1992 Towers Perrin presentation titled "Purchasers, Providers, Protocols, and Outcomes." Material was supplemented by interviews by the author with Business Health Care Action Group members and with Thomas Kuhlman, a Towers Perrin consultant.

9. Alain C. Enthoven, "Consumer-Choice Health Plan," *New England Journal of Medicine* 298, no. 12 (23 March 1978): 650–58.

10. Alain C. Enthoven and Richard Kronick, "A Consumer-Choice Health Plan for the 1990s," *New England Journal of Medicine* 320, no. 2 (12 January 1989): 94–101.

11. The alliance's original name was GroupCare.

CHAPTER TWELVE: CHANGING THE SYSTEM FROM WITHIN

1. Donald M. Berwick, "Continuous Improvement as an Ideal in Health Care," *New England Journal of Medicine* 320, no. 1 (5 January 1989): 53–56.

2. The quotations from Donald M. Berwick, M.D., that follow, when not otherwise credited to his writing, come from his presentation to the Mayo Conference on Quality, 27 October 1995, or from interviews by the author on 25 July 1986, 1 August 1994, and 1 March 1995 or other personal communications.

3. Sang-O Rhee, "Factors Determining the Quality of Physician Performance in Patient Care," *Medical Care* 14, no. 9 (September 1976): 733–51. The same theme is sounded in other articles, including prominently Beverly C. Payne, Thomas F. Lyons, and Evelyn Neuhaus, "Relationships of Physician Characteristics to Performance Quality and Improvement," *Health Services Research* 19, no. 3 (August 1984): 307–32.

4. Robert M. Smoldt, chairman, Division of Planning and Public Affairs, Mayo Clinic, quoted in Walter Parker, "The Mayo Clinic: A Changing Legacy," *St.Paul Pioneer Press and Dispatch,* 13 July 1986, 1. The second part of the quotation from Smoldt comes from an interview by the author on 18 September 1986.

5. Loyal Davis, *Fellowship of Surgeons: A History of the American College of Surgeons* (Springfield, Ill.: Thomas, 1960), 172. Strangely, the archivists at Mayo had no knowledge of the Codman connection.

6. Personal communication from Michael O'Hara, Communications Department, Mayo Foundation, 19 December 1995.

7. Personal communication from John T. Shepherd, M.D., chair, Mayo Historical Committee, 12 December 1995.

8. In 1905 the clinic received its first burst of national publicity from a laudatory profile by the influential reporter Samuel Hopkins Adams. Adams, as discussed in chapter 5, was also the writer whose exposés of dangerous infant formula and of fraudulent claims for drugs helped lead to the establishment of what became the Food and Drug Administration. In later years the muckraking

Adams wrote novels, including one that was made into the 1934 movie *It Happened One Night.*

9. The biographical material that follows was taken from "Highlights in the Life of Walter A. Shewhart" and "Tributes to Walter A. Shewhart," which appeared after his death in *Industrial Quality Control* 24, no. 2 (August 1967): 109–17.

10. For younger readers, it is worth noting that before the 1984 breakup of AT&T, almost all telephones were owned by "Ma Bell" and rented to its customers.

11. The description that follows is based on Lloyd S. Nelson, "The Legacy of Walter Shewhart," in *Quality Progress* 12, no. 7 (July 1979): 20–28.

12. David W. Hays argues in the May 1994 issue of *Quality Progress*—the renamed *Industrial Quality Control*—that quality expert Frank Gilbreth, whose work intrigued Ernest Amory Codman, invented the graphic comparisons of statistics in 1923. Although that claim may be true, it is clear that few in industry realized what Gilbreth had done (including, most probably, Shewhart). Shewhart deserves his historical status as the developer and popularizer of this industrial tool.

13. Walter A. Shewhart, *Statistical Method from the Viewpoint of Quality Control,* ed. W. Edwards Deming (Lancaster, Pa.: Graduate School of the Department of Agriculture, 1939), 149.

14. Ibid., iv.

15. Ibid.

16. Mary Walton, *The Deming Management Method* (New York: Perigree, 1986), 18–21.

17. Nancy Mann, "Why It Happened in Japan and Not in the U.S.," *Chance: New Directions for Statistics and Computing* 1, no. 3 (1988): 8–15.

18. Ibid., 19.

19. Ibid., 20, 246.

20. Material that immediately follows comes from an interview by the author with Paul B. Batalden, M.D., 30 November 1995.

21. W. Edwards Deming, *Out of the Crisis* (Cambridge: Massachusetts Institute of Technology, Center for Advanced Engineering Study, 1986), 23–24.

22. Thomas Frist Jr., "TQM at HCA," *Health Systems Review,* May–June 1992, 15–18.

23. Mary Walton, *Deming Management at Work* (New York: Putnam, 1990), 92–94.

24. Avedis Donabedian, "Evaluating the Quality of Medical Care," *Milbank Memorial Fund Quarterly: Health and Society* 44, pt. 2 (July 1966): 166–203.

25. Frist, "TQM at HCA."

26. Donald M. Berwick, "Do We Really Need a Framework in Order to Improve?" *Joint Commission Journal on Quality Improvement* 19, no. 10 (October 1993): 449–50.

27. David Blumenthal, preface to *Improving Clinical Practice,* ed. David Blumenthal and Ann Scheck (San Francisco: Jossey-Bass, 1995), xi.

28. Presentation by J. Wesley Long, in "Report of Hospital Conference Held

at Chicago, October 22–23, 1923, and Survey of Hospitals of Fifty Beds and Over for the Year 1923," *Bulletin of the American College of Surgeons,* January 1924, 63–67.

29. The account of the efforts by the carotid endarterectomy quality improvement team is taken from an interview by the author with David Piepgras, M.D., 13 April 1995; from Julia Utz, "A Continuous Improvement Case Study: The Carotid Endarterectomy Length-of-Stay Team," *Mayo Alumni,* fall 1995; and from presentations made by various Mayo physicians and leaders to the Mayo Conference on Quality, Rochester, Minnesota, 27 October 1995. Gilbert Korb Jr. was also interviewed on 13 April 1995.

30. Mayo also had a separate period for patients who received angiograms as outpatients.

31. Korb was a stroke victim who also had heart problems. As described in chapter 9, Winthrop-University Hospital patient Art Segal had a heart problem and was also treated for a potential stroke. In both cases the secret to ultimate success was a careful workup.

CHAPTER THIRTEEN: THE EARLY WORM GETS THE BIRD

1. Institute for Clinical Systems Integration Business Plan, 18 November 1992, 1–8.

2. Joyce Orsini, "Recollections about Deming," *Quality Progress,* March 1994, 31–36.

3. U.S. General Accounting Office, *Management Practices: U.S. Companies Improve Performance through Quality Efforts,* Report GAO/NSIAD-91-190 (Washington, D.C.: U.S. Government Printing Office, 1991).

4. George C. Halvorson, *Strong Medicine* (New York: Random House, 1993), 184–88.

5. George C. Halvorson, "It's Time Buyers of Health Care Demand Results," *Minneapolis–St. Paul Star Tribune,* 13 January 1992.

6. James Reinertsen, "The Point Is Transformation, Not 'Doing Continuous Improvement,'" *Joint Commission Journal on Quality Improvement* 19, no. 10 (October 1993): 451.

7. Ibid.

8. Lloyd Dobyns and Clare Crawford-Mason, *Quality or Else: The Revolution in World Business* (Boston: Houghton Mifflin, 1991).

9. Interview by the author with Robert Marder, M.D., formerly with the Joint Commission on Accreditation of Healthcare Organizations and currently with Chicago's Rush-Presbyterian-St. Luke's Medical Center, 12 April 1994.

10. Interview by the author with Thomas Granitir, director of quality systems, American Hospital Association, 12 April 1994.

11. Although no one tracks precisely who has done what with guideline implementation, I base this assessment on more than two years of on-site research, my own reading of the medical and trade press, and conversations with some of the nation's most knowledgeable users and developers of guidelines.

12. Norbert Goldfield, "Ambulatory Encounter Systems: Implications for Payment and Quality," *Journal of Ambulatory Care Management* 16, no. 2 (1993): 33–49.

13. Osler L. Peterson et al., "An Analytical Study of North Carolina General Practice," *Journal of Medical Education* 31, no. 2 (December 1956): 1–165.

14. Jonathan P. Weiner et al., "Variation in Office-Based Quality: A Claims-Based Profile of Care Provided to Medicare Patients with Diabetes," *JAMA* 273, no. 19 (17 May 1995): 1503–8.

15. Joel Arthur Barker, *Future Edge: Discovering the New Paradigms of Success* (New York: William Morrow, 1992), 75.

CHAPTER FOURTEEN: MONEY, MANAGED CARE, AND MOM

1. Henry J. Aaron and William B. Schwartz, *The Painful Prescription: Rationing Hospital Care* (Washington, D.C.: Brookings Institution, 1984), 81, 83, 114.

2. Anne M. Stoline and Jonathan P. Weiner, *The New Medical Marketplace: A Physician's Guide to the Health Care System in the 1990s* (Baltimore: Johns Hopkins University Press, 1993), 44.

3. Bob Herbert, "Torture by H.M.O.," *New York Times*, 15 March 1996, sec. 1, p. 15.

4. "New on the Exchange," *Time*, 12 February 1996, 11.

5. Ellen E. Spragins, "Beware Your HMO," *Newsweek*, 23 October 1995, 54–56.

6. William Sherman, "Ex–New Yorker Is Told: Get Castrated So We Can $ave," *New York Post*, 18 September 1995, 5.

7. Marcia Angell and Jerome P. Kassirer, "Quality and the Medical Marketplace—Following Elephants," *New England Journal of Medicine* 335, no. 12 (19 September 1996): 883–85.

8. Thomas R. Mayer and Gloria Gilbert Mayer, "HMOs: Origins and Development," *New England Journal of Medicine* 312, no. 9 (28 February 1985): 590–94. This brief history is largely taken from that article and from Emily Friedman, "Capitation, Integration and Managed Care: Lessons from Early Experiments," *JAMA* 275, no. 12 (27 March 1996): 957–62.

9. "Reduced Fees and Increased Risks," *JAMA* 24 (1895): 290, quoted in "*JAMA* 100 Years Ago," *JAMA* 273, no. 8 (22 February 1995): 604.

10. "Report of Commission on Medical Care Plans," *JAMA* 169, no. 3 (17 January 1959), special supplement.

11. From 15 September and 15 August 1949 issues of the *New York State Journal of Medicine*, quoted in Richard Carter, *The Doctor Business* (New York: Doubleday, 1958), 55–56. This was not a fringe opinion. In 1952 the AMA House of Delegates promptly passed a resolution that read: "Any system of medicine that offers complete coverage and relieves the recipient of making any direct contribution for his own medical care will lower his sense of responsibility for his own health care and that of his family."

12. The figures come from Louis S. Reed and Willine Carr, "Independent Health Insurance Plans in 1968, Preliminary Estimates," *Research and Statistics Note*, 6 October 1969, and from a survey of group practice in the United States by Mary McNamara and Clifford Todd conducted on behalf of the American Medical Association and published in "The Coronary Drug Project: Initial Findings Leading to Modifications of Its Research Protocol," *JAMA* 214, no. 7 (16 November

1970): 1303–13). The survey is quoted in Rosemary Stevens, *American Medicine and the Public Interest* (New Haven: Yale University Press, 1971), 422–25.

13. Mayer and Mayer, "HMOs: Origins and Development," 593.

14. The first plan to win federal qualification was in Tacoma, Washington, the birthplace of prepaid care.

15. Joann S. Lublin, "Unhealthy Start: Prepaid Medical Plans Run into Difficulties as Enrollment Falters," *Wall Street Journal,* 11 February 1975, 1.

16. Michael Millenson, "Managing Health Care," *APF Reporter* 9, no. 4 (fall 1986): 20–23.

17. Harold S. Luft, "How Do Health Maintenance Organizations Achieve Their 'Savings'? Rhetoric and Evidence, *New England Journal of Medicine* 298, no. 24 (15 June 1978): 1336–43.

18. Frances C. Cunningham and John W. Williamson, "How Does the Quality of Health Care in HMOs Compare to That in Other Settings? An Analytic Literature Review: 1958 to 1979," *Group Health Journal* 1 (winter 1980): 4–25.

19. *The Health Maintenance Organization Industry Ten Year Report, 1973–1983: "A History of Achievement, a Future with Promise"* (Washington, D.C.: National Industry Council for HMO Development, [1984?]), 19. The AMA report referenced in this publication was issued in 1980.

20. Medicare bundled sets of symptoms together into diagnosis-related groups, or DRGs, which became a shorthand term for prospective payment.

21. Richard D. Lyons, "A.M.A. Fears Rationing of Services," *New York Times,* 18 June 1984.

22. Sharon McIlrath, "Congress Hears DRG Horror Stories," *American Medical News,* 8 March 1985.

23. Jennifer Bingham Hull, "Medicare Payment Plan Is Blamed for Hasty Release of Aged Patients," *Wall Street Journal,* 25 June 1985, B1.

24. McIlrath, "Congress Hears DRG Horror Stories."

25. "Half of MDs Feel Pressure to Discharge Patients Early," *American Medical News,* 5 December 1986.

26. Author's notes from 12 March 1987 session of the annual meeting of the Federation of American Health Systems in Orlando, Florida. The video featured a hospital administrator from Huntsville, Alabama, claiming, "Our ability to provide quality care each year is less and less." I found this administrator after the video was over and asked whether she felt the quality of care her hospital now provided was inadequate because of the tightened Medicare reimbursement. No, she replied, *her* hospital was still providing high-quality care—at least for the present—but the stories she had heard about *other* hospitals showed there was a real problem.

27. Douglas B. Sherlock, *The Response of Providers toward the Emerging Buyer's Market* (New York: Salomon Brothers, May 1985), 11.

28. Arthur Owens, "Working at Full Capacity? A Lot of Your Colleagues Aren't," *Medical Economics* 56, no. 7 (2 April 1979): 63–71.

29. InterStudy and Census Bureau figures reported in *Trends in U.S. Health Care 1992* (Chicago: American Medical Association, 1992), 144–45.

30. The federal Office of Health Maintenance Organizations commissioned

auditors Touche Ross and Company to study the financial performance and investment potential of the HMO industry in a report titled *The 1983 Investor's Guide to Health Maintenance Organizations* (Washington, D.C.: U.S. Government Printing Office, n.d.).

31. *Health Maintenance Organization Industry Ten Year Report, 1973–1983,* 21–23.

32. Sherlock, *Response of Providers toward the Emerging Buyer's Market,* 1.

33. Kenneth S. Abramowitz, *Health Maintenance Organizations: Strategic Analysis/ Financial Forecast* (New York: Sanford C. Bernstein, July 1986), 5.

34. Tessa Richards, "HMOs: America Today, Britain Tomorrow; Medicine American Style and the Growth of HMOs," *British Medical Journal* 292 (1 February 1986): 330–32.

35. William B. Schwartz and Daniel M. Mendelson, "Hospital Cost Containment in the 1980s: Hard Lessons Learned and Prospects for the 1990s," *New England Journal of Medicine* 324, no. 15 (11 April 1991): 1037–42.

36. Interestingly, in a January 1970 *Fortune* article on the health care crisis by reporter Edmund K. Faltermayer, famous Harvard Medical School economist Rashi Fein was quoted as estimating that "at least 10 percent" of medical expenses were wasted, while Howard Ennes, an executive with Equitable Life, put the number at 40 percent. Perhaps it took an insurer to know waste when he saw it.

37. "PPS 'Reduces Inefficiencies' without Sacrificing Quality of Care: Study," *Hospital Week,* 22 November 1985, 2; *Impact of the Prospective Payment System on Quality and Access for Medicare Beneficiaries: Final Report* (Boston: Massachusetts Department of Public Health, Division of Health Care Quality, June 1988); S. Allison Mayer-Oakes et al., "The Early Effect of Medicare's Prospective Payment System on the Use of Medical Intensive Care Services in Three Community Hospitals," *JAMA* 260, no. 21 (2 December 1988): 3146–49. In addition, a series of studies printed in *JAMA* during 1990 also failed to find significant evidence of harm.

38. Bruce Vladeck, "Hospital Prospective Payment and the Quality of Care," *New England Journal of Medicine* 319, no. 21 (24 November 1988): 1411–13.

39. Personal communication to the author on 2 December 1988 from a spokeswoman for Senator John A. Heinz.

40. David Burda, "What We've Learned from DRG's," *Modern Healthcare,* 4 October 1993, 42–44.

41. Ann Landers, "That Must Have Been Some Splinter!" *Chicago Tribune,* 25 November 1990, sec. 5, p. 3.

42. D. M. Kessner, C. K. Snow, and G. Singer, *Contrasts in Health Status* (Washington, D.C.: National Academy of Sciences, 1974), quoted in Cunningham and Williamson, "How Does the Quality of Health Care in HMOs Compare?" 8.

43. Marc A. Rodwin, *Medicine, Money, and Morals* (New York: Oxford University Press, 1993), 135.

44. Millenson, "Managing Health Care."

45. Michael L. Millenson, "Health-Care Debate Rages; Cost-Paring: Good Business or Bad Medicine?" *Chicago Tribune,* 14 June 1987; and Michael L. Millenson, "Growing Pains Afflict HMOs," *Chicago Tribune,* 16 June 1987.

46. The exact rendition of "we have no idea" read as follows: "The use of

some, but not all, financial incentives, as well as the type of HMO, does influence the behavior of physicians toward patients. It remains to be determined how these factors affect the quality of care." See Alan L. Hillman, Mark V. Pauly, and Joseph J. Kerstein, "How Do Financial Incentives Affect Physicians' Clinical Decisions and the Financial Performance of Health Maintenance Organizations?" *New England Journal of Medicine* 321, no. 2 (13 July 1989): 86–92.

47. Their version of "we have no idea" read: "Generalizations must be made with caution." Robert H. Miller and Harold S. Luft, "Managed Care Plan Performance since 1980: A Literature Analysis," *JAMA* 271, no. 19 (18 May 1994): 1512–19.

48. Millenson, "Managing Health Care."

49. David Mechanic, "Professional Judgment and the Rationing of Medical Care," *University of Pennsylvania Law Review* 140, no. 5 (May 1992): 1713–54.

50. Personal communication from Donald White, director of media relations, American Association of Health Plans, 23 May 1996. Based on extrapolation of data from AAHP and InterStudy.

51. "Health Benefit Costs Rose 2.1% in 1995," news release on *Foster Higgins National Survey of Employer-Sponsored Health Plans,* 30 January 1996. The survey included 2,764 respondents in 1995 using a national probability sample of public and private employers to reflect the demographics of all United States employers with at least ten employees.

52. *Health Maintenance Organization Industry Ten Year Report, 1973–1983,* 13.

53. Charles Marwick, "Health Plan Accountability Still a Long-Term Goal," *JAMA* 276, no. 1 (3 July 1996): 10–11.

54. Alan L. Hillman, "Health Maintenance Organizations, Financial Incentives, and Physicians' Judgments," *Annals of Internal Medicine* 112, no. 12 (15 June 1990): 891–93.

55. Testimony of Sharon Levine, M.D., associate executive director for physician and professional support services for the Kaiser Permanente Medical Group, before the Senate Committee on Labor and Human Resources, 12 September 1995. See p. 5 of written statement submitted to the committee.

56. Michael Millenson, "Double and Nothing" (poster), *Physician's Weekly,* 6 December 1993.

57. A ban on abortions or partial abortions is different from telling doctors and hospitals how they should go about "treating" new mothers; that is, by keeping them in the hospital for forty-eight hours if they want to stay.

58. Susan A. Beebe et al., "Neonatal Mortality and Length of Newborn Hospital Stay," *Pediatrics* 98, no. 2 (August 1996): 1–5.

59. George J. Annas, "Women And Children First," *New England Journal of Medicine* 333, no. 24 (14 December 1995): 1647–51.

60. John E. Ware et al., "Differences in Four-Year Health Outcomes for Elderly and Poor, Chronically Ill Patients Treated in HMO and Fee-for-Service Systems: Results from the Medical Outcomes Study," *JAMA* 276, no. 13 (2 October 1996): 1039–47.

61. Paul M. Ellwood Jr. and George D. Lundberg, "Managed Care: A Work in Progress," *JAMA* 276, no. 13 (2 October 1996): 1083–86.

62. Joseph Cardinal Bernardin, "Managing Managed Care," speech presented to the International Association of Catholic Medical Schools, Loyola University, 13 May 1996; official text from the Archdiocese of Chicago.

CHAPTER FIFTEEN: MEDICINE IN THE INFORMATION AGE

1. Mark Braly, "Managed Care: Who's the Customer?" posted in mid-1996 to World Wide Web site "Empower! The Managed Care *Patient* Advocate." Braly, who identifies himself as the editor of the site, says he is from Davis, California.

2. Jay Katz, *The Silent World of Doctor and Patient* (New York: Free Press, 1984), 2, 207.

3. The legal details in this account of the evolution of informed consent are taken from Katz, *Silent World of Doctor and Patient,* 48–84.

4. William Kates, "Spock's Secret: 50 Years Later, 'Baby and Child Care' Is Helping Parents Raise Children in the 21st Century," *Daily Southtown,* 17 October 1996, D1.

5. Based on presentation made by Albert G. Mulley Jr. to a meeting of the Healthcare Forum on 16 February 1994 in Pasadena, California, and on subsequent interviews by the author.

6. Howard Brody, *The Healer's Power* (New Haven: Yale University Press, 1992), 16–17, 88–89.

7. Andy Grove, "Taking on Prostate Cancer," *Fortune,* 13 May 1996, 55–72.

8. The history of John E. Wennberg's involvement in this area is taken from interviews by the author and from "Outcomes Research," *Dartmouth-Hitchcock Medical Center Research* 3, no. 2 (1991): 1–6.

9. Michael L. Millenson, "Patients Now Offer 2d Opinions: Experimental Videos Assist Decisions on Surgical Need," *Chicago Tribune,* 27 November 1988. Portions of this narrative are based on interviews I conducted for the *Tribune* article but that did not appear in it.

10. Timothy E. Quill and Howard Brody, "Physician Recommendations and Patient Autonomy: Finding a Balance between Physician Power and Patient Choice," *Annals of Internal Medicine* 125, no. 9 (1 November 1996): 763–69.

11. Portions of the anecdote that follows are taken from Michael L. Millenson, "Balancing High-Tech, 'High-Touch' Care," *Chicago Tribune,* 31 May 1993, A1. Other portions are from previously unpublished notes for that article.

12. The SUPPORT Principal Investigators, "A Controlled Trial to Improve Care for Seriously Ill Hospitalized Patients: The Study to Understand Prognoses and Preferences for Outcomes and Risks of Treatments (SUPPORT)," *JAMA* 274, no. 20 (22–29 November 1995): 1591–98, and Joanne Lynn et al., "Perceptions by Family Members of the Dying Experience of Older and Seriously Ill Patients," *Annals of Internal Medicine* 126, no. 2 (15 January 1997): 97–106.

13. Klemens B. Meyer et al., "Monitoring Dialysis Patients' Health Status," *American Journal of Kidney Diseases* 24, no. 2 (August 1994): 267–79. Also, interview by the author with Klemens B. Meyer, M.D., 12 May 1994.

14. Marilyn Bergner et al., "The Sickness Impact Profile: Validation of Health Status Measure," *Medical Care* 14, no. 1 (January 1976): 57–67.

15. Don Riesenberg and Richard M. Glass, "The Medical Outcomes Study," *JAMA* 262, no. 7 (18 August 1989): 943.

16. Michael L. Millenson, "Project May Spur Better Health Care," *Chicago Tribune,* 18 August 1989, sec. 1, p. 4.

17. Paul M. Ellwood Jr., "Shattuck Lecture—Outcomes Management: A Technology of Patient Experience," *New England Journal of Medicine* 318, no. 23 (9 June 1988): 1549–56.

18. Michael L. Millenson, "Quality Medical Treatment—by the Numbers," *Chicago Tribune,* 9 May 1993, sec. 1, p. 1.

CHAPTER SIXTEEN: POWER TO THE POPULATION

1. Michael L. Millenson, "Flood Lifts Insurer's Low Profile," *Chicago Tribune,* 3 May 1992, sec. 7, p. 1.

2. The HMO, which was called Harvard Community Health Plan until a recent merger, has a clinical relationship with the Harvard Medical School, but the two organizations are separately owned and operated.

3. National Asthma Education Program, Expert Panel Report, *Executive Summary: Guidelines for the Diagnosis and Management of Asthma,* Publication 91-3042A (Bethesda, Md.: National Institutes of Health, 1991), 43. See also Associated Press, "Deaths from Asthma on the Increase," *Chicago Tribune,* 8 December 1994, sec. 1, p. 12.

4. Michael Von Korff et al., "Essential Elements for Collaborative Management of Chronic Illness," paper presented at "Requirements for Effective Chronic Disease Management," conference sponsored by Robert Wood Johnson Foundation, Seattle, Washington, 26–28 June 1996, 4.

5. Doug Levy, "Chronic Care Crisis Looms: More Ill; Fewer to Care for Them," *USA Today,* 13 November 1996, D1.

6. Interviews by the author and internal reports from the Medical Director's Office of Harvard Pilgrim Health Care.

7. Associated Press, "New Guidelines on Asthma Care," *New York Times,* 26 February 1997, B11.

8. David M. Eddy, "Clinical Quality Improvement: Political and Practical Milestones," speech presented at a meeting of the Healthcare Forum in Chicago, 24 August 1994.

9. Dianne Hales, "The Mathematical Approach," *American Medical News,* 20 March 1981, 21.

10. Interview by the author with Edward F. Scanlon, M.D., 23 August 1994.

11. David Lawrence, "The Ultimate Purpose of Clinical Improvement: Healthier Communities," speech presented at a meeting of the Healthcare Forum in Pasadena, California, 17 February 1994.

12. Five women researchers who combined and reanalyzed the key breast cancer screening studies over the past thirty years reiterated that point in a 1995 *JAMA* article. See Karla Kerlikowske et al., "Efficacy of Screening Mammography: A Meta-analysis," *JAMA* 273, no. 2 (11 January 1995): 149–54.

13. Sarah A. Fox, Albert L. Siu, and Judith A. Stein, "The Importance of Physician Communication on Breast Cancer Screening of Older Women," *Ar-*

chives of Internal Medicine 154, no. 18 (26 September 1994): 2058–68; quotation on 2058.

14. Susan Love, "The Untold Truth behind the Mammogram Dispute," *Los Angeles Times,* 13 March 1994, M6.

15. David M. Eddy, "Rationing Resources While Improving Quality: How to Get More for Less," *JAMA* 272, no. 10 (14 September 1994): 817–24; quotation on 818.

16. My trip with a survey team for the National Committee for Quality Assurance was the first time the committee has allowed a reporter to accompany surveyors. Because of the sensitive nature of the material disclosed to NCQA, I agreed not to identify the plan surveyed and to let the NCQA review the material for factual accuracy before publication. No other constraints were put on either selection or interpretation of material, or on use of information about NCQA gathered from other sources. As a reporter for the *Chicago Tribune,* I have covered NCQA since 1991. This section is based on my interviews with NCQA officials and on presentations they have made since that time.

17. Susan M. Pisano, "Anything but Boring," *HMO Magazine* 36, no. 1 (January–February 1995): 7. At the time Pisano wrote, she was executive editor of *HMO Magazine,* an official publication of the Group Health Association of America. GHAA cofounded NCQA with the American Managed Care and Review Association. Since then the two groups have merged into the American Association of Health Plans, and the magazine's name was changed to *Healthplan.*

18. Interview by the author with Margaret O'Kane, executive director, National Committee for Quality Assurance, April 1991.

19. David T. Kearns and David A. Nadler, *Prophets in the Dark: How Xerox Reinvented Itself and Beat Back the Japanese* (New York: HarperBusiness, 1992), 122–23. Although Xerox is sometimes credited with inventing the business definition of benchmarking, the *Oxford English Dictionary* cites an article in the *Economist* of 18 May 1963: "Foreign firms have failed to get orders unless they have offered a price advantage of at least 50 percent. This is the 'bench-mark.' "

20. The quotations attributed to Patricia Nazemetz are based on an interview by the author with her on 14 December 1995 and on comments Nazemetz made at various trade conferences and in NCQA materials.

21. HEDIS was originally known as the HMO–Employer Data and Information Set and was developed with staff-model HMOs that belonged to a consortium called the HMO Group. Others on the original development list in addition to Xerox and the HMO Group included Bull HN Information Systems, Digital Equipment, GTE, benefits consultants Towers Perrin, and the Washington Business Group on Health. The name of the measures was changed to Health Plan–Employer Data and Information Set to reflect the possible use of the standards with other types of managed care plans.

22. William A. Schaffer, F. David Rollo, and Carol A. Holt, "Falsification of Clinical Credentials by Physicians Applying for Ambulatory-Staff Privileges," *New England Journal of Medicine* 318, no. 6 (11 February 1988): 356–58.

23. Stephen L. Isaacs, "Consumers' Information Needs: Results of a National

Survey," *Health Affairs* 15, no. 4 (winter 1996): 31–41, and Susan Edgman-Levitan and Paul D. Cleary, "What Information Do Consumers Want and Need?" *Health Affairs* 15, no. 4 (winter 1996): 42–56.

24. "Leap of Faith over the Data Tap," *Lancet* 345, no. 8963 (10 June 1995): 1449–50.

EPILOGUE: A CELEBRATION OF MEDICINE'S FUTURE

1. Ronald L. Goldman, "The Reliability of Peer Assessments of Quality of Care," *JAMA* 267, no. 7 (19 February 1992): 958–60.

2. *American Medicine: Expert Testimony out of Court,* vol. 1 (New York: American Foundation, 1937), 160–61.

3. Arthur M. Schlesinger Jr., "The Challenge of Change," *New York Times Magazine,* 27 July 1986, 20–21.

4. Samuel O. Thier, "Health Care Reform: Who Will Lead?" *Annals of Internal Medicine* 115, no. 1 (1 July 1991): 54–58.

5. Codman's work has been rescued from invisibility in the past decade or so, as, to a lesser extent, has the work of Lembcke. That "rescue," however, is mostly confined to the health policy and health services research communities. Although the Professional Activity Study is known as a source of hospital medical records, its original intent—quality-based comparisons of doctors and hospitals—has been lost in time. The National Halothane Study's clinical results are well known; the study's unexpected implications for the quality of everyday care in hospitals constitute the kind of trivia question a handful of older health services researchers might be able to answer.

6. Richard Malmsheimer, *"Doctors Only": The Evolving Image of the American Physician* (New York: Greenwood, 1988), 1, 45.

7. Everett M. Rogers, *Diffusion of Innovations,* 3d ed. (Detroit: Free Press, 1983), 1, 14–15.

8. From "Anesthesia, Literature," a review by E. S. Siker of Emanuel M. Papper's *Romance, Poetry and Surgical Sleep: Literature Influences Medicine,* Contributions in Medical Studies 42 (Westport, Conn.: Greenwood, 1995). The review is contained in *JAMA* 275, no. 7 (21 February 1996), 567.

9. Thomas S. Kuhn, *The Structure of Scientific Revolutions,* 2d ed. (Chicago: University of Chicago Press, 1970), 100.

10. William Campbell Felch and Donald M. Scanlon, "Bridging the Gap between Research and Practice," *JAMA* 277, no. 2 (8 January 1997): 155–56.

11. The distinction between reform and revolution comes from the nineteenth-century British writer Edward George Earle Bulwer-Lytton. He is best known today for a sentence borrowed by Snoopy in the comic strip *Peanuts:* "It was a dark and stormy night."

12. Phillip B. Crosby Sr., "The Price of Noncomformance," *Group Practice Journal* (March–April 1986): 37–42.

13. Phillip R. Kletke, David W. Emmons, and Kurt D. Gillis, "Current Trends in Physicians' Practice Arrangements: From Owners to Employees," *JAMA* 276, no. 7 (21 August 1996): 555–60.

14. Paul Starr, *The Social Transformation of American Medicine* (New York: Basic, 1982), 342–43.

15. David C. Goodman et al., "Benchmarking the U.S. Physician Workforce: An Alternative to Needs-Based or Demand-Based Planning," *JAMA* 276, no. 22 (11 December 1996): 1811–17.

16. Walt Bogdanich, *The Great White Lie: How America's Hospitals Betray Our Trust and Endanger Our Lives* (New York: Simon and Schuster, 1991), 29.

17. David Brailer and R. Lawrence Van Horn, "Health and the Welfare of U.S. Business," *Harvard Business Review* 71, no. 2 (March–April 1993): 125–32.

18. Charles R. Buck, "Terms and Trends in Quality Assurance," *Trustee,* September 1975, 32–34.

19. Steven A. Schroeder, "Outcomes Assessment 70 Years Later: Are We Ready?" *New England Journal of Medicine* 316, no. 3 (15 January 1987): 160–62.

20. Messages posted 21 November 1996 on sci.med.informatics. I have withheld the names of the discussants, since they did not intend to speak publicly for their organizations.

21. Robert S. Ledley and Lee B. Lusted, "Reasoning Foundations of Medical Diagnosis," *Science* 130, no. 3366 (3 July 1959): 9–21.

22. Thomas J. Watson, Jr., quoted in "Editorial Viewpoint: Living with Computers," *AMA News,* 18 April 1966, 4.

23. Joel Arthur Barker, *Future Edge: Discovering the New Paradigms of Success* (New York: William Morrow, 1992), 7.

24. Xinhua News Service, "President Asks Medical Personnel to Improve Quality," 9 December 1996, via Individual Inc.

25. As a former reporter at the *Chicago Tribune,* I can attest that the presence of informed journalists at the *Tribune, Boston Globe, Fort Lauderdale Sun-Sentinel,* and similar newspapers does not influence the national agenda.

26. Reliable quality of care measurement requires advances in risk adjustment and a host of other areas. Without minimizing the significance of this effort, it is important to emphasize that the primary barrier is not technical, but organizational. Technical barriers certainly need to be addressed, though, in any sort of discussion with health care professionals.

27. Peter L. Bernstein, *Against the Gods: The Remarkable Story of Risk* (New York: John Wiley, 1996), 6–7.

28. Kenneth I. Shine, "Beyond the Crisis: Preserving the Capacity for Excellence in Health Care and Medical Science," address by president, Institute of Medicine, to New York Academy of Sciences seminar, 14–15 February 1994.

29. Terence D. Murphy, "Medical Knowledge and Statistical Methods in Early Nineteenth-Century France," *Medical History* 25 (1981): 301–19.

INDEX